Evidence-based
Health Promotion

Edited by
Elizabeth R. Perkins
Ina Simnett
and
Linda Wright

JOHN WILEY & SONS

Chichester · New York · Weinheim · Brisbane · Singapore · Toronto

Copyright © 1999 by John Wiley & Sons, Ltd, The Atrium, Southern Gate,
Chichester, West Sussex PO19 8SQ, England
Telephone (+44) 1243 779777

Email (for orders and customer service enquiries): cs-books@wiley.co.uk

Reprinted September 2000, March 2001, February 2002, September 2003

Other Wiley Editorial Offices

John Wiley & Sons Inc., 111 River Street, Hoboken, NJ 07030, USA

Jossey-Bass, 989 Market Street, San Francisco, CA 94103-1741, USA

Wiley-VCH Verlag GmbH, Boschstr. 12, D-69469 Weinheim, Germany

John Wiley & Sons Australia Ltd, 33 Park Road, Milton, Queensland 4064, Australia

John Wiley & Sons (Asia) Pte Ltd, 2 Clementi Loop #02-01, Jin Xing Distripark, Singapore 129809

John Wiley & Sons (Canada) Ltd, 22 Worcester Road, Etobicoke, Ontario M9W 1L1

Wiley also publishes its books in a variety of electronic formats. Some content that appears in print may not be available in electronic books.

Library of Congress Cataloging-in-Publication Data

Evidence-based health promotion / edited by Elizabeth R. Perkins,
    Ina Simnett and Linda Wright.
        p. cm.
    Includes bibliographical references and index.
    ISBN 0–471–97851–5
    1. Primary care (Medicine) 2. Evidence-based medicine. 3. Health
promotion. I. Perkins, Elizabeth R. II. Simnett, Ina.
III. Wright, Linda.
    RA427.9.E94 1999
    613—dc21   98–30820
                                                          CIP

British Library Cataloguing in Publication Data

A catalogue record for this book is available from the British Library

ISBN 0–471–97851–5

Typeset in 10/12pt Palatino by Mayhew Typesetting, Rhayader, Powys.
Printed and bound in Great Britain by Biddles Ltd, Guildford and King's Lynn
This book is printed on acid-free paper responsibly manufactured from sustainable forestry, for which at least two trees are planted for each one used for paper production.

Contents

About the Editors

Elizabeth R. Perkins MA PhD Cert Ed is an independent researcher and trainer who has practised in the field of health care and health promotion since the mid-1970s, first as part of a university-based research project, then within a health promotion department, and more recently on a freelance basis. She is particularly interested in helping practitioners develop their skills and evaluate their own practice, and sees research as a learning process for all concerned – funders, practitioners, users and researchers themselves. Her continuing commitment to encouraging practitioners to write up their own work for publication started in the 1980s when she edited the Nottingham Practical Papers in Health Education. She has herself published extensively, both in book form and in the professional press associated with the wide range of groups with whom she has worked.

Ina Simnett MA (Oxon) DPhil Cert Ed has worked since 1989 as a freelance health promotion consultant. She contributed to a number of health promotion open learning materials and she has published extensively in the health promotion literature. She is the co-author, with Linda Ewles, of the most popular text on health promotion: *Promoting health – a practical guide* (fourth edition, Baillière Tindall, 1998). Her book *Managing health promotion* (Wiley, 1995) has also been well received. Ina started her career as a research physiologist, took 'time out' to rear three daughters, then worked in the NHS for 26 years, first in health education and health promotion and later in management training. She retired in 1998 and is now busy as a grandmother and promoting her own health.

Linda Wright BSc MSc works as a freelance health promotion consultant. She has a first degree in Genetics and a Masters degree in Community Medicine. During her 20-something years in health promotion, she spent ten years managing an NHS health promotion service in the North East of England, was a lecturer in health promotion at the University of Durham and worked for Tacade for five years. She has written and co-authored a number of health promotion resources, including several training manuals on alcohol and drug education. She is currently writing up her PhD on alcohol and youth work at the University of Durham, in between earning a living, bringing up two lively lads and riding her pony.

List of Contributors

John Balding is Director of the University of Exeter, Schools Health Education Unit.

Liz Batten is a researcher, writer, trainer and consultant in behaviour and health. She is also Honorary Senior Research Fellow in the Department of Psychology at Southampton University.

Kathy Brummell is a Lecturer Practitioner currently working between Nottingham Community Health NHS Trust and the University of Nottingham. She previously worked as a health visitor (public health) in the Nursing Development Unit at Strelley Health Centre in Nottingham.

Robin Burgess is Chief Executive of CAN: changing people's lives, a charity providing counselling, education and training concerning drugs, mental health, homelessness and offending and based in Northamptonshire. He has been involved for eight years in developing resources on substance misuse for use with offenders in custodial and community settings.

Sandy Burnham is Deputy Health Promotion Manager with Borders Community Health Services NHS Trust.

Jacki Gordon At the time of the study reported on in her contribution to this book, Jacki worked as a health promotion officer for the Greater Glasgow Health Board. She has continued working within health promotion, now with a remit for mental health.

Dominic Harrison is the Health Promotion General Manager for the North West Lancashire Specialist Health Promotion Unit which covers Blackpool and Preston areas. Since 1992 he has been involved with the WHO European Health Promoting Hospital Project and is now the English National Health Promoting Hospitals and Trusts Network Co-ordinator. He has recently undertaken work in central and eastern Europe advising on the development of national infrastructures for health promotion and has contributed to a number of publications including a recent *British Medical Journal* article on evidence-based health promotion.

Sue Hepworth is a chartered psychologist working as an independent social researcher. She particularly enjoys applied research focusing on improvements in material, physical or psychological well-being. Since moving to the Peak District in pursuit of the rural idyll, she has been challenged by the hinterland realities of rural poverty, and unequal access to health care, low cost housing, training and employment.

Frances Hudson worked for 20 years with school-age mothers and their families, running a special educational unit for Avon LEA. She is the co-author (with Bernard Ineichen) of *Taking it lying down: sexuality and teenage motherhood* (Macmillan, 1991). Currently she works as a freelance counsellor, researcher and trainer, specialising in young people and sexual health issues.

Tony Jeffs teaches in the Community and Youth Work Studies Unit, Department of Sociology and Social Policy at the University of Durham. He has written extensively about youth work issues, informal education and community schooling. He is a member of the editorial board of *Youth and Policy*.

Lesley Jones runs her own consultancy providing advice and training in management, communications and health promotion. She previously worked within the NHS, building up and managing thriving health promotion services in Wales, London and Yorkshire. Lesley recently completed an MSc in Training and Development with Leicester University.

Ruth Joyce worked within the education and health services for over 25 years and was one of the early appointments of drug education co-ordinators working for Cambridgeshire Education Authority. She has since taken up the post of Head of Education and Prevention with the Standing Conference on Drug Abuse.

Terry Lawrence is Senior Health Development Adviser in the Department of Public Health and Epidemiology at Birmingham University. Her background is in Sociology, Education, Research and Health Promotion. She is currently managing a programme of three randomised controlled trials, which is applying the transtheoretical model and its applications to population groups of smokers in the West Midlands.

Linda Lawton began her professional career as a science teacher before becoming a health promotion specialist. She has a first degree in Biology, a Masters degree in Health Education and has recently completed her MBA. She has now worked in health promotion in the NHS for 17 years, including a five-year stint as manager of a health promotion department. She has also worked in purchasing and commissioning mental health services. Linda is currently based in the Public Health Department of Warwickshire Health Authority, with responsibility for health promotion.

Beth Lindley is a youth and community work practitioner based in South Bank, Middlesbrough. She has been working mainly in the detached field since qualifying in Sheffield as part of the Community Work Apprenticeship Scheme in 1989.

Margaret MacVicar has practised as a nurse, midwife and health visitor, and is now a lecturer in nursing in the School of Health Studies at Bell College of Technology, Hamilton, Scotland.

Alison McCamley-Finney is a Senior Lecturer in the School of Health and Community Studies at Sheffield Hallam University. She has undertaken applied drug research in a range of areas including HIV risk behaviour and injecting practices and young people and drug use. She is particularly interested in methodological issues relating to drug research.

Anne McClelland is currently a practising health visitor and a member of the Rotherham Health Visitor Development Group. She has wide research experience within and outside the health service and is at present looking at the health consequences of domestic violence for women and children.

Majella McFadden is a Lecturer in the School of Health and Community Studies at Sheffield Hallam University. She has spent the last six years, including three in Northern Ireland, researching various aspects of women's sexual identities and practices.

Alison Mitchell is currently working as a Clinical Nurse Specialist in Breast Care within the Dudley Group of Hospitals NHS Trust, and has been in her present post for five years. She has previous experience within the fields of midwifery, research and health promotion and she is undertaking an MSc in Health Promotion at the University of Central England, Birmingham.

Alysoun Moon Following careers in nursing and teaching, Alysoun specialised in health education and promotion research and development with children in school settings. She has worked as a trainer, nationally and internationally, and is the author and co-author of a number of health education resources for primary, secondary and special school pupils and teachers.

Elizabeth R. Perkins is one of the editors of this book and information about her can be found in About the Editors (p ix).

Sally Perkins is an independent consultant who has been working on health issues since the mid-1980s, with a particular interest in custody, communicable diseases, drugs and sexual behaviour. She has been a member of the National AIDS and Prisons Forum since 1989, when she was the Forum's first convener, and has been a facilitator, trainer and training designer for the Prison Service Directorate of Health Care. Sally is the regular contributor on prisons in the *National AIDS Manual*. Her most recent research has been a study of access to condoms for prisoners in the European Union, for the European Commission, which was presented to an international symposium in 1997.

Jenny Poulter is a nutritionist specialising in food/health promotion. Her background is in research, education and the NHS. Since moving into the freelance field in 1990 she has worked extensively in both the private and public sectors, including input into the last government's Nutrition Task Force Initiative.

Jane Powell is the Cardiac Rehabilitation Co-ordinator at the Princess Royal Hospital NHS Trust, Telford, Shropshire. Jane is responsible for the overall co-ordination and monitoring of the programme.

David Regis is a former teacher who now works as a researcher in the University of Exeter, Schools Health Education Unit.

Kenny Richardson is Area Health Promotion Manager for Borders Community Health Services NHS Trust. Needs assessment is a fundamental way of working for this Health Promotion Department and is used in every setting from primary care to local communities.

Heather Roberts works for the School of Community Health Sciences, University of Nottingham, where she was Director of the Trent Health Lifestyles Survey from 1991–1995. Her previous experience was in community-based surveys within Trent Region, in adult education and within the voluntary sector.

Robbie Robertson At the time of the study, Robbie was a GP practising in an inner city Glasgow practice. He has since retired from general practice and is a half-time senior tutor at the University of Glasgow, Department of General Practice.

Liz Rolls Following secondment to the Health Education Authority from the Cheltenham and Gloucester College of Higher Education, to act as Professional Development Manager, during 1995 to 1997 Liz managed the health promotion and co-ordination aspects of the UK-wide activity which led to 'National Occupational Standards for Health Promotion and Care'. She now acts as consultant to HEA's Piloting National Occupational Standards for Health Promotion and Care project, while continuing to teach at the Cheltenham and Gloucester College of Higher Education.

Graham Simmonds is a health promotion specialist who has worked for Avon Health Promotion Service for five years. He is currently completing his PhD on the 'Get Moving!' project at the University of Bristol.

Ina Simnett is one of the editors of this book and information about her can be found in About the Editors (p ix).

Mark K. Smith is the Rank Research Fellow and Tutor at the YMCA George Williams College, London. His writing and teaching is mainly around informal and community education. He compiles *the informal education homepage* (www.infed.org).

Margaret Swan At the time of the study reported in her contribution to this book, Margaret worked as a health promotion officer for the Greater Glasgow Health Board. Since then she has become a full-time parent and has returned to health visiting part-time.

David Wall has been a General Practitioner in Sutton Coldfield since 1975. He has also worked as a GP trainer, course organiser, GP tutor, Associate Adviser and Regional Adviser in the West Midlands. He is now Deputy Regional Postgraduate Dean of Medical Education for the West Midlands.

Maggie Wark has worked in health promotion for the last 20 years. She has, at different times, managed two specialist health promotion departments, and also set up the Postgraduate Diploma/MSc in Health Promotion at the University of Central England in Birmingham. She has been working freelance for the last four years. During that time she has administered the Society of Health Education and

Promotion Specialists Audit Scheme and has developed her interest in the possible positive mental health effects of colour consultancy.

Dale Webb has worked in the health promotion field for six years, first as a health promotion specialist, and then as a researcher. His research interests include evidence-based health promotion and the epistemology of health care evaluation. He is also currently engaged in a two-year study which is seeking to develop a consumer definition of quality in the provision of general practice and genito-urinary medicine services for gay men.

Anne Wise is a former teacher who now works as a researcher in the University of Exeter, Schools Health Education Unit.

Linda Wright is one of the editors of this book and information about her can be found in About the Editors (p ix).

Acknowledgements

John Balding, Anne Wise and David Regis The distribution map of smokers is reproduced by permission of C.A. Jordon, Gateshead and South Tyneside Health Promotion Service.

Liz Batten thanks the hospital, community and research midwives who administered the questionnaires, and their managers in North Staffordshire Maternity Hospital, Walsgrave Maternity Hospital and Wordsley Maternity Hospital for permitting the study on smoking in pregnancy to take place. Thanks also to her colleagues, Sue High of the Department of Social Statistics at Southampton University, Professor Hilary Graham of the Department of Applied Social Science, University of Lancaster and Professor Joe Rossi and Dr Laurie Ruggiero of the Cancer Prevention Research Centre, University of Rhode Island, for their support and consultancy throughout this project. Most of all, thanks to all the women who took the time to complete the questionnaire. The study on smoking in pregnancy reported here was funded by West Midlands NHS Executive Research and Development Directorate.

Kathy Brummell Thanks go to the many people who have supported this work both locally and nationally. Of particular importance are the people who live in the Strelley area, and the health visitors and managers who were involved with the Nursing Development Unit.

Margaret MacVicar Acknowledgements to Bell College of Technology, Hamilton, Scotland. Also to the students whose words are invaluable to me, to my colleague Rosemary McKendrick, and the late Stuart Alvey, formerly of Lanarkshire College of Nursing and Midwifery.

Anne McClelland wishes to be cited as author on behalf of the Rotherham Health Visitor Development Group. Acknowledgements for support to Rotherham Priority Health Trust, Parkgate Women's Health Group and Rotherham Health Authority.

Alison Mitchell The Dudley Breast Health Care Project was jointly co-ordinated by the author, Alison Mitchell, and Kate O'Hara, Women's Health Adviser at Dudley Health Promotion Service. Kate, Women and Theatre and all those women who attended the project must be thanked for their wonderful contributions, openness and enthusiasm, making the whole project a success.

Heather Roberts' section draws on her experience as Director of the Trent Health Lifestyle survey. This was funded by North Derbyshire Health Authority and

Trent Regional Health Authority, without whose support it would not have been possible.

Maggie Wark The project on the use of colour analysis as a technique for improving self-esteem in breast cancer patients was kindly supported by Dudley Health Authority via the *Health of the Nation* special reserve fund.

The Editors wish to thank Deborah Reece and Michael Osuch for support and practical help in enabling meetings of contributors. We also thank our partners for moral and practical support.

Chapter 1

Creative Tensions in Evidence-based Practice

Elizabeth R. Perkins, Ina Simnett and Linda Wright

WHY THIS BOOK?

This book is about 'the art of the possible'. It is therefore much more about reality than rhetoric. It aims to increase the skills and confidence of health promoters to work in an evidence-based way. Success in the achievement of the targets of the renewed national health strategy *Our Healthier Nation* (Secretary of State for Health, 1998) will depend in part on the commissioning and implementation of effective health promotion programmes. We need good evidence about how best to do this.

It was against this background that we, the editors, began to consider the need for a book about evidence-based health promotion. We realised that evidence-based health promotion is problematic and that practitioners were going to need support and encouragement. We thought that there was a need to clear up some of the confusion and present a picture of how an evidence-based approach to health promotion could be applied. This book is not a textbook on how to do evidence-based health promotion practice; such a book would be out of date before it was published, as new evidence emerges all the time. Instead, it is something more complex and more reflective, an examination of what it could mean to be an evidence-based practitioner.

We hope that this book will help you to:

- Know and understand what being an evidence-based practitioner means to you.
- Have the courage of your convictions to put this into action.
- Stand your ground and fight off unrealistic expectations.
- Encourage you to develop a network, so that you know what is going on and have support in a difficult task.
- Explore and remain open-minded.

Whilst few would argue about the principle that all health promotion practice should have its basis in sound evidence, there is lively discussion about exactly

Evidence-based Health Promotion. Edited by Elizabeth R. Perkins, Ina Simnett and Linda Wright.
© 1999 John Wiley & Sons Ltd.

what this means and what are the best ways of achieving it. This book aims to contribute to the debate and help to inform practice in three areas:

- assessing existing evidence
- collecting new evidence
- providing practicable solutions about what to do when there isn't any direct evidence.

The purpose of the book is to enable a wide range of health promotion practitioners to think more broadly about what 'doing the right thing' and 'doing things right' mean, and to use this thinking to inform their practice ('doing the right things right'). In a nutshell, it is about how to become an 'evidence-based' health promotion practitioner. To achieve this we show what practitioners are currently doing to incorporate an evidence-based approach into their practice. So the book is about 'good enough' practice, not 'best practice' (we don't know what best practice is yet). We hope that it will help to improve health promotion practice, especially through helping practitioners and managers from different backgrounds, inside and outside the health service, to work together.

HOW THIS BOOK WAS WRITTEN

We set about designing this book in an unconventional way. Many edited books have contributions written by people who do not meet to discuss the book, and may never have met at all. The editors' task is to develop a coherent pattern, both through their recruitment of contributors and through their editorial overview in the introduction. This can be difficult, and is the reason why some edited books can read more like an issue of a journal than a coherent whole. We wanted to improve on this model by providing opportunities for contributors to meet, thus enabling them to see for themselves where their contribution fitted in with those of others and what were the opportunities for confirmation and contrast with the work of others. With help from our commissioning editor, Deborah Reece, we borrowed space at the Wiley office in London to do so. These meetings made it possible for us to put our health promotion values into action through the process of developing the book. Everyone involved, whether as an editor or as a contributor, had an opportunity to contribute ideas about how the book as a whole should develop.

We also departed from the norm for edited books in our choice of contributors. We thought that if we were to produce a book which would be genuinely helpful to 'ordinary' health promoters and their managers, working in neighbourhoods where things are far from perfect and resources distinctly limited, then the book should include contributions from some of these people for others like themselves. So, we set about finding such people, who were struggling with attempting to take an evidence-based approach, and who had the courage to write about it. We wished to illustrate the enormous range of different ways in which health promotion can be practised, and the number of different types of practitioner involved, and thus asked for a lot of short contributions rather than a few long ones. Even so, there will be many groups who are unrepresented! However, the range includes health promotion specialists, clinicians, teachers, health visitors and youth workers, those involved with primary and secondary prevention, commissioners, managers, researchers and practitioners. . . . Most chapters have several contributors. Some contributions are short case studies. Others provide different perspectives to an issue under discussion. In this way we have been able to involve a wide range of contributors (nearly 40 in all) and have a wide ranging debate, whilst retaining a clarity of purpose.

Some of the contributors to this book have not had their names in print before; others are well-established researchers and writers. So the book includes writing at a range of academic levels, and one way in which readers can use this book is to recognise the level of evidence-based practice where they would feel comfortable working. Some sections aim to help readers to think about underlying issues for their practice. Other sections are personal accounts and views of practitioners about their experiences at the 'coal-face'. No attempt has been made to impose a corporate view or style on the contributors. The opinions expressed are those of the individual authors. We believe that the variations in writing styles enhance the book and make for more exciting reading. We hope that, like us, you recognise that they have the ring of truth about them. They will help you, like Star Trek, to boldly go where no one has gone before!

Using This Book

This book has an introductory chapter which discusses the creative tensions around evidence-based health promotion, and sets the scene in considering the kind of attitudes and practices which we, the editors, think are helpful to its development. The remainder of the book is divided into three parts, concerned respectively with theories, settings and methods. Each part has five chapters and an editorial overview from one of us; most chapters have several contributions and an introductory page to show how they all fit together. If you are a person who likes to read books from cover to cover, we suggest you read this chapter and Part I, and then choose according to your interests whether to explore evidence about work in settings first, in Part II, or how to collect evidence, in Part III. If you work in one single setting, like a school or a hospital ward, and know it well, you may want to start with methods, in Part III; if you work in a lot of different settings, you may want to read Part II first.

Many people, however, use edited books only to read the bits which directly relate to their practice setting. If you have got this far with the introduction, we suggest you resist the temptation to turn instantly to youth work or cardiac rehabilitation. Instead, consider using the rest of this chapter, and Part I, to orientate yourself to the more general issues, against which you can set the more specific contributions on the kind of practice which is of most interest to you. Many health promoters wrestle with issues which are actually problems for others too, but which they feel are unique to their own work. This book may show you that you are not alone, and some of the ways forward which others have found may help you too, even if they work in a different field or in a different way from you.

WHAT IS EVIDENCE-BASED HEALTH PROMOTION PRACTICE?

Evidence-based practice has become rather like motherhood and apple pie – a 'good thing'. Opposition would be rather like thinking the unthinkable. However, ideas which receive this treatment can become very ill-defined and eventually subject to serious logical error – so that since evidence-based practice is a good thing, and important, other good things must be assimilated to evidence-based practice in order for them to be treated as important. Both inspiration and values, for example, can be immensely important in shaping practice, and will do this better if they are not confused with evidence. Health promotion work is at particular risk from this tendency, because most health promoters query the specialised use of the word evidence which is currently in use in purely clinical contexts, where the specified hierarchy of evidence includes only quantitative studies (NHS Executive, 1996). Health promotion needs the results of both quantitative and qualitative research to inform its practice, and health promoters are likely to argue for an extended, rather than restricted, use of the word evidence. However, the status of evidence and the reliance which can be placed on it depends on the degree of rigour involved and the extent to which the investigator is systematic in the collection and analysis of data and its limitations. Alison McCamley-Finney and Majella McFadden, in their discussion of qualitative methods in Chapter 15 Section 15.1, illustrate this well.

What can be identified as common ground?

- On one level, evidence-based health promotion is an attitude of mind similar to research-mindedness, a tendency to ask repeatedly 'How do we know? Who says so?' This questioning approach to practice can be applied to a number of different kinds of evidence, from experience to statistics, and will seek neither to dismiss nor to over-rate its source material. It provides a defence against practices which have become institutionalised on the basis of little or no evidence (like four-hour feeds for babies (Fisher, 1986; Royal College of Midwives, 1988)) or tend to be extended beyond their research-based legitimacy because they 'feel' right (like arousing fear to try to persuade people to change their behaviour (Hovland et al., 1963; Schramm, 1960; and more recently on drugs, Power, 1989)).
- Evidence-based health promotion also involves a willingness to contribute to building up the evidence base for health promotion, even if only in a modest way; the contributors to this book are doing just that. Being willing to write up work which has involved the systematic collection or use of evidence involves taking the risk of peer and public criticism, but it also enables other people to

learn, both from your successes and from your failures. In a culture where criticism is constructive, sharing your work with others enables you to benefit from the experience and reading of others. Building up such a culture is a task to which all health promotion practitioners can contribute. A start was made in this direction with the Nottingham Practical Papers in Health Promotion in the early 1980s, when most of the members of one (admittedly large) health promotion unit wrote up an aspect of their practice to share with other specialist and non-specialist colleagues. Other professional groups have other approaches: the Nurse Education Tomorrow conference, associated with the journal *Nurse Education Today*, provides a forum for many nurse teachers to present research in progress and have it discussed, rather than having to go straight for publication without the opportunity for comment from their peers. A similar forum in the addictions field is provided by the 'New Directions' conferences.

- Evidence-based practice can also encourage an attitude of modesty in action. This can helpfully counteract the fashions in health promotion, which, as in other fields of professional practice, frequently benefit from a critical examination: how extensive *are* the emperor's new clothes? It can also be directed against unreasonable demands for the working of health promotion wonders, like reducing smoking to single figures single-handed, or proving that community development works on a budget of £2,500. Working within your perceived limitations can in itself be evidence-based, like a refusal to walk on water – after all, even anecdotal accounts of this particular capacity are rare!

Sometimes it is easier to achieve a working understanding of a portmanteau word like evidence by defining what it is not.

EVIDENCE-BASED HEALTH PROMOTION IS NOT:

- The property of PhDs
- A bright idea
- Using your intuition without checking it against other ways of knowing
- Saying 'I've worked here for 25 years and I know!'
- A moral framework, like the assumption in much of the early 'evidence' about young people's drinking behaviour that *all* youthful drinking is inevitably problematic (Sharp & Lowe, 1989)
- Using casual conversations, anecdotes and stories to support major initiatives (*Yes, we did a needs assessment – I talked to a couple of nurses and then we wrote a pack*)
- Growing a bright idea with a few colleagues and then going out and implementing it

- Carrying on doing things without questioning *(But we've always given out tooth-brushes . . . Does it improve their dental health? But we've always done it . . .)*
- Something you use to bolster up what you're already doing – operating defensively
- Reinventing the wheel by researching work well-documented elsewhere
- Hugging your work to yourself rather than opening it to scrutiny
- An excuse for doing nothing (though it might be a good reason for doing nothing in a particular context)
- Just an attitude of mind – it involves action!

The identification of common ground, and drawing some boundaries round it, shows some of the problems likely to occur. These will get easier to manage as evidence-based practice spreads and more people have more experience with the skills required. At a deeper level, there are perennial tensions which are unlikely to go away, and which practitioners and managers will find it helpful to recognise in advance as general problems, not specific to their situation.

LIVING WITH TENSIONS

The Tension Between Reflection and Action

Becoming evidence-based does not involve turning yourself into an academic. Evidence-based practice needs to retain a practical focus, and to build on reflective practice without inducing paralysis. It uses the skills built up in reflective practice – thinking about what you do, questioning whether it is the best way of handling that particular situation – and extends them by finding out what other people's views and experience might bring to bear on the problem in hand.

The thinking process cannot go on for ever. At some point a decision will have to be made about what to do next. This means that there will always be a question about how much evidence is 'good enough' – to act, to advise others to act, or to purchase services. In the present state of knowledge about health promotion, conclusive evidence is frequently not available. Furthermore, busy practitioners, even armed with this book, will not be able to be sure that they have assembled and assessed all that might be available if they had more resources at their disposal.

> Practitioners have to learn how to work with imperfect knowledge: they cannot wait for the results of a piece of research before they act, they must act with what is available. Practitioner research, therefore, deals with ambiguity and messy contextual dependent problems. . . . It follows, therefore, that practitioner research draws heavily on 'insider' knowledge and experience. . . . (Reed & Proctor, 1995, p 15).

Similarly, if you undertake small-scale research to find out for yourself, you can expect to end up with more questions, as well as, hopefully, at least some of the answers you wanted. As in so many situations in the real world (cf Janis and

Mann, 1977), evidence-based health promotion will involve acting on imperfect knowledge and thus running the risk of subsequently being shown to have got it wrong. Evidence-based practice, therefore, is not a flak-jacket for health promoters – though it may stop some bullets. What is 'good enough' evidence for an intervention in any given situation will depend on:

- the nature of the risk of being wrong (and who runs it)
- the extent to which mistakes can be corrected in the light of evidence which emerges later – that is, how flexible the intervention can be.

This dilemma needs far more discussion, in print as well as in person. How do practitioners decide what evidence is good enough for their purposes? How can a small-scale local study be good enough to act on, but not good enough to publish?

The Tension Between Evidence and Practice

The naïve model of evidence-based practice is as follows: the research says X works, practitioners go and implement X. This model is full of problems. Failure to implement research is a recurring theme in the literature on professional practice in all areas of health care (Blackburn et al., 1997; Haines & Jones, 1994; Maguire, 1990). A forest of explanations has been identified for this evidence–practice gap. Practitioners can be accused of a failure to read relevant evidence, information overload, and difficulties in extracting and synthesising relevant findings from the morass of research. Researchers can be blamed for a failure to disseminate to practitioners, or to communicate their findings in forms which meet health promotion practitioners' needs and priorities (Crossthwaite & Curtice, 1994).

The tension between evidence and practice can also be explained by factors which are unrelated to the failures of either practitioners or researchers. There is the lack of acknowledgement of the uniqueness of practice contexts and the processes of social, organisational and educational change. Where research does say unequivocally that X works, and it frequently does not, this often applies only in a set of experimental conditions which are not reproduced in most real life settings. In addition, there is plenty of evidence that practice has its own independent set of dynamics which may ignore research-based innovations (e.g. Ford & Walsh, 1994; Hunt, 1987; on nursing). Health promotion continues to feature models of individual behaviour change (like the Stages of Change theory – see Chapter 4) as a framework for promoting healthier lifestyles. It has even extended these models, which see change as a process, to justify targeting of initiatives within groups or communities, despite ethical issues of equity (Whitehead, 1997). Yet at a community or organisational level, changing practice to take account of new research evidence is often viewed as an event rather than a process. Change takes time!

There is extensive empirical evidence that organisational and educational change is indeed a process, with several identifiable phases, from dissemination and adoption, through implementation, to institutionalisation and ultimately outcomes (Fullan, 1991). Each phase has its own set of dynamics which determine the likelihood of progression to the next phase. Movement from dissemination through to successful implementation takes years rather than months. This time frame is frequently ignored by planners and funders, meaning that health promotion practitioners are increasingly being set up to fail by being expected to achieve implementation and successful outcomes within a year – or even less!

Research projects suffer from the same form of short-term thinking. The bulk of studies are accounts of innovative health promotion programmes and evaluation of their impact. Dissemination and implementation research is still in its infancy for all aspects of health care. Until more attention is paid to how research evidence can be put into practice, the evidence–practice gap is bound to persist. Where implementation and dissemination studies have been conducted in health promotion, the results have been of practical value, for example Basch (1984) on disseminating and implementing health education programmes in schools, and Blackburn et al. (1997) on disseminating research findings on women's smoking. However, it does appear that the results of such studies are setting- and context-specific, so that the features which enable successful implementation of research evidence in schools may not be the same as those operating within other settings, like the NHS or the criminal justice system.

This therefore means that managers or practitioners wishing to implement research findings in their work environment have no firm guidance available about what is guaranteed to work. You may initially collect evidence on an issue with a fairly open mind, to seek insights on the right way forward. Once you have done this, and made the best assessment you can, you will need to change the focus – thinking politically, and seeing your evidence as a tool, or a collection of tools, which will suit some tasks and not others. If you are trying to initiate change from the 'bottom up' you will need allies as well as evidence. If you are trying to implement change from the 'top-down' or from the 'outside-in', you will need to become attuned to a different kind of evidence, on the nature of real life in the situation you are trying to change (see Part II). Many practitioners and managers will have experience of trying to implement research-based ideas and hitting a brick wall – or a soggy marsh. Before you jump into the marsh, it is worth considering the following:

- Changing practice is exhausting. How many other changes has this work group been expected to absorb recently? How conservative are they? How much can you ease the process for them?
- Changing practice involves accepting that you may, at least, have ceased to be right, and have possibly not been right for some time. This is uncomfortable for many people. How defensive is this community? How threatening is the presentation of the new approach to their self-esteem?
- Implementing research on one area of practice may disrupt others. This can make a change which is fairly small in itself unmanageable without commitment at a higher level than you may have achieved. For example, a

community centre considering a non-smoking policy will need to be aware of the groups who may cease to use it if such a policy is implemented – Alcoholics Anonymous? The Job Club? The Probation Service's groups for young offenders? Could the centre's use become limited to mother and toddler groups and the local asthma group? Insiders may make a different judgement from outsiders about whether the change produces gains or losses to their health and well-being.

- Reflective practitioners in any area of work will have their own insights and hunches about what could be developed and changed. Where research supports these, it is likely to be well received.
- In any situation there are other values that matter besides research.
  - Implementing research could threaten, or be perceived to threaten, relationships with clients or colleagues – diverting resources from an ineffective service to an effective one is usually unpopular. Why else do doctors still prescribe cough medicine?
  - On a broader front, evidence showing that a social services office or a family planning clinic on a deprived estate is poorly attended is often seen as a justification for closure and provision of the service more centrally. However, opposition to closure could be based on an argument that the evidence could be used as a starting point for identifying ways to improve attendance and maintain a local service, which will be easier for local people to use and local professionals to work with.
  - Choices between two proposals chasing the same resources will not be made solely on the basis of the quality of the proposals and their supporting evidence. Values and power both come into play. Some proposals – like, perhaps, a drop-in centre for prostitutes as an access point for health promotion – are just not popular with local residents, and evidence of the effectiveness of such proposals may not be enough to win over the opposition. Local response can still be more or less sophisticated versions of 'Not in my back yard!' If the local politicians are powerful, or there is an alternative proposal around which causes less contention, the evidence-based proposal may well not succeed.

The Tensions Between Different Types of Knowledge

Thus far we have been considering evidence which is collected using the methods of the social or natural sciences. Much discussion of evidence-based health care restricts serious consideration to research within the scientific paradigm, based on hypothesis testing and relying almost exclusively on quantitative methods (e.g. NHS Executive, 1996). Social science, and qualitative methods, may be accepted as relevant to some questions and useful in complementing the more familiar quantitative approaches (Muir Gray, 1997; see Chapter 2 for further discussion of this point). However, knowledge collected in these ways is not the only kind available. Philosophers argue for a range of forms of knowledge, which have their own tests for truth. Hirst (1974), thinking within an educational framework, argued for seven basic forms: philosophy, religion, literature and the fine arts, history, mathematics, the physical sciences and the human sciences, and was prepared to add to these moral knowledge. Carper (1978), much quoted in the nursing literature, identified four separate ways of knowing about nursing: empirics, where knowledge is drawn from observation; ethics, or moral knowledge; the art of nursing, or aesthetics; and personal knowledge, the individual's insight into how he or she functions (see Margaret MacVicar, Chapter 13, Section 13.2, for further discussion of this). The recognition that health care is not solely associated with knowledge derived from observation, or the natural and human sciences, explains why attempts to introduce evidence-based practice into clinical areas have been uneasily associated with assertions of the value of clinical judgement (e.g. Sackett et al., 1996; Walsh, 1996). An article in *Health Service Journal* (Stewart, 1998), following others on the difficulties of introducing evidence based practice elsewhere, provocatively suggests that evidence-based management might be worth considering too. A recurring theme is the extent to which the activity under discussion is an art or a science.

It is easy to dismiss claims for professional judgement as professional protectionism, when they are made by groups to which you are unsympathetic. However, the real issue is not the group which makes the claim, but the level of rigour with which clinical judgement, professional intuition, or practitioner knowledge is cultivated and pursued (see Meerabeau, 1995, for a review covering a range of disciplines). This is partly a matter of personal qualities – we all know professionals in a particular field of work who are insightful and whose judgement we would trust implicitly, while their equally experienced colleagues may show no similar flair for identifying the crucial angle or the right way forward. It is also, however, partly a matter for professional training, and the current emphasis on reflective practice for a number of groups shows a concern to develop these qualities more systematically.

Reflective practice is not, however, a complete solution. It is interesting to note the ways to which the concept has been adapted since it was developed by Schon (1983; 1987). He saw it as a training process involving a skilled professional mentor as an integral part of it, and a safe place to practise which did not involve real clients. The realities of current professional training are often far from the individual support that Schon saw working well. Reflective practice as it is currently offered tends to depend heavily on reflective diaries, and looks more like a way of pulling oneself up by one's own bootstraps, for novices and experienced staff alike. This method demands the commitment of the individual to what is a time-consuming process, and one for which staff in post will have no time allocated. Furthermore, the less support which is available from others, the more practitioners are exposed to the twin evils of an over-critical assessment of their own work, which is demoralising, or a blinkered failure to see the places where improvement in perception or action is needed. Reflective practice may indeed deepen understanding of a particular way of working, but it can also operate to exclude the challenge that will extend a practitioner's range and deepen insight into others' perspectives. If it is used as a complete answer to the problems of developing and sharpening professional intuition and practitioner knowledge, it may induce complacency rather than stimulate rigour.

Practitioner knowledge needs to be recognised alongside knowledge collected through more conventionally recognised means (Benner, 1984; Meerabeau, 1995; Schon, 1987). Those who ignore it in pursuit of evidence-based practice based purely on evidence collected through scientific or social scientific methods will probably find that their schemes fail. This will partly be for political reasons, since practitioners resent having their knowledge dismissed, but also because real understanding is being excluded from the frame. The most obvious area where this will be so is in the knowledge of work in settings, where practitioners' knowledge of what can be made to work and what cannot will be profound. They may well also have a considerable knowledge of their clients, though this will vary and may need supplementing with more independent access to clients' views. Part II provides examples of practitioners spelling out their own knowledge of particular work in settings and choosing to supplement this by investigating clients' views more systematically.

However, practitioner knowledge should not be elevated to an exclusion of the claims of evidence collected from other sources. Williams and McIntosh (1996) described their experience of designing and evaluating the use of an information pack for women with abnormal cervical smears. The pack was based on a needs assessment and the final version was well received by both women and by the general practices involved in this stage of the study, showing improvements in a variety of outcome measures. Despite this, and an official launch, actual use of the material was very limited indeed, with many practice nurses denying that their practice had received it. Discussion with practice nurses suggested that there was a fear that providing more information and support to patients would increase work overload:

> There was no evidence that the consumer-led and researched nature of the material influenced its use. Some nurses held the view that the amount of information given to women should be restricted. However, this belief is not supported by the research on which the material was based (Willliams & McIntosh, 1996, p 28).

Mark Twain said that it wasn't the things folk don't know that are the problem – 'it's the things that they know that ain't so'. Practitioner knowledge is vulnerable to distortion by self-interest; it needs balancing by knowledge derived from formal research.

Holding the tension between knowledge gained in different ways, so that one does not dominate or exclude others, is a difficult task. Evidence-based practice in health promotion needs to address itself explicitly to this.

Tensions Between Values and Evidence

Nutbeam (1996) identifies three distinct types of health promotion programmes, planned, responsive or reactive, which use evidence in different ways and to different extents. *Planned* programmes are top-down; they can be based on the best available evidence on health needs, effective interventions and ways of supporting them organisationally. *Responsive* programmes involve communities in defining their own health problems and choosing the methods of intervention; research evidence is therefore only one element in the planning process. *Reactive* programmes are responses to a crisis, and frequently involve a demand for a rapid and high profile public response. The use of research evidence is usually limited to the selection of effective mass communication techniques. Values, including political values, affect the choice of programme and thus the way and extent to which evidence can be used in planning. Different types of programme have different criteria for success, which in turn affect the kind of evaluation required.

Many health promoters feel that a primary value for them is to work creatively with the clients and communities they serve, fostering empowerment by taking their priorities seriously (see Ina Simnett's comments in Chapter 7 for a statement of this case in the context of work in settings). Evidence-based health promotion, in this context, would involve collecting evidence about what health issues were priorities for local communities, and what methods were acceptable ways forward. There is also evidence that involving communities, as in the responsive model outlined above, is more likely to result in a good response to programmes and sustained effects (Bracht et al., 1994, and see the discussion from this perspective by Dominic Harrison in Chapter 6, Section 6.1). Social capital theory builds on the pioneering work in an educational context of Friere (1972), so it has a long pedigree as well as many current adherents.

It is important to recognise, however, that those who support other models of health promotion also have a claim to values. Ovretveit, an eminent management researcher and trainer, commented on the difficulty of convincing clinicians 'that efficiency is also important to caring and that inefficiency is unethical' (Ovretveit, 1996). He could have the same problem with health promoters who want to go with the flow of local opinion on tackling one issue, when the health statistics for the area show many higher priorities in terms of health gain, with better tested methods for tackling them. And what about politicians who want to run fear campaigns in the face of the evidence (see p 4) that scare tactics arc only effective in very limited contexts? Politicians like campaigns such as these because they are popular – the dividing line between this and following a smaller community's lead is not always as clear as it might be.

In practice, evidence and values intertwine like strands of DNA. Values affect the evidence we choose to collect, the conclusions we draw from it, and how we respond to the evidence collected by others. They affect what we choose to act on and how we choose to act on it. Evidence-based health promotion offers no escape from the chronic practical problem of working with people with different value systems from one's own – though it may add some new material around which creative compromises can be made.

Tensions Between Inspiration and Evidence

If everyone waited for the evidence before they did anything new, practice would never progress. More fundamentally, the capacity to have new ideas relies on the willingness to move out of the fundamentally rationalist framework within which the collection and assessment of evidence takes place, and free-wheel. The stories about Newton and the apple, and Archimedes in his bath, continue to circulate because they exemplify an important truth. A better documented, more recent, example, is Kekule's discovery of the ring structure of the benzene molecule, which came to him in a dream of a snake with its tail in its mouth (Meerabeau, 1995). The contribution of the right brain to creative thinking is well documented (e.g. Blakeslee, 1980; Bruner, 1962; Ornstein 1975) and this understanding has informed the production of handbooks for enhancing personal and professional creativity (e.g. Buzan, 1989; Capacchione, 1988; Ealy, 1995).

The unsolved problem here is how to link the conditions which foster creative new ideas with the ability to sift ideas to identify which of them are good ones. We do not know how many baths Archimedes had before the crucial one, and how many of them caused him to have bright ideas that burnt out. We do know that Kekule played about with a lot of possible structures before he dreamt of the right one, and that he carefully checked his inspiration against his data before announcing it to the world. It is important not to get so bogged down in evidence that we can neither think nor act creatively; but it is also important that we do not inflict our inspirations on the world of practice (and next year's budget!) without some reality checking against the evidence.

SKILLS FOR EVIDENCE-BASED HEALTH PROMOTION

Evidence-based health promotion starts from skills and qualities which many health promoters have already. It complements reflective practice by adding the experience of others, presented in various forms. A practitioner needs to be, or to become, both questioning and a good listener.

Instead of limiting these skills to the people and situations immediately to hand, evidence-based practitioners and managers will extend their range. They will include in their interests the research of others, in other areas, and possibly in other professional fields beside their own. They may also extend the ways in which they ask questions locally, making more systematic enquiries and possibly undertaking small-scale research themselves. It may be useful to see four different ways of relating to evidence:

- Looking for existing evidence
  - reading the literature
  - checking the files
- Digging for new evidence
  - planning a project
  - collecting data
- Questioning evidence
  - what have I really learnt?
  - does this apply here?
  - what is good enough to act on?
- Acting on evidence

The first two are activities which can be pursued separately; the third is an attitude of mind which you will need to cultivate whatever else you do in relation to evidence. The fourth is implicit in any discussion of evidence-based practice – the point is to work out what to do! Part III of this book discusses a range of techniques in more detail; the rest of this introduction provides an overview of the issues.

Reflective Practice

Developing the ability to think on your feet, or reflect-in-action, is one of the roots of evidence-based practice. Reflecting-*in*-action means listening to what is said and observing what is happening, as you work. At the same time you try to make sense of what is happening and use this information to help you to make decisions about what to do and how to behave. In this way, a reflective practitioner is continually trying out mini-experiments, which create small changes and provide new understanding about the situation. Mark Smith points out that:

> . . . in this, we do not closely follow established ideas and techniques – textbook schemes. We are not following a plan like technicians. . . . We may have our own routines or ways of doing things but these have to be held in tension with each situation (Smith, 1994, p 129).

As a reflective practitioner you will therefore be constantly gathering, assessing and using evidence as part of the way that you think.

As well as thinking 'on your feet', to be a reflective practitioner you also need to think about your work afterwards, to reflect-*on*-action. This will allow you to think about why you acted and felt the way you did, what was happening to others, what you didn't notice at the time that might have been helpful, and what you have learned which might help you to decide what to do in future. When you do this, you are drawing conclusions from what you have observed, about your own reactions and those of others. This is assessing evidence. It may not be very good evidence – after all, you only have your own point of view, and you were not just observing, you were doing things as well, so your observation may have been hampered by this – but it is still evidence. Developing your skills in reflective practice is therefore a good basis for developing further your skills in handling evidence; Linda Wright discusses this in more detail in Chapter 12.

EXAMPLES OF LEVELS OF REFLECTIVE THINKING

The following are extracts from the course diaries of students participating in an alcohol education module as part of a Diploma in Community and Youth Work course.

No reflection   1.   We played a card game on alcohol facts.
↓

2. We played a card game on alcohol facts. I did not learn much that was new to me.
↓

3. We played a card game on alcohol facts and I feel there are still gaps in my knowledge about alcohol as a drug, particularly its effects on young people.
↓

4. We played a card game on alcohol facts. I don't think the game covered the information in a systematic way, so permitting gaps in my understanding. Perhaps the tutor could have picked up on more of the queries and difficult areas after we'd finished playing the games.
↓

Good reflection   5.   We played a card game on alcohol facts. I need to learn more about alcohol 'facts'. I will read the leaflets and handouts the tutor gave me and see if they are enough. If necessary I will ask her to recommend a book from the reading list. It seems to me a lot of the so-called 'facts' are based on very little evidence.

Source: Wright, L. (1998). Unpublished Material for PhD thesis.

Reflective practice on its own, however, is not enough. It is limited in scope (see also the discussion of practitioner knowledge, earlier in this chapter, p 11) and can reinforce rather than challenge professional habits. The selective nature of memory can easily encourage a self-protective bias, 'rather like looking at myself and seeing how good I am' (Kirkham, 1997, p 259). The catalyst which triggers a willingness to see things in a new way and consider doing things differently as a result may come from a variety of sources, at least some of which will be external. Although it is currently much favoured as a method of professional development, its weaknesses need to be borne in mind as well as its advantages.

It can thus provide only some of the foundation material from which practitioners can develop evidence-based practice. A willingness to listen to others, both in person and on paper, also has roots in classic health promotion practice and can be carried forward into a more formal concern with evidence.

Reading Other People's Work

Increasing numbers of professionals have had training in research awareness, either as part of basic professional preparation, in degree or higher degree work, or in short focused courses. Much first stage teaching about research is focused on the ability to read research critically, so that students may be less at risk of believing everything they read. While these skills are important, they are only a part of becoming research-minded (see Margaret MacVicar's discussion in Chapter 13, Section 13.2). It is also easy for exercises in critiquing research papers to turn into criticism in the narrow sense, so that weaknesses rather than strengths are given prominence. In evidence-based practice it is important to be able to see what use can be made of a study, and this requires the ability to see strengths as well as weaknesses. This is especially important because the one can at times be the mirror image of the other, as when particular research methods are good at providing one kind of information but not another. It is also important to be able to make sense of a mass of material, often coming from different theoretical perspectives, and this is rarely a part of first stage research awareness (French, 1998).

There are four key problems which the practitioner faces here:

- Defining the issue on which the evidence should throw light
- Allocating time to find and assess published literature
- Finding the material
- Reviewing the material once found.

The first two of these require skills which are needed in a number of health promotion contexts; developing objectives and time management are discussed in Ewles and Simnett (1998). The second two are discussed in more detail elsewhere in this book (see Dale Webb, Chapter 3, Section 3.1, and Elizabeth Perkins, Chapter 13, Section 13.1). The challenge for practitioners is to listen as carefully to pieces of paper as they do to individuals and groups in front of them – for pieces of paper are also a guide to the needs of others and the best ways of meeting them.

An evidence-based practitioner or manager will read published material with a dual focus, assessing it both for its quality as a piece of research and its applicability to the problem in hand. This may yield good results in the shape of a clear way forward with research support. It may, however, produce a jungle of findings which are not immediately compatible, from studies which make different assumptions about the nature of health, the nature and purpose of health promotion, and the nature of research. If this is the case, your path through the jungle will need to be chartered with care, and with clear attention to your own perspective on these matters, as well as the nature of the problem you are investigating.

What Do You Do if There is No Evidence?

Another scenario is that the jungle may not be where you want it, but over there. For example, there are a lot of research studies about family support by home visiting services, but comparatively few on family support through group work, which could be the topic you wanted to investigate (Perkins, 1998). Quite often, questions of concern to health promoters have not attracted the kind of research funding that permits studies of really high quality – whatever criteria you use. Evidence-based practice should not involve a commitment to trudge along all the time in the ruts worn by other people's vehicles – but on what basis can you depart from them and strike out somewhere new? For example, should you, or should you not, run groups on health promotion topics in Greyton for adults with physical disabilities, and if so, what kind? The literature you have found does not help you decide. What do you do?

The first way out of this dilemma is to recognise that there is very rarely really good evidence which tells you what will work in your precise circumstances. Serious research is likely to have been done elsewhere, on a population which may or may not be appropriate for generalisations to be made to your patch. If you feel that your efforts to collect evidence are unfruitful, you have probably defined what you want in a way that excludes studies which might guide you, even if they are not close enough to make you and others feel secure. You may need to consider more theoretical material; see Chapter 2 for a discussion of the uses of theory.

As an example, consider the Stages of Change model, discussed in Chapter 4 by Terry Lawrence and Liz Batten (Sections 4.1 and 4.2) and used in Chapter 11 by Lesley Jones and colleagues (Section 11.1) and in Chapter 16 by Graham Simmonds (Section 16.2). This model is well-researched enough for there to be an extensive dissemination programme based on it, Helping People Change courses abound in the UK at present. Using this model, without further local research, can be an acceptable way of being an evidence-based practitioner, in the current state of knowledge. However, this does not mean that we know all there is to know about the uses of this model (or that it will remain proven as a good way to work indefinitely!). New research studies are being commissioned to test out its applicability in different circumstances, as Liz Batten's section (4.2) in Chapter 4 illustrates. Most people using this model do not have local evidence that it works in their circumstances. You can transfer this experience to help you with your own problem; you may have to move up to a more general level of evidence than the one you would prefer.

This changed approach ought to produce more material, though you will continue to need to assess its quality as well as deciding how conclusive you find its guidance. If you are still in doubt about the support within the evidence for your idea, you could turn to your principles and values for guidance. Tony Jeffs and Mark Smith, in Chapter 9, Section 9.1, make a powerful case for values rather than evidence as the driving force for practice. Values alone, however, are not enough on their own for evidence-based practice. If you want to try out your idea despite

> **'I HAVE FOUND NOTHING ON HEALTH PROMOTION GROUPS FOR ADULTS WITH PHYSICAL DISABILITY IN GREYTON.'**
>
> That's a pity. Ask yourself instead:
>
> - What is special about Greyton? Would evidence from any town of a similar size do as well? What do I need to check in other studies?
> - Is there anything on any kind of group work with these clients?
> - Is there anything on health promotion work with these clients which might give me ideas on groups? Did these projects consider group work and decide not to? Why? Or don't they mention it?
> - What about theoretical material on how people learn to cope with disability? What does this contribute to the assessment of your idea?

the lack of support in the literature you have found, and remain an evidence-based practitioner, you need to plan to collect some evidence. You could do a needs assessment, pilot and evaluate, or use an action research model. Any of these need to be designed so that the findings can challenge you (see Maggie Wark in Chapter 3 (Section 3.3), Chapter 14 on needs assessment, Linda Wright on evaluation in Chapter 16 (Section 16.3), and the earlier discussion in this chapter on the tension between inspiration and evidence, p 13).

Finally, it is worth remembering that you do have the option of doing nothing about this particular idea, and turning your attention to areas where the evidence is better. Practitioners with a commitment to health promotion can feel they have a moral obligation to tackle everything; sometimes it may be better to focus on a more promising, because better researched, issue than to pioneer in all directions.

Collecting Evidence Yourself

Undertaking a local study can be both a way of finding out what you need to know and a political move to involve and convince others. Sometimes you may decide that the national evidence for a particular course of action is compelling, and that there is no need for you to reinvent the wheel locally. If you can convince stakeholders that this is the case, all that may be needed is low level monitoring of the initiative to see that it is running according to plan. In other cases you may need a clearer understanding of local needs, or a more detailed evaluation focusing on more speculative aspects of the plan, either because you yourself need extra information or because you know that others will require a more rigorous approach. You may wish to limit the risk of inappropriately designed initiatives by building in a formative evaluation or adopting an action research approach from the beginning. 'Bottom up' innovation can often recruit support through a well designed local study which shows that there is a local need or that current practice is not working as expected.

If you need, for whatever reason, to undertake a local study, you will be faced with immediate issues about the quality of the work you can undertake. What is 'good enough' small-scale needs assessment and evaluation? This problem is not new minted as part of evidence-based health promotion (cf Perkins, 1987); it has been around since practitioners in health promotion started to think about using research techniques to answer their questions about their own practice (see Part III for detailed discussion). Some general principles are worth considering:

- Practitioner research, evaluation or needs assessment is properly focused on improving specific areas of practice, not on making general statements about the way the social world works (Reed & Proctor, 1995). Using this framework to define the questions you want answered will help you keep the project manageable and greatly increase the chances that you can use the results.
- You need to cut your coat according to your cloth. Attempts to prove that health promotion works, with an evaluation budget of £7,500, are bound to fail. Establishing clear, small-scale, specific objectives for the project which can shape the research will both help to keep you sane and limit the amount of hostile criticism that over-blown studies are prone to attract.
- If in your field there are established ways of doing needs assessment or evaluation, consider using their methods locally; you should save time on design and be contributing to a growing body of knowledge. This will also help you to explore with colleagues the extent to which your area is different from others.
- If there are no blueprints for the kind of work you want to do, or those that exist fit your objectives very imperfectly, be realistic about the resources, both human and financial, that you have at your disposal. If you do not have the skills or the time to do the work alone, you should either negotiate for extra help or abandon the idea of a local study. Unreliable evidence can be worse than no evidence for planning purposes, and it is also likely to be a political liability.

PRACTICE NOT PARALYSIS

Evidence-based health promotion is problematic. It is full of creative tensions which can be exciting but which can also be uncomfortable. It provides no refuge from criticism, because there are so many points of view which have some intellectual, political or practical legitimacy; someone will always be able to suggest that the task could be done differently, and by their standards, better. The Labour government's white paper, *The New NHS* (Secretary of State for Health, 1997) and the green paper, *Our Healthier Nation* (Secretary of State for Health, 1998) have changed some of the criteria by which health care and health promotion are to be assessed, and also encouraged a debate on indicators which can only be healthy. This is unlikely, however, to be concluded in a way that disposes of the tensions; miracles, after all, take a little longer. This means that health promoters, of whatever kind and with whatever interest in matters theoretical, can expect to carry on living with multiple expectations, multiple realities, and multiple definitions of what counts as evidence, in what contexts and for what purposes. They will also be expected, and expect themselves, to carry on practising health promotion.

It is difficult to carry on working in the knowledge that, while it may be the best you can do, it will not be right by everyone's standards. For example, at some point someone may come up with findings which you as well as others would treat as evidence that you should be doing something else. Practitioners in this situation need support, both through pooling knowledge and through sharing the strains of living with uncertainties. This book is intended to open up the issues for debate, to encourage the development of skills to help with the problems of assessing, collecting and managing evidence, and to encourage practitioners to find common ground with others, perhaps outside their own immediate field. The promotion of evidence-based practice, like the promotion of health, is not a task for individuals but for communities. Building professional communities to tackle this will be an essential part of the job.

REFERENCES

Basch C E (1984) Research on disseminating and implementing health education programs in schools. *School Health Research*, 54, 57–66.
Benner P (1984) From novice to expert: excellence and power in clinical nursing practice. Menlo Park, CA: Addison-Wesley.
Blackburn C, Graham H & Scullion P (1997) Evaluation of disseminating research on women's smoking to health practitioners. *Health Education Journal*, 56, 113–124.
Blakeslee T R (1980) The right brain: a new understanding of the unconscious mind and its creative powers. London: MacMillan Education.
Bracht N, Finnegan J R, Rissel C, Weisbrod R, Gleason J, Corbett J & Veblen-Mortenson S (1994) Community ownership and program continuation following a health demonstration project. *Health Education Research*, 9, 243–255.
Bruner J S (1962) On knowing: essays for the left hand. Cambridge, MA: Harvard University Press.
Buzan T (1989) Use your head. Third edition. London: BBC Books.
Capacchione L (1988) The power of your other hand: a course in channeling the inner wisdom of the right brain. North Hollywood, CA: Newcastle Publishing.
Carper B (1978) Fundamental patterns of knowing in nursing. *Advances in Nursing Science*, 1(1), 13–23.
Crossthwaite C & Curtice L (1994) Disseminating research results – the challenge of bridging the gap between health research and health action. *Health Promotion International*, 9, 289–296.
Ealy C D (1995) The women's book of creativity. Dublin: Gill and MacMillan.
Ewles L & Simnett I (1998) Promoting health. Fourth edition. London: Ballière Tindall.
Fisher C (1986) On demand breastfeeding. *Midwife Health Visitor and Community Nurse*, 22, 194–198.
Ford P & Walsh M (1994) New rituals for old: nursing through the looking glass. Oxford: Butterworth-Heinemann.
French B (1998) Developing the skills required for evidence-based practice. *Nurse Education Today*, 18, 46–51.

Friere P (1972) Pedagogy of the oppressed. Harmondsworth: Penguin.

Fullan M G (1991) The new meaning of educational change. London: Cassell.

Haines A & Jones R (1994) Implementing findings of research. *British Medical Journal*, 308, 1488–1492.

Hirst P H (1974) Knowledge and the curriculum: a collection of philosophical papers. London: Routledge and Kegan Paul.

Hovland C I, Janis I L & Kelley H H (1963) Communication and persuasion. Yale: Yale University Press.

Hunt M (1987) The process of translating research findings into nursing practice. *Journal of Advanced Nursing*, 12, 101–110.

Janis I L & Mann L (1977) Decision making: a psychological analysis of conflict, choice and commitment. New York: Free Press.

Kirkham M (1997) Reflection in midwifery: professional narcissism or seeing with women? *British Journal of Midwifery*, 5(5), 259–262.

Maguire J H (1990) Putting nursing research findings into practice: research utilisation as an aspect of the management of change. *Journal of Advanced Nursing*, 16, 614–620.

Meerabeau L (1995) The nature of practitioner knowledge. In: K Reed & S Proctor (Eds), Practitioner research in health care: the inside story. London: Chapman & Hall.

Muir Gray J A (1997) Evidence-based health care: how to make health policy and management decisions. New York: Churchill Livingstone.

NHS Executive (1996) Clinical guidelines. London: HMSO.

Nutbeam D (1996) Achieving best practice in health promotion: improving the fit between research and practice. *Health Education Research*, 11(3), 317–326.

Ornstein R E (1975) The psychology of consciousness. Harmondsworth: Penguin.

Ovretveit J (1996) Ethics: a counsel of perfection? *IHSM Network*, 3(13), 4–5.

Perkins E R (1987) Good enough evaluation? In: G Campbell (Ed), Health education: youth and community. Lewes: Falmer Press.

Perkins E R (1998) Public health approaches to family support: how good is the evidence? *British Journal of Community Nursing*, 13(6), 297–302.

Power R (1989) Drugs and the media: prevention campaigns and television. In: S MacGregor (Ed), Drugs and British society. London: Routledge.

Reed J & Proctor S (Eds) (1995) Practitioner research in health care: the inside story. London: Chapman & Hall.

Royal College of Midwives (1988) Successful breastfeeding. London: RCM.

Sackett D L, Rosenberg W M C, Gray J A M, Haynes R B & Richardson W S (1996) Evidence based medicine: what it is and isn't. *British Medical Journal*, 312, 71–72.

Schon D (1983) The reflective practitioner: how professionals think in action. London: Temple Smith.

Schon D (1987) Educating the reflective practitioner: towards a new design for teaching and learning. San Francisco: Jossey-Bass.

Schramm W (Ed) (1960) Mass communications. Illinois: University of Illinois Press.

Secretary of State for Health (1997) The New NHS: modern, dependable. London: The Stationery Office.

Secretary of State for Health (1998) Our Healthier Nation: a contract for health. A consultation paper. London: The Stationery Office.

Sharp D & Lowe G (1989) Adolescents and alcohol – a review of the recent British research. *Journal of Adolescence*, 12, 295–307.

Smith M (1994) Local education. Buckingham: Open University Press.

Stewart R (1998) More art than science? *Health Service Journal*, 108, 28–29.

Walsh D (1996) Evidence-based practice: whose evidence and on what basis? *British Journal of Midwifery*, 4(9), 454–457.

Whitehead M (1997) How useful is the 'Stages of Change' model? *Health Education Journal*, 56(2), 111–112.

Williams S & McIntosh J (1996) Problems in implementing evidence-based health promotion material in general practice. *Health Service Journal*, 55, 24–30.

Part I

Recent Theories and New Aproaches to Practice

Edited by Elizabeth R. Perkins

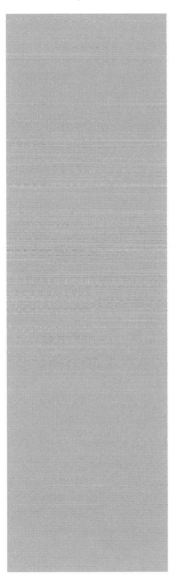

Chapter 2

The Role of Theories in Health Promotion Practice

Elizabeth R. Perkins

WHAT IS THEORY FOR?

Everyone has a set of personal theories about the way the world works – or should work. This is a set of assumptions on which we base our daily lives, about how people behave and relate to each other, about what information in our environment is important for us to take in and what we can screen out, and about how we fit into our world. They are frameworks which help us make sense of the world as we experience it, and also tell us what to do. They are personal and evolve as we experience new things; some may be inconsistent with others, but because they are our own theories this tends not to worry us. We rarely make these explicit, and may notice them only when some event seriously challenges what we take for granted. Since theories intertwine with values, it can be most disconcerting when people not only fail to behave as we expect, but show that they do not even wish to do so – their set of theories about the world are different from ours.

As professionals, we carry our personal theories, moral judgements and value systems into the workplace, and add some more. Initial training is likely to provide both explicit and implicit statements about the way we should organise our working lives, mentally as well as physically. It provides a body of knowledge, with some guidance about how to turn this into a set of operational principles. This guidance can vary both in its quantity and in its quality. When we start work, we may well find that some of the theory we were taught in training and the ways we were taught to apply it do not work very well – most professions have some form of theory–practice gap (Lipsky, 1980). We absorb alternative ways of thinking about the world of work from those around us who are more experienced. These are likely to be more immediately practical theories, and we may settle down comfortably to get on with the job. Theories, after all, are supposed to relate to the world of practice. If we cannot use them to make sense of life as we experience it, they are not good theories for us in our current situation.

Evidence-based Health Promotion. Edited by Elizabeth R. Perkins, Ina Simnett and Linda Wright.
© 1999 John Wiley & Sons Ltd.

Implicit theories are fine in a stable world. They become a problem:

- when major changes take place in our external environment
- when new people come into it who do not know, understand or share our theories or behave in ways that challenge them
- when people with whom we spend time with change
- when people who have authority over us, like employers, change their theories about how the world should work
- when we, in our turn, go forth to new areas and find that our assumptions are not shared.

The clash of implicit theories can cause a lot of messed up communication.

> A small child came to his mother and said 'Mummy, where did I come from?' His mother, being a parent who believed in answering children's questions, had prepared for the need to give informal sex education, and launched into a careful explanation of conception and birth. The little boy listened patiently but looked more and more baffled. When his mother stopped, he said 'Yes, but Mummy – was I born in Birmingham or Devon?'

When faced with clashing implicit theories, it can be difficult to state our assumptions so that they can be discussed and the distress caused by clashes of theories reduced. If our own theories clash with those introduced by employers or other authority figures, it can be even more difficult; see Robin Burgess in Chapter 10, Section 10.1, for an exploration in relation to work with offenders. The problem is further compounded if we are faced with incompatible theories, both of which we are supposed to apply – managing one's own inconsistencies is always a lot easier than incorporating those of others. The pressure to develop evidence-based practice, for example, is not easy to reconcile with the importance of responding to the needs of clients and communities (see Chapter 1).

Theory as developed by academics carries a particular kind of authority, but it is also easy for busy practitioners to dismiss it as coming from, and belonging in, an ivory tower. In fact it can have a variety of possible applications for practitioners:

- It may state your own implicit position, better than you would have managed if challenged.
- It may state the position of a person or a group of people you have never understood properly, so that suddenly their behaviour starts to make sense.
- It may state a position which you find foreign, and possibly uncomfortable.
- It may provide a way of bridging the gap between your position and those of others, so that you can recognise the common ground as well as the differences.

This part of the book offers a range of perspectives on health promotion. Chapter 3 is concerned with perspectives on evidence; Chapters 4, 5 and 6 draw on psychological, educational and social systems approaches to health promotion. This is not the full range of positions; these have been chosen to show different approaches to the use of evidence, and to reflect developments in health promotion which are of current interest. Each chapter pulls out for attention different features of the world of health promotion, and shows how practice could change to pay more attention to them. The more theoretical sections in each chapter are coupled with sections which use this kind of theoretical perspective to collect evidence. To any one reader, one or more of the chapters is bound to feel somewhat uncomfortable, because it is written from a perspective which is not shared. How, then, can this part of the book be used?

THOUGHT EXPERIMENTS WITH THEORIES

Some of the discomfort created by alternative theoretical positions arises because we behave as if we had to have one theory and one only, which covers all situations. Furthermore, we can get very attached to theories, and feel as if, like the RSPCA say about dogs, they should be for life, not just for Christmas. Yet many theories have been developed for particular situations and do not extend well to cover the whole of life – or even professional life. It is worth being prepared to try a new theory on for size and see how it feels and whether it works. You don't have to stick with it for life, just see whether it helps with this job, these people, or this situation. You can always discard it if it is too uncomfortable or doesn't help – but think out what is the matter first.

> If you are in Wales, you will find a contour map more use than a street plan. If you are in London, it will be the other way round. What kind of map will help you in your current situation?
>
> *(from Bill Palmer, one-time chair of the Shiatsu Society)*

Ideas to Try

- If you find the perspective in a particular chapter or section comfortable, look at the implications of this theory for your own practice. The theory will suggest practical consequences. Can you apply it? How does it fit with your current approaches? Does anything need to change?
- Research in another setting may have implications for you. The theory behind the research should help you to see how far it is transferable. What does the theory and the research say about why things happen? What does it suggest (or can you deduce) about how far the results will generalise? What does it suggest are the most important aspects – and would you find them in your own setting?

- If you are moving into a new area of work, or an area where you have difficulty, consider what theory would best suit the situation. Think about the task you have to do, the setting in which you are working, the client(s) you are working with. Can you try working from a theory which suits the situation, even if it is not the one you personally prefer?

- If you find one of these chapters really uncomfortable, try not to shut the book at this point or skip to somewhere more congenial. Work out what it is that you find so unacceptable. Try not to blame the style – after all, all our contributors are committed to communication! Theories tend to arise from real situations and develop beyond them – is the theory you dislike more suitable for some other situation? The discomfort is telling you something about your own perspective as well as the writer's. Can you use the discomfort to get a clearer picture of your own position?

RESEARCH PARADIGMS

Responding to Research

Research methods can provoke the same gut reaction as theories about health promotion – an instinctive sense of comfort or discomfort. Of course if you are inexperienced in reading research papers, practically anything can feel alien and uncomfortable, but as familiarity increases, people develop a sense of what they like and dislike reading which can be independent of the quality of the work, and even of the conclusions drawn. People react emotionally not only to the content of evidence but to the kind of evidence it is. Some loathe tables or figures and never read them if they can help it; others find it difficult to credit any paper without some. Some find quotations from interviews a waste of their time; others warm to them and see them as a sign of contact with the real world of practice. This emotional preference is not just about presentation. It relates to and reflects preferences for the kind of questions particular types of research set out to answer, the types of understanding they offer, and the kind of relationships they imply between the different people involved in producing research (Baum, 1995; Milburn et al., 1995; Reason & Rowan, 1981; Secker et al., 1995). One of the reasons why the debate about qualitative versus quantitative research methods is so interminable and can become so bitter is that not everyone wants to settle for a peaceful compromise which says 'horses for courses'. For some the issue is fundamentally about the nature of truth, and whether there is one single truth which we can pursue with the right instruments, or whether there are multiple truths which are in principle equal. This is a debate about the proper view of the world, not about the right tools for a particular job, and in such a clash of research paradigms compromises are not acceptable.

Power is also a complicating factor. Quantitative methods were there first; they are the normal methods used by the scientific community, and when the social sciences started to establish themselves they used similar methods and hoped to be respected in the same way. Given the respect which scientific methods have accrued, quantitative methods are understandably popular with decision-makers; the production of a mass of figures is a good way of being taken seriously, even in a position that is actually rather weak. In health care and health promotion, quantitative methods are also associated with doctors, both through clinical trials and epidemiology, and doctors are the most powerful single professional group. Qualitative methods therefore have both a shorter history and a weaker political base. Explaining unfamiliar research processes to powerful stakeholders who may find them emotionally alien is not a straightforward process, and sometimes the protagonists emerge feeling battered, with little real communication having taken place.

Why do many health promotion people prefer qualitative to quantitative research? It is a good approach for understanding the point of view of particular groups, and health promoters are well aware that it is important to think about their clients' starting point before trying to improve their knowledge, affect their attitude or change their behaviour. In addition, qualitative social science has had a tradition of exploring the position of the underdog, and this suits the politics of many health promotion specialists. Part III in this book therefore discusses a number of qualitative approaches in some detail. However, it is easy to become trapped in a particular perspective which does not suit all situations, and in this part it so happens that many of the case studies have a quantitative bias. We did not plan this, but it adds to the potential challenge of the contributions in this part.

Building Theory

Theories are developed from research, logic and experience; they need to be tested against experience and research. One way of looking at academic research studies is to divide them into two groups: those which are designed to use existing theory and test it, and those which are set up to develop new theory which can be tested in its turn. Most health promotion work which uses explicit theory draws on research and theory building which has been undertaken in established academic disciplines like psychology and sociology, or within better established fields of practice, like education. It is also worth considering the possibility, however, that health promotion work can contribute to the development of theory, either for use in health promotion or for more general use. For example, every time a trainer uses a model to present a way of looking at a small aspect of the world, a low-level theory is being suggested. Some of these are home-grown, developed as a way in which trainers can communicate their understanding of their own experience to the group in front of them. This is theory building. Good trainers will have tested this theory in some way, however informally, before launching it on the world of their trainees, perhaps by discussion with colleagues, perhaps by checking it against personal past experience or reading, perhaps even against a small-scale piece of research.

The rigorous approach to theory building developed by Glaser and Strauss (1967) and elaborated by Strauss and Corbin (1990) can be seen as having parallels with the modest model building of an experienced and conscientious trainer. Glaser and Strauss developed a new way of developing theory, known as 'grounded theory', where theory is grounded in the evidence collected, usually, though not necessarily, from qualitative studies. Such work can provide a good understanding of the ways in which particular groups think and behave (see Chapter 15 for a worked example). There is also scope, in a grounded theory study, for practitioners who are part of the group being researched to contribute their own understanding of the way their professional world works, and to become part of the process of theory generation about it. The practitioner knowledge set out in Part II of this book provides material not only to guide practice but also, potentially, for the development of theory – though this book does not take on that task!

Health promoters and health promotion specialists can continue to use work undertaken from within other disciplines indefinitely, if they so choose; most small-scale studies will inevitably and properly be focused on practice, not on theory (Reed & Proctor, 1995). An example of a study of the role of health promotion specialists which takes a more theoretical approach can be found in Nettleton and Burrows (1997). The option of contributing to theory, as well as borrowing it, is open, and those who commission health promotion research, at least, would do well to bear it in mind.

USING THE IDEAS IN THIS PART OF THE BOOK

One way to use this part of the book is simply to read sections for interest – not necessarily all in one sitting! This is a good way to approach theory; a relaxed attitude means you are more likely to hear what writers are saying in their own terms, rather than instantly looking for applications to your own situation. A new idea can be relevant in several different ways, and if you are only looking in one direction it is easier to miss possibilities elsewhere.

Those who prefer a more focused approach may well be starting from a version of the dilemma outlined in Chapter 1 (p 17) – the would-be evidence-based health promoter who can find no evidence that helps. In this situation, you could try some of the following:

- Decide whether your basic approach is one-to-one, training and education, or working with organisations or communities. Read the theoretical parts of Chapters 4, 5 or 6 for guidance, and the case studies for some ideas on how others have taken this approach forward.
- Even if you are sure which chapter covers your basic approach, put this on hold for a while. Read one or both of the alternatives and see what insights these may give you. Might there be an alternative way of approaching your situation? You can still return to your original choice if you want. You may be

able to enhance your familiar ways of working through understanding gained by trying on a different perspective and seeing how it would work.

- If you have already been introduced to one of these perspectives – Stages of Change through a *Helping People Change* course, perhaps – read the relevant chapter for more background. Introductory courses have to simplify, and if you are responsible for planning an initiative, it may be really important to have more than the basic idea of what to do.
- If you have no local studies to guide you, and you are aiming to do something new, you are almost certainly going to have to collect some local evidence. Before you turn to Part III of this book to consider methods, needs assessment or evaluation, read Chapter 3, and Dominic Harrison's section in Chapter 6 (Section 6.1), and think about what kind of evidence you, and others involved in the project, will value and take seriously.

Reading theory can give you inspiration. It can also provide support, if you find writers who have struggled with the kind of intellectual problems which your practice generates, and have found ways forward. Theory may show you the way to evidence-based practice in your particular situation, though it cannot provide blueprints for what to do. It can help to find others who have tried to apply the theory in their situation and are prepared to communicate about the snags. The chapters in this part of the book provide examples of this.

REFERENCES

Baum F (1995) Researching public health: behind the qualitative–quantitative methodological debate. *Social Science and Medicine*, 40(4), 459–468.

Glaser B G & Strauss A L (1967) The discovery of grounded theory: strategies for qualitative research. New York: Aldine Publishing.

Lipsky M (1980) Street-level bureaucracy: dilemmas of the individual in public services. New York: Russell Sage.

Milburn K, Fraser E, Secker J & Pavis S (1995) Combining methods in health promotion research: some considerations about appropriate use. *Health Education Journal*, 54, 347–356.

Nettleton S & Burrows R (1997) If health promotion is everybody's business, what is the fate of the health promotion specialist? *Sociology of Health and Illness*, 19(1), 23–47.

Reason P & Rowan J (1981) Human inquiry: a sourcebook of new paradigm research. Chichester: John Wiley.

Reed J & Proctor S (1995) Practitioner research in health care: the inside story. London: Chapman & Hall.

Secker J, Wimbush E, Watson J & Milburn K (1995) Qualitative methods in health promotion research; some criteria for quality. *Health Education Journal*, 54, 74–87.

Strauss A & Corbin J (1990) Basics of qualitative research: grounded theory and procedures and techniques. Newbury Park, CA: Sage.

Chapter 3

Evidence

Elizabeth R. Perkins

INTRODUCTION

Becoming an evidence-based practitioner inevitably involves thinking about what kind of evidence is required to guide practice or to answer questions, and this is not a simple matter. This chapter includes two theoretical discussions on evidence in a health promotion context, and two case studies which illustrate different points in the development process where evidence can support the growth of new practice. Both concern mental health and both use quantitative methods to evaluate new initiatives.

This first section, *Current approaches to gathering evidence*, is written from a research perspective, and explores the difficulties posed in applying the dominant model of reviewing health care interventions to health promotion. It argues for the importance of exploring the philosophical assumptions behind different research approaches in order to identify appropriate designs, methods and outcome measures for health promotion.

The second section, *The challenge of evidence-based practice*, complements the first by looking at the issues from a practitioner's perspective.

The third section, *Improving mental health in women with breast cancer*, is an example of a 'bright idea' about the possible therapeutic value of colour analysis for women recovering from breast surgery. The idea was developed as a pilot project and evaluated to see whether further development seemed warranted. The project's focus on mental health, rather than five-year survival rates, was matched by the use of a measure of self-esteem to assess the effects of the process.

The fourth section, *Parenting support groups*, is an example of a practical initiative based more securely on established knowledge, and evaluated by means of a randomised controlled trial. The project was set up as a response to GP concern about frequent consultations by mothers of young children, and is unusual in that both the practical work and the research were conducted from within a health promotion department. Outcome measures were related to mental health, not to the patterns of consultation which had prompted the project.

Evidence-based Health Promotion. Edited by Elizabeth R. Perkins, Ina Simnett and Linda Wright.
© 1999 John Wiley & Sons Ltd.

Section 3.1

Current Approaches to Gathering Evidence

Dale Webb

INTRODUCTION

In recent years a view has emerged that the dominant approach to health care evaluation in the NHS is inappropriate to determining effective health promotion. This section of the chapter will explore the key elements of concern that have been expressed by those working as researchers and practitioners in the health promotion field. Principally, there are three sets of considerations:

- How appropriate to health promotion evaluations are the research designs considered by the dominant approach to offer the 'best evidence' of effectiveness?
- What has been the development of systematic reviews of health promotion and which way should they be going?
- What assumptions about health promotion are made by those who argue that health promotion must be understood through the dominant approach to health care evaluation?

This section will be divided into three parts and will consider:

- the dominant approach to health care evaluation
- limitations in applying this approach to health promotion research
- ways in which effective health promotion may be determined.

THE DOMINANT MODEL OF HEALTH CARE EVALUATION

The dominant model for reviewing health care interventions is that established by the Cochrane Collaboration (1994). It is basically a bio-medical model, in which the ultimate effectiveness of interventions is expressed as 'hard' outcomes such as changes in mortality and morbidity, and behavioural outcomes. Accumulating scientific proof of the effectiveness of a clinical intervention can be complex, and can involve:

Evidence-based Health Promotion. Edited by Elizabeth R. Perkins, Ina Simnett and Linda Wright.
© 1999 John Wiley & Sons Ltd.

- clinical trials
- combining clinical trials into a meta-analysis
- undertaking systematic reviews.

Each of these will be described briefly.

Clinical Trials

The 'gold standard' of clinical trials is the randomised controlled trial (RCT). An RCT is an experiment with a group of patients that seeks to determine which outcomes are obtained with a particular intervention. Of course, it is always possible that a clinical outcome may be a consequence of some factor other than the intervention. This possibility is 'controlled for' by incorporating into the design of the trial a second group, the 'control group', who do not receive the intervention. Patients are randomly assigned to either the intervention or the control group: through randomising the allocation of patients to intervention and control groups it becomes likely that factors which might influence an outcome, for example socio-economic differences, are equally distributed, and therefore cancel each other out. Measurements are taken of the intervention and the control groups before and after the intervention, the intervention groups are exposed to the intervention, and the results are compared within groups and between them. Thus, as factors capable of influencing outcomes are equally distributed among groups, and as the only difference between the two groups is the application of the intervention, the RCT provides the best assurance that outcome differences can be attributed to the intervention and not to extraneous factors.

1. Experimental studies	2. Observational studies
1a. Randomised controlled trials	2a. Cohort (prospective) study
1b. Controlled trials (non-randomised)	2b. Case-control (retrospective) studies
1c. Quasi-experimental design	2c. 'Before' and 'after' studies (no controls)
	2d. Descriptive studies

A research evidence hierarchy (adapted from Lawrence et al., 1989).

The 'stronger' research designs are those which are best able to attribute outcomes to an intervention through the use of a control or comparison group. Thus, although it is recognised that other study designs are possible, the RCT is taken as the most persuasive.

Meta-analysis

Since the late 1970s meta-analysis has emerged as a powerful tool for synthesising the results of independent trials. In essence it is an overview of clinical trials in a particular area of treatment, in which the results are presented in the form of a numeric summary. Given that in many spheres of medical research studies may provide conflicting results, meta-analysis offers a scientific method for resolving conflict. A particular strength of this sophisticated method is its ability to undertake analysis of sub-groups of data in ways that RCTs, given their sometimes small sample sizes, cannot do. This increases the ability to arrive at definite conclusions about the presence or absence of an intervention effect (Schell & Rathe, 1992). By using meta-analysis cumulatively, it is possible to demonstrate the year in which the combined results of RCTs achieve a given level of statistical significance (Elliot et al., 1992).

Systematic Reviews

Increasingly, systematic reviews of the literature on clinical effectiveness are being undertaken to provide clinicians, managers and policy-makers with a more efficient means of accessing information about effective interventions. Systematic reviews are intended to provide a synthesis of research findings in given areas and present the results in ways which are manageable. Systematic reviews can seek to establish whether research findings are consistent, can be generalised across target groups and settings, or determine whether they vary by particular sub-sets (Mulrow, 1995). In the UK one of the main producers of systematic reviews of health care interventions is the Centre for Reviews and Dissemination (CRD), which is funded by the NHS Executive and health departments of Wales, Scotland and Northern Ireland.

A CRITIQUE OF THE DOMINANT APPROACH

Having described key aspects of the dominant approach, what are the limitations in applying it to health promotion? By way of introducing the arguments, consider the following:

- *What is being measured? – types of outcome*: Health promotion is concerned, not just with preventing disease, but with encouraging positive health and well-being. Its goals include enhanced community empowerment and social change. If a local health promotion department is working with community groups to develop greater community skills and sense of empowerment, then determining whether the intervention has worked should involve determining whether the community felt empowered. However, there is evidence that current purchasing arrangements for health promotion are principally concerned with measuring effectiveness through changes in morbidity, mortality and individual behaviour (Webb, 1997). So, the same local health promotion department may actually be asked to determine how many people stopped smoking as a consequence of the intervention. Thus, there is often disagreement about what constitutes an appropriate outcome for an intervention.

- *Whose activity is being measured? – the problem of attribution*: Health is a multi-dimensional concept. The reasons why people have good or poor health are complex and can involve individual, environmental, cultural, legal, fiscal and other factors. The efforts of those working in a voluntary agency or specialist health promotion department may form only part of the reasons why a particular outcome is observed. Thus, it is not always possible to attribute health outcomes to the specific activities of a local department as opposed to, for example, the impact of a health issue raised in a BBC soap opera or a secular trend.
- *Over what period is measurement taking place? – the problem of time-lag*: Many areas of health promotion activity (such as reducing the incidence of coronary heart disease) require health promotion efforts which may span decades. Relating a specific health outcome to a particular health promotion input may be problematic, but it often becomes impossible when the time-scale between health promotion input and health outcome is so lengthy.
- *Can it be measured? – the problem of quantification*: Health promotion interventions may have benefits which are impossible to quantify. For example, a smoking intervention may lead to reductions in coronary heart disease, a range of cancers and obstructive airways disease. It may also lead to a decrease in the prevalence of disease among passive smokers and may also affect the next generation, through a decrease in neo-natal dysmaturity (Burns, 1996). Therefore, it is likely that some research will under-estimate the overall effect of an intervention.

These issues are crucial to health promotion research, and the dominant approach to evaluation makes assumptions about them which need to be challenged. Having set out some of the issues involved, let's consider the use of RCTs in evaluating health promotion.

The Use of Randomised Controlled Trials to Evaluate Health Promotion Interventions

The appropriateness of experimental designs to health promotion research has come under a lot of scrutiny in recent years. Three main objections are described:

- their use in evaluating complex interventions
- their use in evaluating community-based initiatives
- their focus on 'what was the outcome?' and not on 'how was it achieved?'

Complex Interventions

Many health promotion interventions are dynamic and complex, and combine different approaches. It has been suggested that such interventions may be too complex to standardise fully (Bonell, 1996), such that they can never be repeated exactly the same way twice. We know that the quality of a health promotion intervention may depend on the individual characteristics of the person providing it – such inter-personal aspects of health promotion may be impossible to standardise. So, an RCT evaluator has two choices:

- first, try and break down the intervention into simpler components so that it is analysable. However, this results in an intervention which is unrealistic to everyday health promotion practice and hence causes what is known as validity problems (that is, the intervention would not be a true reflection of the phenomenon being studied).
- second, treat the intervention as 'black box', in which we know what goes in (the intervention), we know that something comes out, but we're not sure what happens in the middle. This would mean that outcomes could not confidently be assigned to the particular intervention being evaluated.

Neither of these choices is particularly satisfying.

Community-based Initiatives

It has been suggested that the RCT is not an appropriate tool for measuring the effectiveness of community-based health promotion (Nutbeam et al., 1993). The main reason is that the allocation of participants to intervention and control groups would be impractical. In such a context, an intervention would have to avoid using the media and other formal structures through which information is distributed because a control group would have the same access to such information as the intervention group. It would need to be designed in such a way that the intervention group had no contact with the control group. However, given that community-based health promotion uses community infrastructures, and that people invariably mix in social settings, such a design would be both artificial as well as impractical (Nutbeam et al., 1993; Sanson-Fisher et al., 1996). In RCT terms, if a control group in this circumstance had access to the intervention (for example, an intervention participant talking to a control participant, who is a friend, in the local supermarket) it would be referred to as 'contamination'. The results would be seen to be contaminated. However, in health promotion terms this would be referred to as a good diffusion of the intervention throughout the community.

The Focus on 'What' not 'How'

It is widely acknowledged that RCTs are not well suited to explaining how something happens, rather than what happens (Pawson & Tilley, 1997). However, understanding how something was implemented, and what effect this has on outcomes, is absolutely crucial to health promotion. This is of particular importance when considering systematic reviews, given that purchasers and providers need to know why and how a particular approach worked before considering whether it would be an appropriate approach to adopt locally. Without this information, purchasers and providers cannot make informed views about the local applicability of evidence.

Finally, it is worth noting that several other problems exist in the use of experimental designs in clinical design. Lipsey et al. (1985) have suggested that much experimental research is of poor design, low statistical power, and involves ad hoc measurements. Sackett et al. (1991) have remarked that RCTs can be unjustifiably expensive, given the large scale often required to produce statistically meaningful results.

The Use of Quasi-experiments

One of the solutions proposed to these problems has been the advocacy of quasi-experimental designs. These designs do not allocate *individuals* to intervention or control group, but instead allocate *localities* to intervention locality or comparison locality. A famous example of this is Kelly et al.'s (1992) study of HIV prevention peer education with gay men. It used a number of US cities as intervention and comparison groups. The cities were of sufficient distance apart to avoid any contamination (or diffusion) of the intervention, and the population group deemed to be relatively immobile socially (that is, they weren't travelling large distances for their recreation) to make this approach feasible. The outcomes among gay men in the intervention cities were markedly different to those in the comparison towns, and Kelly et al. concluded that their peer education approach was effective.

However, this approach is less promising in the UK because, as Bonell (1996) observes, towns with comparable populations of gay men tend to be geographically close to one another. Further, this population is characterised by a high degree of social and sexual mobility, so that even a randomisation by town is unlikely to produce an internally valid design, as contamination of the results is likely to occur.

There have been attempts to use quasi-experimental designs in the UK, the most famous of which is the Heartbeat Wales study. This intervention, in Wales, used a reference area in England to act as comparison. The researchers hypothesised that some diffusion of ideas would occur, but that it would dilute rather than compromise the study. However, the speed and extent of the contamination by diffusion to the reference area led them to conclude that if a quasi-experimental design is used it should include a process evaluation which is set in the comparison area in order to determine the precise mechanisms through which contamination by diffusion occurs (Nutbeam et al., 1993).

Systematic Reviews of Health Promotion

The art or science of undertaking systematic reviews of health promotion has been a developing one, as was recently acknowledged at a conference on reviews of effectiveness hosted by the HEA (Meyrick, 1997). Some reviewers subscribe, at least overtly, to the Cochrane hierarchy of evidence. Oakley et al.'s (1996) review of sexual health promotion with gay and bisexual men synthesised the evidence from RCTs alone, whilst at the same time describing a number of evaluations that did not meet their stringent inclusion criteria. Hodgson and Abbasi's (1995) systematic review of mental health promotion acknowledged the value of quasi-experimental designs and qualitative approaches yet chose to review only RCTs and 'good' quasi-experimental studies.

However, others are beginning to move away from this model. The International Union of Health Promotion and Health Education (IUHPE) undertook a series of reviews that incorporated non-experimental/quasi-experimental designs (Veen et al., 1994). These reviews were not systematic, but chose to include 10–15 studies for each of the topic areas. In stark contrast to reviews that have followed the Cochrane approach these gave considerably more attention to the characteristics of the health promotion intervention than to the research design (see later).

More recently, the HEA (Health Education Authority), which has already com-missioned a series of reviews, has committed itself to ensuring that future reviews include methodological development as a key function of the review (Meyrick, 1998). That is to say, review teams will need to be reflexive about the approaches they take and make adjustments to existing approaches to systematic reviews of health promotion.

In addition to the need for systematic reviews to incorporate less stringent inclu-sion criteria for research designs is the criticism that they have been predominantly concerned with the quality of the research design, and have not considered in detail the range and quality of the interventions in each study (Speller & Webb, 1997). If systematic reviews fail to make critical distinctions between different health promotion interventions in any given area, they may risk a loss of credi-bility and validity (Webb, 1997). For example, Speller et al. (1997) cite a review undertaken by the NHS Centre for Reviews and Dissemination on brief inter-ventions in excessive alcohol consumers. This review (CRD, 1993) concluded that brief interventions were effective in reducing alcohol consumption by over 20% for those with raised consumption levels, and that such interventions were as effective as more expensive specialist treatments. In considering the literature on brief interventions the review team decided that the variety of brief intervention tech-niques described were of similar duration and had common features, and, there-fore, could be considered together. However, even a quick glance at the summary table that had been included in the review reveals that the interventions varied considerably in nature. The failure to develop rigorous health promotion inter-vention criteria to the study provided misleading evidence which led to the influencing of treatment policy and purchasing decisions, and which, in the short term, may have adversely affected funding for specialist services (Heather, 1994).

Finally, it may be argued that systematic reviews of health promotion often contain studies that do not reflect everyday health promotion practice. Take two studies from a recent review on adolescent smoking (Stead & Hastings, 1995). One was a school-based programme in Vermont, USA, that incorporated a mass media intervention. The media aspect involved 36 different television broadcasts and 17 radio broadcasts over a four-year period, and is considered to be one of the most expensive youth-based smoking interventions ever undertaken. The second was a general health promotion programme aimed at middle schools in Wisconsin, in which instructors received 80 hours of training. It is difficult to imagine the use of such programmes in most localities of the UK, given their cost and labour intensity. Thus, how can health promotion specialists and purchasers make meaningful decisions about what constitutes an effective approach when the studies included in the reviews often do not reflect practice-based research?

DETERMINING EFFECTIVE HEALTH PROMOTION

If health promotion is going to gather evidence of its effectiveness then it will need to do the following:

- clarify its philosophical position in relation to the bio-medical model
- state the case for a broader range of research designs than is usually deemed acceptable within the dominant approach to health care evaluation
- advocate new ways for the systematic review process in health promotion to develop.

Understanding Health Promotion as a Different Kind of Endeavour than Clinical Practice

Thus far, we have seen how the debate about effectiveness and health promotion has been largely concerned with issues relating to research methods. However, beyond this there are underlying philosophical problems that need to be examined in order to develop better ways of determining effective health promotion. What we need to do is look at the *epistemology of health promotion and health care evaluation*. When people say that 'the bio-medical model doesn't work for health promotion' what does it mean?

Medical science understands the human body as a complex physical system which becomes dysfunctional when affected by disease. Health and illness are constructed as distinct and separate states. Although it is accepted that the origins of disease are both social and physical, the focus of medical science lies predominantly with the latter. Its use of the pathogenic as an explanation for health and disease leads to a concern with eliminating those pathogens from the human body or minimising their effects. In order to understand how different curative interventions affect a particular pathogen, evaluative medical research uses experimental designs that test a specific hypothesis and seek to reduce uncertainty about the links between variables, as is manifested in the RCT.

Many of the assumptions of the bio-medical model appeal to positivism, which underpins the dominant approach to health care evaluation in the NHS (Fox, 1991). This philosophy assumes that there are universal, discoverable laws about the world which can be understood through a mechanical explanation of cause and effect. It argues that accounts of the physical and social world can be represented accurately and reliably, with a minimum of researcher bias (Charlton, 1993). Positivism argues that it offers a unifying theory of the social world.

There are several problems with seeing health promotion in this way. First, as was stated earlier, health promotion has multiple determinants, and is a multi-dimensional concept. It emphasises the social and mental aspects of health as well as the physical, and views health as something more than a state in which disease is absent. Whereas the human body may be seen as a relatively closed system, the social body is an open system, subject to influence by multiple factors. Thus, there is a difference between biological explanations of health and illness and health promotion style socio-environmental and historical accounts. Health promotion suggests that there are diverse means through which positive health can be achieved, and that the community has an important role in shaping health promotion strategies. So, our conception of what health is, and the means to achieve it, depend on specific social and cultural processes. If health promotion is characterised in this way, there can be no single, objective and universal notion of what health promotion is. Health promotion therefore seeks to permit multiple perspectives rather than focusing on a single goal or desirable outcome.

Recently, it has been suggested that health promotion should be understood as a postmodern endeavour. There isn't space here to look at postmodernism in any detail, but basically, it is a school of philosophical thought that has developed in the last couple of decades. Postmodernism provides a powerful critique of all research paradigms. With regard to health care evaluation and health promotion, postmodernists argue the following:

- *Can there be universal indicators of success?* Postmodernists would argue against universal indicators of success because they fail to take account of the unique circumstances of different communities. Community-based health promotion takes place in different communities where there are very different conditions. So, developing measures of success of community empowerment requires appreciating that the baselines (how empowered the communities felt before the interventions) and the processes (how a sense of community empowerment developed) in different communities are not going to be comparable (Hayes & Willms, 1990). A postmodern view is that there is no absolute truth about health and that positive health is a quality defined by individuals and groups, not imposed by external forces.
- *What about attributing health outcomes to health promotion inputs?* Postmodernists would argue that it is often not possible to understand what happens in a causal way. Given everything that has been said about the multiple factors affecting people's health, and the time-scales often involved before some outcomes are

seen, it is not possible to relate particular health outcomes to specific inputs. Instead, postmodernists talk about things being 'intertextual': what this means in health promotion is that the different factors that can affect health are, to some extent, interdependent with each other. Thus, a postmodern approach to health promotion does not attempt to attribute specific behavioural and other outcomes to a particular intervention, but rather to understand the relationships between the different social processes that affect health.

- *What research methods work best in health promotion evaluations?* Postmodernists would argue against a hierarchy of research methods. Given its commitment to different perspectives, or truths, there can be no single method which is universally 'best' for discovering those truths. This view thus leads to a re-evaluation of the role of qualitative research methods in health promotion (see later).

So, if we are to provide better ways of determining effective health promotion than at present we need to look at the philosophical assumptions underlying the debate in order to resolve tensions about research methods and outcomes.

The Role of Qualitative Research Designs in Evaluating Health Promotion

Having suggested a number of ways in which experimental research designs are sometimes inappropriate to evaluate health promotion it is important to consider the role of qualitative, sociological research methods. Qualitative methods are well suited to illuminating the processes involved in implementing an intervention, helping us to understand how something worked and why it worked. But their value goes beyond that. Qualitative approaches are able to explore the different meanings that individuals attach to health, and to different interventions. This is important, given that health promotion is committed to the idea that there are many different definitions of health and that the role of health promotion is to help meet some of the diverse needs and aspirations of different communities, as can be seen in the Ottawa Charter.

However, it is important to be clear that it is not a question of incorporating qualitative research methods into the existing Cochrane hierarchy, for two reasons. First, qualitative methods can be as important as experimental designs in answering certain questions. Second, it is problematic to talk about a hierarchy of qualitative approaches – how can one compare a case study against an ethnographic investigation? The point is that different research methods are more appropriate at some times than at others *depending on the question they're trying to answer.* What is important is to develop standards for the design, implementation and reporting of qualitative studies in health promotion. Work is underway at the Health Education Authority with a small multi-disciplinary team of social science researchers who are attempting to develop a consensus on what constitutes a rigorous approach to qualitative research (Meyrick & Gillies, 1998).

Taking Forward Systematic Reviews

Although systematic reviews have the potential to provide a powerful synthesis of what is and isn't effective, a number of adjustments will need to be made if these reviews are to provide health promotion with better evidence than at present:

- The inclusion criteria should be broadened to include rigorous observational studies.
- Inclusion criteria should focus not just on the quality of the research design but on the quality of the intervention. Although it might be argued that the inclusion of such criteria would further complicate the review procedure, and its reporting, the results could be represented quite simply:
  quality of research design (good, reasonable, poor) X *quality of intervention* (good, reasonable, poor) X *intervention result* (effective, partly effective, ineffective, not known).
- The review process needs to be more transparent so that, in considering local applicability, practitioners can more easily assess generalisability.
- It should be acknowledged that the systematic review process is a subjective one, in so far as different reviewers will interpret data in different ways, and even if disputes are taken to an arbitrator, the validity of the results may be questionable.
- Greater attention should be given to the reporting of process detail, which would allow for a more informed consideration of local applicability of an approach judged to be effective.

CONCLUSION

This section of the chapter has suggested that a central problem in gathering evidence on effective health promotion lies in the application of the dominant bio-medical model of evaluation to health promotion. That model brings with it a hierarchy of evidence built on a set of philosophical assumptions. In applying the dominant model, the methodological approaches sometimes used to measure the effectiveness of health promotion may be inappropriate to what we understand as a socio-environmental model of health. This may result in misleading judgements about what is effective, which in turn offers poor counsel to policy-makers, health care purchasers and providers alike. It has been suggested that by exploring the philosophical assumptions behind different research paradigms, we can find more appropriate terms for the debate, and suggest ways forward in identifying appropriate methodological approaches to determining effectiveness. This involves a re-examination of: the contexts in which experimental designs are appropriate; the value of qualitative research methods; the types of outcomes which are appropriate measures of success; and, methods for undertaking systematic reviews.

REFERENCES

Bonell C (1996) Outcomes in HIV prevention: report of a research project. London: The HIV Project.

Burns H (1996) Purchasing cost effective health care. Presentation at Making a Difference: Investing in Effective Health Promotion Conference, Durham.

Centre for Reviews and Dissemination (1993) Brief interventions and alcohol use. *Effective Health Care*. York: CRD.

Charlton B (1993) Medicine and postmodernity. *Journal of the Royal Society of Medicine*, 83, 497–499.

Cochrane Collaboration (1994) Report. Oxford: UK Cochrane Centre.

Elliot M, Lau J et al. (1992) A comparison of results of meta-analyses and randomised control trials and recommendations of clinical experts. *Journal of the American Medical Association*, 268, 240–248.

Fox N (1991) Postmodernism, rationality and the evaluation of health care. *Sociological Review*, 39, 709–744.

Hayes M & Willms S (1990) Healthy community indicators: the perils of the search and the paucity of the find. *Health Promotion International*, 5(2), 161–166.

Heather N (1994) Interpreting the evidence on brief interventions for excessive drinkers: the need for caution. *Alcohol and Alcoholism*, 30(3), 287–296.

Hodgson R & Abbasi T (1995) Effective mental health promotion: literature review. Cardiff: Health Promotion Wales.

Kelly J, St. Lawrence J et al. (1992) Community AIDS/HIV risk reduction: the efforts of endorsement by popular people in three cities. *American Journal of Public Health*, 82, 1483–1489.

Lawrence R, Friedman G, DeFriese G et al. (1989) Guide to clinical preventive services: an assessment of the effectiveness of 169 interventions – report of the US Preventive Services Task Force. Maryland: Williams and Wilkins.

Lipsey M, Crosse S et al. (1985) Evaluation: the state of the art and the sorry state of the science. *New Directions for Programme Evaluation*, 27, 7–28.

Meyrick J (Ed) (1997) Reviews of effectiveness: their contribution to evidence based practice and purchasing in health promotion. Conference Proceedings. London: Health Education Authority.

Meyrick J (1998) Personal communication. February 10.

Meyrick J & Gillies P (1998) Recognising the contribution of qualitative studies to systematic reviews and the search for evidence in health promotion: not widening the goal posts but changing the field of play (unpublished consultation paper). London: Health Education Authority.

Mulrow C (1995) Rationale for systematic reviews. In: I Chalmers & D Altman (Eds), Systematic reviews. London: BMJ Publishing Group.

Nutbeam D, Smith C et al. (1993) Maintaining evaluation designs in long term community based health promotion. *Journal of Epidemiology and Community Health*, 47, 127–133.

Oakley A, Olivers S et al. (1996) Review of effectiveness of health promotion interventions for men who have sex with men. London: EPI Centre, London University Institute of Education.

Pawson R & Tilley N (1997) Realistic evaluation. London: Sage.

Sackett S, Haynes R et al. (1991) Clinical epidemiology: a basic science for clinical medicine. Oxford: Radcliffe Medical Press.

Sanson-Fisher R, Hancock L et al. (1996) Developing methodologies for evaluating community-wide health promotion. *Health Promotion International*, 11(3), 227–236.

Schell C & Rathe R (1992) Meta-analysis: a tool for medical and scientific discoveries. *Bulletin of the Medical Library Association*, 80(3), 219–222.

Speller V & Webb D (1997) Looking at the quality of health promotion interventions in the systematic review process: redressing the balance. In: J Meyrick (Ed), Reviews of effectiveness: their contribution to evidence based practice and purchasing in health promotion. London: Health Education Authority.

Speller V, Learnmouth A & Harrison D (1997) The search for evidence of effective health promotion. *British Medical Journal*, 315, 361–363.

Stead M & Hastings G (1995) Developing options for a programme on adolescent smoking in Wales. Technical report no. 16. Cardiff: Health Promotion Wales.

Veen C, Vereijken A et al. (1994) An instrument for analysing effectiveness studies on health promotion and health education. Development, use and recommendations. Utrecht: International Union for Health Promotion and Health Education.

Webb D (1997) Measuring effectiveness in health promotion. Southampton: University of Southampton.

The Challenge of Evidence-based Practice

Liz Rolls

The planning and delivery of care within the primary care-led NHS must be evidence-based (NHS Executive, 1996). The framework for evidence-based care has arisen as a logical extension of evidence-based medicine, defined by Sackett (1996) as:

> . . . the conscientious, explicit and judicious use of current best evidence in making decisions about the care of individual patients. The practice of evidence based medicine means integrating individual clinical expertise with the best available external evidence from systematic research (p 71).

However, Kendall (1997), suggests that evidence-based *care* must be distinguished from evidence-based *medicine* because, she argues '. . . care extends beyond the purely medical' (p 24).

As an activity, health promotion presents both challenges *to* and is challenged *by* the need to provide and use evidence in a number of ways.

THE CHALLENGE OF THE NATURE OF HEALTH PROMOTION TO EVIDENCE-BASED CARE

Health promotion is a reflective and responsive activity in which practitioners work at a high level of complexity, making decisions based on competing needs and conflicting knowledges. Furthermore, 'it requires an ability to critically appraise, to synthesise sophisticated levels of knowledge and to work within a framework of, amongst other things, empowerment, negotiation and the building and maintenance of intersectoral alliances' (Rolls, 1997, p 203). It draws its knowledge base from disciplines such as psychology, sociology, media studies, medicine and social theory and it is undertaken by a wide range of practitioners working with diverse populations in a number of settings in the health services and beyond. The range of definitions and models, such as those described by

Evidence-based Health Promotion. Edited by Elizabeth R. Perkins, Ina Simnett and Linda Wright.
© 1999 John Wiley & Sons Ltd.

Beattie (1991), Caplan and Holland (1990), Ewles and Simnett (1998), Naidoo and Wills (1994), Tones et al. (1990) and WHO (1984) are an attempt to make visible these underlying and often competing philosophical perspectives. This diversity and complexity, however, contributes to the contested nature of health promotion and to what counts as evidence of best practice and best outcomes.

THE CHALLENGE OF THE NATURE OF EVIDENCE TO HEALTH PROMOTION

Using evidence drawn from bio-medicine and epidemiology as a basis for determining health promoting activity and outcomes and using bio-medical health outcomes as evidence of health promotion effectiveness is problematic.

Firstly, problems arise from an inappropriate reliance on quantitative research methodologies to derive both the evidence on which professional practice will be based *and* on which judgements of effectiveness will be made. Quantitative methodologies, including experimental design, rest on the notion of the possibility of neutral, objective, scientific research. Smith and Cantley (1985) term this the *presumption of the experimentalist ideal*. This presumption obscures the difficulties of such research, in particular:

- the difficulties associated with the random assignment of clients
- the ethical and administrative objections to randomisation (de Raeve, 1994)
- that inputs are rarely stable
- that awareness of difference introduces bias
- that it is almost impossible to exclude extraneous variables
- the research is unable to say why changes detected have occurred (Newell, 1992).

In addition, and of significance to health promotion:

- generalisation from the results can be hazardous (Newell, 1992)
- there are problems of using randomised control trials in social and process-based settings (Newell, 1992; Oakley, 1990)
- arguing for the possibility that reliable and valid data can be generated suggests an 'underlying assumption that the social world can be described in terms of univocal facts' (Ashworth, 1995, p 367).

Secondly, the way in which outcomes are used as evidence of effectiveness is often inappropriate and questionable. The Department of Health suggests that 'Outcome measurement shows not only change, but relates that change to identifiable actions, resources and events . . . [and] allows the effectiveness of policies to be evaluated' with health objectives, 'not in terms of process but of improvements in health' (DOH, 1992, p 43). However:

- there is no agreed taxonomy to measure health outcomes
- there are difficulties in describing and therefore measuring the characteristics which impact on desirable outcomes
- the development and utilisation of health outcome measures remains disparate (Long, 1995).

In particular, there is often an inability to specify the process of care and the criteria of evaluation are not always clear or appropriate (Jelinek, 1992). Nor does the use of epidemiologically based outcomes as evidence of health promotion activity take account of the problems of time-scale in the attribution of interventions (Long, 1995).

THE NEED FOR APPROPRIATE EVIDENCE IN HEALTH PROMOTION

The *Health of the Nation Strategy for Health* (DOH, 1992) relies on health promotion as part of its delivery and has placed health promotion firmly within the legitimate remit of all those engaged in activities for health. Indeed, within initiatives such as the Healthy Alliances movement, key health workers are embracing their health promotion role and function as well as identifying and developing the health promotion skills required to contribute to meeting the *Health of the Nation* targets (DOH, 1993). Furthermore, the recommendations of the White Paper 'Working for Patients' (DOH, 1989) seek a greater accountability for the quality and efficiency of the provision of services and activities, including those around the promotion of health.

Evidence-based activity, therefore, is important in establishing legitimacy, for as Hasenfield (1992) argues, all forms of welfare or human service must be perceived as legitimate by not only their clients but also by regulators, resource providers and other 'stakeholders' (McLeod, 1994).

There is, thus, a need to derive *appropriate* evidence on which to:

- base health promotion activities and practice
- determine the effectiveness of health promotion activities, practices and services which takes account of the variety of perspectives and practitioners within health promotion and the issues and problems identified earlier.

It is important to evaluate health promotion services and activities *on their own terms* and not by a different set of values and criteria than those by which they themselves are underpinned or by a different set of outcome measures than those which are intended. Furthermore, the contribution of a number of practitioners and sectors to health outcomes also needs to be taken into account.

REFERENCES

Ashworth P (1995) The meaning of participation in 'participant observation'. *Qualitative Health Research*, 5(3), 366–387.

Beattie A (1991) Knowledge and control in health promotion: a test case for social policy and social theory. In: J Gabe et al. (Eds), The Sociology of the Health Service (pp 162–202). London: Routledge.

Caplan R & Holland R. (1990) Rethinking health education theory. *Health Education Journal*, 49, 10–12.

Department of Health (1989) Working for patients. London: HMSO.

Department of Health (1992) The Health of the Nation. London: HMSO.

Department of Health (1993) The Health of the Nation – targeting practice – The contribution of nurses, midwives and health visitors. London: The Stationery Office.

de Raeve L (1994) Ethical issues in palliative care research. *Palliative Medicine*, 8, 298–305.

Ewles L & Simnett I (1998) Promoting health: a practical guide. Fourth edition. London: Baillière Tindall.

Hasenfield Y (Ed) (1992) Human devices as complex organisations. London: Sage.

Jelinek M (1992) The clinician and the randomised control trial. In: J Daly, I McDonald and E. Willis (Eds), Researching health care: designs, dilemmas, disciplines (pp 76–89). London: Tavistock/Routledge.

Kendall S (1997) What do we mean by evidence? Implications for primary health care nursing. *Journal of Interprofessional Care*, 11(1), 23–34.

Long A (1995) Assessing health and social outcomes. In: J Popay & G Williams (Eds), Researching the people's health (pp 157–182). London: Routledge.

McLeod J (1994) Doing counselling research. London: Sage.

Naidoo J & Wills J (1994) Health promotion: foundations for practice. London: Baillière Tindall.

Newell D (1992) Randomised controlled trials in health care research. In: J Daly et al. (Eds), Researching health care: designs, dilemmas, disciplines (pp 47–61). London: Routledge.

NHS Executive (1996) Primary care led NHS: briefing pack. London: NHSE.

Oakley A (1990) Who's afraid of the randomized controlled trial? In: W Roberts (Ed), Women's health counts (pp 167–194). London: Routledge.

Rolls E (1997) Competence in professional practice: some issues and concerns. *Educational Research*, 39(2), 195–210.

Sackett D L et al. (1996) Evidence based medicine: what it is and what it isn't. *British Medical Journal*, 312, 71–72.

Smith G & Cantley C (1985) Assessing health care: a study in organisational evaluation. Milton Keynes: Open University Press.

Tones K, Tilford S & Robinson Y (1990) Health education; effectiveness and efficiency. London: Chapman & Hall.

World Health Organisation (1984) Health promotion: a WHO discussion document on concepts and principles. Geneva: WHO.

Section 3.3

Improving Mental Health in Women with Breast Cancer

Maggie Wark

BACKGROUND TO THE PROJECT

The promotion of positive mental health and prevention of mental ill-health are difficult areas for health promotion. The causes of mental ill-health are probably less well understood than those of physical disorders, and the measurement of changes in mental health status can also prove difficult for most health promoters, especially within the usual constraints of time and money.

Positive mental health has been extensively linked to increased survival rates in cancer patients including breast cancer patients. Indeed, Fallowfield and Clark in their book *Breast cancer* (Fallowfield & Clark, 1991) states:

> It should be obvious that any therapeutic approach that dismisses or ignores the substantial impact that psychological factors have on good outcome and long-term adjustment is both poor medicine and poor science.

The nature of most psychological morbidity in women with breast cancer is depression and anxiety. It is estimated that between 25% and 50% of cancer patients suffer some psychological morbidity. The causes of this morbidity are many and complex, as might be expected. In general, however, they fall into the following categories: fear of the disease and its consequences, fear of the treatment, especially of mutilation (both in women who have had mastectomy and those who have had the more conservative lumpectomy), unhappiness about altered body image, and sexual dysfunction (Anderson, 1988; Darbyshire, 1986; Denton & Baum, 1983; Maguire et al., 1978; Price, 1992).

Traditional responses to emotional distress following breast surgery are self-help groups, counselling by specialist breast-care nurses, and, for more disturbed

Evidence-based Health Promotion. Edited by Elizabeth R. Perkins, Ina Simnett and Linda Wright.
© 1999 John Wiley & Sons Ltd.

patients, therapy from clinical psychologists or psychiatrists. It appears that little has been done to address problems directly associated with altered body image at a basic physical level.

There is, however, one programme called 'Look Good, Feel Better' which was developed in the USA a couple of years ago, and later extended to the UK. It involves providing make-up lessons to small groups of women who have breast cancer, and giving them a free pack of cosmetics to take away. The evaluation of this programme reports success in reducing anxiety, and producing improvements in mood and perceptions of attractiveness in the short-term (Manne et al., 1994).

Colour and image consultancy teaches people, both men and women, the styles and colours of clothes which enhance their individual body shape and colouring. The consultation specifically focuses on parts of the body which the client is unhappy about, and gives advice on how best to draw attention away from these to other body areas or to camouflage them. Colour and image consultation is often seen as being rather trivial. Typically consultations are aimed at helping business people to present a more appropriate business image, or create a good impression with clients; or at helping bored middle-class housewives avoid expensive mistakes while choosing their wardrobe. As far as I am aware, colour and image consultancy has not, until now, been used as a therapeutic tool.

Whilst training to become a colour and image consultant, I was immediately struck by the possible positive mental health benefits the process might have for patients who had suffered body image trauma both in terms of the educational value of the process, and in the ability to empower patients in a very direct and visible way. This, plus an interest in breast cancer, led to the development of the project.

THE 'LOOKING WELL!' PROJECT

In discussion with two local breast-care nurses, it was decided to develop a pilot project to assess the effectiveness of colour and image consultancy in improving the body image and self-confidence of a small group of women who had under-gone surgery for breast cancer.

Funding was obtained from Dudley Health, the local purchasing authority, for a pilot project to test 50 patients. The project involved the active co-operation of the two breast-care nurses, having first checked with all surgeons involved in breast surgery that the project and its methodology were acceptable to them.

Recruitment of Women

From a pre-determined date, all women who have breast surgery in Dudley are informed about the project via one of the breast-care nurses at the point of dis-charge from hospital. The colour and image consultant also gave a talk about the project and what to expect during the consultation to the local breast cancer support group.

It is then up to the women themselves to make direct contact with the consultant if they wish to take up the option of a free consultation. Places are allocated on a first-come-first-served basis. No attempt is made to pre-select women in respect of age, recency or type of surgery, or treatment regime.

Information is given to patients just before they leave hospital. This is not ideal, but is the only opportunity the breast care nurses have to see every woman who has had surgery. Therefore, if a patient decides to take up the offer of the consultation quickly, she may be able to have it within three to four weeks of surgery. To date, a couple of women have responded this quickly.

The Consultation

Consultations are done on an individual basis at a mutually convenient time, and patients are encouraged to bring along a friend. The consultation takes place in a small, private room familiar to the patients within a large local acute hospital. The process is informal and the emphasis is on the patient enjoying the process as well as learning how to make the most of their appearance.

The consultation is in two parts. The colour analysis involves testing 150 different colours against the skin, hair and eyes of the patient. It lasts about an hour, and the emphasis is on teaching the patients to recognise for themselves which colours suit them best. After the colour analysis, the patient goes for a break to the nearby hospital canteen, then returns for the second half of the consultation — the image analysis. This lasts about one-and-a-half hours. It involves taking some vital statistic measurements to ascertain the patient's basic body shape. Having done this, detailed advice on all aspects of dress from hair to hem line, from spectacles to shoes is given. Again, the consultation aims to teach the woman the basic rules of shape and scale which apply to her, and how judicious use of shape and colour can produce a slimming or figure enhancing effect. Each patient is given a swatch wallet with samples of all her best colours, and a 'stylefax' of individual style and image information to take away.

EVALUATION

After some discussion with health promotion colleagues (who specialise in mental health promotion) and a clinical psychologist, it was decided to use an adapted form of the 'Ideal-Self Inventory' (ISI) developed by Norton et al. in 1995 as a basis for pre- and post-consultation questionnaires.

The ISI test, as described by Norton et al., consists of two stages. Stage one asks the patient to identify ten characteristics, using either a word or short phrase, which would describe her *ideal self*, and for each characteristic to list its opposite, which describes her *not ideal self*. Stage two asks the patient to rate herself on a seven-point continuum between the ideal and the not ideal. The seven points are then scored from 7 (nearest to the *ideal self*) to 1 (nearest to the *not ideal self*). By adding the scores, an overall self-esteem score, ranging from 70 (high self-esteem) to 10 (low self-esteem) is produced, as well as a profile for each characteristic.

After discussion with the breast-care nurses, it was felt that stage one might cause many of the patients difficulty, and so we decided to pre-determine the ten characteristics, and simply to ask each patient to rate herself on the same ten characteristics both before and after the consultation. The list below was partly adapted from a list of characteristics in Norton et al.'s paper, and partly brainstormed by the breast-care nurses and me. The ten characteristics chosen were as follows:

- attractive/unattractive
- confident/unconfident
- happy/unhappy
- focused/unfocused
- satisfied/unsatisfied
- carefree/troubled
- sociable/unsociable
- healthy/unhealthy
- in control/out of control
- independent/dependent

In order to see if there were any lasting effects, it was decided to send out the post-questionnaire four weeks after the colour and image consultation. It was felt that four weeks provided a reasonable interval between pre- and post-test. Within this period, many of the women were going through considerable emotional turmoil: some had a positive cancer diagnosis, some had started their treatment. Patients were also asked to what extent they felt any increase in self-confidence was due to the consultation.

Preliminary Results

By the end of the first year (November 1997), 19 women had taken up the option of the consultation. This represents 11% of those to whom it was offered. Of these, all except one returned their pre-questionnaire, and 14 had returned both pre- and post-questionnaires, to date. The comments below relate only to those 14 women who returned *both* pre- and post-questionnaires within the first year of the project. This is a very small sample, so firm conclusions should not be drawn from the data. However, this preliminary data may give an indicator of broad trends which might emerge when more data is available.

From the preliminary sample of 14 women, the following has been found:

1. The average age of the women taking up the offer of the consultation was about 50. This is significantly younger than the average age of women undergoing breast surgery in Dudley, according to the breast-care nurses. They estimate the average age of these women to be over 70.

2. Of the 14 women in the sample, nine had mastectomies (64%), five had wide local incisions ('lumpectomy') (36%) and seven also had their lymph glands removed (50%). There does not appear to be any correlation between type of surgery and degree of benefit reported from the consultation which might be expected. Maguire et al. (1978) reports that women who have had mastectomies show significantly higher rates of psychological disturbance than those who have had more conservative surgery, so it might be expected that the women who have had a mastectomy would benefit more than whose who have not.

3. Since their surgery, nine women (64%) of the sample have been put on Tamoxifen, five (36%) have had radiotherapy, and two (15%) have had chemotherapy. Three women had not been told what treatment they required at the time of asking. Again, there does not appear to be any correlation between type of treatment and reported benefit from the consultation.

4. The results of the women's self-assessment on the ten characteristics identified above looks promising. Reported self-esteem increased by an average of over 20% between the pre- and post-consultation questionnaires. Scores range from +36 to –7 (the only one with reduced self-esteem). Furthermore, over 90% of this perceived increase is reported by the women to have been due to the consultation.

5. All of the women said that they enjoyed it, and most provided positive and enthusiastic support for the project in their general comments, e.g.
    - *Patient 1.* '. . . I did feel very low after my operation and was starting to stay in a lot. But now I go out nearly every day if I can. Thank you.'
    - *Patient 5.* 'After the surgery the consultation was something to look forward to. The help and advice . . . was brilliant. When I got home I felt really good and only hope that other people in my position can have the same opportunity. Thank you once again.'
    - *Patient 10.* '. . . This consultation . . . made me feel special.'

DISCUSSION AND IMPLICATIONS FOR EVIDENCE-BASED HEALTH PROMOTION

The project described above does not form a rigorous piece of research, but is a first attempt to explore the usefulness of a tested process applied to a new context and different group. The method provides an unusual and enjoyable way of seeking to help a group of women who have been through (or are going through) physical and emotional trauma. There is no known research on the psychological effects of colour and image consultancy, but it seems logical that a process which focuses directly on image and which provides such an individual focus should have the ability to raise self-esteem.

Although the early results appear to indicate a positive improvement in self-esteem in those who took part, a more critical examination reveals that there are a number of unknowns which might be influencing the results:

- No attempt was made in this project to compare the self-selected group with a control group. It would be interesting to know in what ways the test group differs in their response from a control group of women who have had breast surgery but have not taken up the option of the consultation.
- There was no attempt to select the women who were offered the consultation. They vary considerably in age, social class, type of surgery, type and stage of treatment (post-surgery), prognosis, etc. Selection of one or more of these factors to form different test groups from a wider cohort might reveal more specific findings.
- Although a positive effect appeared to be identified four weeks post-consultation, it is not known if this is sustained, for example, after six months or a year.
- It is possible that the improvements identified may be due to the individual attention given to each woman – about three-and-a-half hours – and not to the consultation itself.
- Alternatively, the effect identified might be a function of normal healing and not due to the consultation.
- It is always good practice in assessing changes in mental health indicators to use more than one validated measurement tool in the evaluation process.
- It would be interesting to see the effect of giving only the colour analysis, or only the image consultation as opposed to the whole package.

It seems logical, therefore, to build on the Dudley project by developing a bigger, more rigorously evaluated project which seeks to get a clearer picture of what is happening and, if possible, why. A proposal for a regional pilot to address these questions is in the process of being developed.

REFERENCES

Anderson J (1988) Coming to terms with mastectomy. *Nursing Times*, 84(4), 41–44.
Darbyshire P (1986) Body image – when the face doesn't fit. *Nursing Times*, 82(39), 28–30.
Denton S & Baum M (1983) Psychological aspects of breast cancer. In: R Margalese (Ed.), Contemporary issues in clinical oncology. London: Churchill Livingstone.
Fallowfield L & Clark A (1991) Breast cancer. London: Tavistock/Routledge.
Maguire G P, Lee E G, Bevington D J, Kuchemann C S, Crabtree R J & Cornell C E (1978) Psychiatric problems in the first year after mastectomy. *British Medical Journal*, 1, 963–965.
Manne S L, Girasek D & Ambrosino J (1994) An evaluation of the impact of a cosmetics class on breast cancer patients. *Journal of Psychiatric Oncology*, 12(1/2), 83–97.
Norton L S, Morgan K & Thomas S (1995) The ideal-self inventory: a new measure of self-esteem. *Counselling Psychology Quarterly*, 8(4), 305–310.
Price B (1992) Living with altered body image: the cancer experience. *British Journal of Nursing*, 1(13), 641–645.

Section 3.4

Parenting Support Groups

Jacki Gordon, Robbie Robertson and Margaret Swan

The stimulus for this piece of work was the common observation by a GP (RR) and his primary care team that they were seeing the same young children time and time again, often for complaints considered to be of a minor nature. He observed that the mothers of these frequent attenders appeared to be highly stressed with many experiencing feelings of isolation, and believed that they were experiencing coping difficulties. A successful proposal to the Greater Glasgow Health Board resulted in the recruitment of two health promotion officers (JG and MS) whose remit was to enhance the coping of mothers whose children were frequent users of primary care services.

Following an extensive literature review it became apparent that a range of diverse factors may influence mothers' consulting patterns including lack of information, socio-economic status, loneliness, lack of social support, and maternal anxiety and depression (Gordon, 1995).

To meet the aim of enhancing coping in mothers whose children were high-users of primary care services, we agreed to develop a one-year intervention with the following objectives:

- to set up support groups
- to enhance maternal mental health
- to provide advice on the management of minor illnesses
- to provide advice on the management of children's behaviour.

Here we are going to focus on just one of these objectives – that of maternal mental health – and describe how we set up a randomised controlled study to answer the specific question of whether our parenting groups reduced measured anxiety and depression.

At the start of the study we agreed to look at mothers of children under the age of five years who were high-users. To identify the high-users among the 303 under-fives who were registered with the practice, we took a retrospective view of

Evidence-based Health Promotion. Edited by Elizabeth R. Perkins, Ina Simnett and Linda Wright.
© 1999 John Wiley & Sons Ltd.

incidents of help-seeking behaviour for the one year preceding onset of the study. For each of the children we totted up the number of patient-initiated non-routine face-to-face contacts with GPs (including out of hours calls), health visitors, community medical officers, doctors' deputising service and accident and emergency departments. We took care to avoid double-counting by cross-referring dates of consultations.

Next, we divided children into one-year age bands, and further sub-divided with respect to gender. For the age group 0–1 year, there was obviously not the potential to establish consultation over a full year, and so this age group was further subdivided into three-month age bands. Infants less than three months old were excluded from the study as there had been little opportunity for them to establish a high number of consultations. For each age/gender group, we ordered the frequency of number of incidents of help-seeking behaviour for each child and ascertained the median (i.e. the value that divided the distribution in half). Within each age/sex grouping, attendance frequency was positively skewed: there were a minority of children who had a very high consultation frequency which rendered the mean an inappropriate measure to represent the average number of consultations. For the purposes of this study we defined high-usage as two or more visits above the median which identified 98 high-user children. As some of these high-users were from the same family, we grouped the children into 92 high-user families. The GP then wrote to all mothers of the high-user children explaining that two health promoters who were working with his practice to run parenting support groups would visit them at home to find out whether they would be interested in attending. In this letter it was stressed that there would not be enough places for all but that the names of those who were interested would be picked out of a hat.

For those mothers who indicated that they would like to attend (either verbally or by returning a stamped-addressed envelope if the health promotion officers were unable to catch them at home), their child was matched with another high-user child with respect to:

• age
• presence or absence of a chronic condition (e.g. asthma, eczema)
• number of instances of help-seeking behaviour (within the one-year retrospective period).

For those mothers who had two or more children falling into the high-user category, only one child was selected for the study group. Children within matched pairs were then randomly assigned to intervention and control groups, giving 30 matched pairs.

Prior to being notified as to whether they had been successful in securing a place at one of the support groups, all mothers were sent the Hospital Anxiety and Depression Scale (HADS: Zigmond & Snaith, 1983). HADS were printed on to different colours of paper so that we could identify whether a respondent was in the intervention group (i.e. mother of a high-user who would be offered a place in a support group) or a control (i.e. a mother of a high-user who wanted to come to a support group but who had not been allocated a place). In this pre-intervention administration of the HADS, we achieved response rates of 71% and 86% for the intervention and control groups, respectively.

We analysed HADS data in line with Zigmond and Snaith's (1983) recommendation to adopt a score in excess of 10 as a conservative indication of a case of anxiety or depression. Prior to intervention, chi-square tests revealed that there was no significant difference between the intervention and control groups in the prevalence of anxiety (p = 0.9) or depression (p = 0.9). Once we had collected these baseline data, the GP wrote to each mother who wanted to attend a support group informing her as to whether or not she had been allocated a place.

We (JG,MS) ran the parenting support groups on a weekly basis out in the community. Information regarding the intervention is reported elsewhere (Gordon, 1995; Gordon et al., 1995a).

Of the 30 mothers offered places, 25 came along at least once, 17 attending regularly for a period of three months or more. Five of the 17 found jobs which prevented them from continuing to attend. Nine continued coming on a regular basis for one year. (New mothers who were not part of the study group were also referred to the support groups to boost group size.)

Following the full one-year intervention period, HADS were again administered: response rates from the intervention and control groups were 69% and 86%, respectively. Post-intervention data were analysed in two ways (see Table 1). Firstly, scores of all those in the intervention group who completed HADS were compared with those in the control group, reflecting analysis on the basis of 'intention to treat' (column 4). Secondly, those who had attended the last ten week term of the support group at least three times (i.e. the 'attenders') were compared with the control group (column 6).

After the one-year period of intervention, analyses of HADS revealed the following:

- Although a trend was exhibited to less anxiety in the intervention group, this difference was not statistically significant (p = 0.1).
- There was a lower prevalence of cases of anxiety for those who were attending the support groups at the end of the one-year intervention compared with the control group (Fisher Exact Probability = 0.013).
- There was a lower prevalence of cases of depression for those in the intervention group than for the control group (chi-square = 4.85, p = 0.027).
- There was a lower prevalence of cases of depression for those attending the support groups at the end of the one-year intervention period than for the control group (Fisher Exact Probability = 0.035).

Table 3.4.1 Cases of anxiety and depression after one-year intervention period

	Intervention (n = 18)	Control (n = 24)	Chi-square test	Attenders (n = 8)	Fisher Exact Probability
Not anxious	10 (55.6%)	8 (33.3%)		7 (88%)	
			$p = 0.1$		$p = 0.01$
Anxious	8 (44.4%)	16 (66.7%)		1 (12%)	
Not depressed	16 (89%)	14 (58%)		8 (100%)	
			$p = 0.03$		$p = 0.03$
Depressed	2 (11%)	10 (42%)		0 (0%)	

We feel that there should be a debate about which analysis is the 'right' one – analysis according to 'intention to treat' or analysis of attenders.

In a controlled trial it is conventional and conservative to appraise effectiveness using the criterion of 'intention to treat'. However, a controlled trial is essentially a medical methodology appropriate for a medical model in which professionals primarily define need and appropriate treatment, and where the probable outcome of treatment is understood by, or conveyed to, the patient. In contrast to this, our study was a health promotion initiative, and as health promotion subscribes to a 'bottom up' approach in which individuals define their own needs, perhaps a more appropriate analysis should explore the extent to which the intervention successfully met its objectives *for those who chose to participate*. This being the case, it may therefore be more appropriate to place more emphasis on the demonstrable effectiveness of the intervention for both anxiety and depression for those who continued to attend the support groups.

Certainly the qualitative data which we obtained supported the conclusion that the support groups were effective in enhancing mental health as well as meeting our other stated objectives (Gordon, 1995; Gordon et al., 1995a; 1995b).

IMPACT OF THE PROJECT

From the outset, the health promoters impressed upon the mothers that the groups would be running for only one year. However, as the year was coming to a close, the group members were keen that the groups should continue. To this end the health promoters provided them with very basic training on running the groups independently. For one of the groups this was not possible as the premises in which it was running were vandalised, driving out the community project to which it belonged. The other two groups have continued to date (more than three years after the end of the intervention period), and are run by the women with support from Community Education.

Following a presentation of results to health visitors in the area, considerable interest was generated in working with mothers through running support groups. Discussions took place with the local health visitor manager who agreed to release five health visitors to co-work with the health promotion officers in the refinement, delivery and evaluation of materials for groupwork.

The pilot project subsequently moved into its second phase (this time led by MS and another health promotion officer Jackie Bell). The initiative was now widened to include eight practices in the area, and this time mothers of children under the age of two years were invited to participate in support groups of a shorter duration. The feedback from these new mothers largely echoed that obtained in phase one. Similarly, health visitors were enthusiastic about providing support and information to new parents through groupwork (Greater Glasgow Health Board, 1996).

The health promotion officers collaborated with the health visitors in producing a stand-alone parenting pack entitled 'All in the Same Boat'. Considerable interest in this work continued with 70 health visitors from around Greater Glasgow participating in an introductory session on running support groups and on using the pack. Over 100 packs have now been distributed around the city and this resource is now being used by health visitors running parenting support groups.

REFERENCES

Gordon J (1995) Home alone: an evaluation of the effectiveness of support groups for mothers. Unpublished Masters thesis.

Gordon J, Robertson R & Swan M (1995a) 'Babies don't come with a set of instructions': running support groups for mothers. *Health Visitor*, 68(4), 155–156.

Gordon J, Robertson R & Swan M (1995b) Support groups for high-dependency mothers in an inner city area of high deprivation. In: D R Trent & C A Reed (Eds), Promotion of mental health. Volume 4. Aldershot: Avebury.

Greater Glasgow Health Board (1996) Springburn parenting groups phase two: working with health visitors 'It Made Perfect Sense'. Unpublished Report. Glasgow: Health Promotion Department, Greater Glasgow Health Board.

Zigmond A S & Snaith R P (1983) The Hospital Anxiety and Depression Scale. *Acta Psychiatrica Scandinavica*, 67, 361–370.

Chapter 4

Work with Individuals

Elizabeth R. Perkins

INTRODUCTION

For many health promoters, perhaps for the majority, work with individuals is a major part of their health promotion practice. Even for those who do not themselves work directly with patients or clients, there may be a responsibility for training and supporting those who do. How to give advice in such a way that it will encourage healthy behaviour, rather than fall on stony ground or even be counter-productive, is therefore a very important matter. Insights from psychology have been applied to this process for many years. The most comprehensive approach at present is Prochaska and DiClemente's transtheoretical model, commonly known as the Stages of Change. It offers a guide to what kind of advice to give, and at what point, to an individual with a health behaviour which is felt to be in need of modification. The possibilities afforded by the application of this theory has resulted in the promotion, by the Health Education Authority in the UK, of short 'Helping People Change' courses offered to a wider range of professionals, and also in its dissemination through a range of other material designed for professionals.

The first section, *A stage based approach to behaviour change*, provides a detailed account of the model, based on the original research rather than the (probably inevitable) simplifications used in many forms of training material.

The second section, *The Transtheoretical Model: Profiling Smoking in Pregnancy*, considers a range of current applications of the model. It then moves on to focus on a study of pregnant smokers. This was designed to include information on social and economic circumstances as well as on stages of change, and to provide guidance for professionals on the usefulness, or otherwise, of the Stages of Change model as a guide to work with women who smoke during pregnancy.

Evidence-based Health Promotion. Edited by Elizabeth R. Perkins, Ina Simnett and Linda Wright.
© 1999 John Wiley & Sons Ltd.

A Stage-based Approach to Behaviour Change

Terry Lawrence

A significant contribution to the understanding of behaviour change and health promotion practice has been made by theories drawn from psychology. In particular, over the past decade, the work of US psychologists Jim Prochaska and Carlo DiClemente has attempted to provide theoretical constructs for understanding the process of behaviour change itself, along with a model for assessing the pace and preparedness to change. Over numerous years of research, across a wide range of health behaviours, they have defined behaviour change as a dynamic process, developing and evolving through a number of definable stages, and drawing on a range of identifiable psychological processes to initiate and support the desired outcome. As practising clinical psychologists they were first interested in how self-changers managed to change addictive behaviours, for example, stopping smoking. There is ample evidence that people can successfully modify problematic behaviour with and without the help of professional intervention (Lambert et al., 1986; Marlatt et al., 1988; Shapiro et al., 1984; Smith et al., 1980) but such studies throw little light on *how* people change. The question is – are there any themes in the process of change itself which are common to all or most people? Are there basic common principles that can reveal the structure of change occurring with and without intervention?

Concentrating initially on intentional changers (as opposed to societal, developmental or imposed change), Prochaska and DiClemente originally identified four discrete stages through which people pass in linear progression during the process of change itself. The evolving model, sometimes referred to as the 'Stages of Change Model', built on the earlier work of psychologists such as Horn and Waingrow (1966), Cashdan (1973) and Egan (1975). The four stages of change which dominated the first seven years of research were: pre-contemplation, contemplation, action and maintenance. However, continuous work and analysis of behaviour change revealed clusters of people scoring highly on both contemplation and action stage indicators. Thus a fifth, and highly significant stage of change, preparation, was identified (DiClemente et al., 1991; Prochaska et al., 1992).

Evidence-based Health Promotion. Edited by Elizabeth R. Perkins, Ina Simnett and Linda Wright.
© 1999 John Wiley & Sons Ltd.

STAGES OF CHANGE

Pre-contemplation

Pre-contemplation is the stage in which there is no intention to change behaviour in the foreseeable future. Many people in this stage are unaware that they have a problem. Resistance to recognising or modifying a problem is the hallmark of pre-contemplation. When pre-contemplators present for help it is often because they have been forced to do so either by some authority (for example the courts giving drink-drive offenders a sentence which requires them to attend a drink-driver education course; or a GP giving an exercise prescription), or to please, or appease, someone close to them. Those who remain in pre-contemplation may demonstrate change once the pressure is on, but return to the problematic behaviour once the pressure is eased. Studies indicate (McBride & Pirie, 1990; Mullen et al., 1990) that between 50% and 60% of women who give up smoking during pregnancy return to smoking after the baby's birth. These women may be 'temporary quitters' – not so much intending to give up smoking for good, as to put it on hold whilst they are pregnant. Individuals who do not intend to make a particular behaviour change within the next six months are categorised as pre-contemplators. Intending to change is significantly different from 'wishing' or 'wanting' to change. Most of us, if asked, would wish or want to have a top-of-the-range car, but very few of us would be seriously intending to put in motion the prerequisites for obtaining one, which might involve such life changes as selling the house, foregoing holidays and entertainment, working longer hours or making any number of other unacceptable sacrifices. Similarly, many overweight women 'want' to be slim and aspire to look like role model images in magazines, but foregoing the high-fat foods to make the image a reality is very much harder!

Contemplation

Contemplation is the stage in which people are aware that a problem exists and are seriously thinking about tackling it, but have not yet made a commitment to take action. People can be stuck in the contemplation stage for considerable amounts of time, but the majority will assert their intention to change their problematic health behaviour within the next six months. Prochaska illustrates the essence of this stage with an anecdote. The psychotherapist, Alfred Benjamin, was walking home one evening when a stranger approached him and asked for directions to find a certain street. Benjamin gave the stranger specific instructions on how to find it. After demonstrating that he had understood the directions, the stranger thanked Benjamin and headed off in precisely the opposite direction. Benjamin called after him, indicating that he was going the wrong way, to which the stranger replied 'Yes, I know. I am not quite ready yet' (Prochaska et al., 1994, p 42). This describes pre-contemplation – knowing where you want to get to, but not being quite ready to set out on the route. Setting out on the route, of course, means leaving a set of familiar and well established, possibly significant and cherished, circumstances behind, and striking out for the new and unknown. A smoker, deciding to give up smoking, not only has to struggle with possible symptoms of withdrawal from a physical addiction, but also has to cope without a cigarette during those times which are emotionally associated with smoking – perhaps with friends in the pub, or after a meal, or once the children have gone to bed. An important aspect of the contemplation stage is weighing the pros and cons of changing the behaviour. For our smoker, this might mean a pros balance sheet which includes issues such as health improvement, cost savings, feeling proud of the achievement, clothes, breath and car all free of the smell of smoke; whereas the cons list might consist of loss of companionship in sharing a smoke with work colleagues in the 'smoking room', having to find another way to relax, fear of putting on weight. Contemplators appear to struggle with their positive evaluations of the addictive behaviour and the amount of effort, energy and loss it will cost to overcome the problem (DiClemente et al., 1991; Prochaska et al., 1992; Velicer et al., 1985).

Preparation

Preparation is the stage that combines intention and behavioural criteria. Individuals in this stage are intending to take action to change their behaviour within the next month, and indeed, are making plans – or preparations – to do so. Preparations for action might include having already reduced the number of cigarettes they smoke each day, or cutting out a particular cigarette, such as the first one in the morning, or the one after the evening meal, for example. However, although they have started to take small steps towards changing the problematic health behaviour, people in the preparation stage have not fully committed themselves to the overall criteria which characterises action. For smokers this commitment would be total abstinence. For people wanting to reduce their drinking or stick to a low-fat diet, it would be staying within predetermined consumption limits. Preparation is the precursor of action. Before it was identified as a discrete stage in its own right, the common principles were acknowledged by Prochaska et al. and labelled 'decision making'. However, it is now recognised that when individuals slip back into the old habits of problematic behaviour (relapse, or recycle), it may be because they had not initially given sufficient thought and planning to the preparation stage.

Action

In the action stage the new changed behaviour is practised. The behaviour change must be sustained for six months before the individual can be reassured that he or she is no longer practising, but maintaining, the changed behaviour. To sustain the changed behaviour in the action stage requires considerable commitment and energy. During this stage it is apparent to people around that an individual is carrying out a decision to change his or her behaviour – by stopping smoking or refusing sweets, biscuits, chocolates, or alcohol, for example. Whilst external recognition can be helpful it can sometimes also be out of kilter with the needs of the changer.

Maintenance

Maintenance is the stage in which people work to prevent relapse and consolidate the gains achieved during the action stage. Maintenance may last for six months or may be a stage you inhabit for a lifetime. Current thinking is that for some behaviours, particularly acquisition behaviours, such as sticking to a low-fat diet or taking regular exercise, it is never possible to progress from maintenance to termination – that is, to be absolutely certain that you will never slip back to the problematic behaviour, and have just one cream cake or piece of chocolate, or have a week when the exercise regime is forfeited. Initially, research data and theoretical concepts identified maintenance as a static stage. It has subsequently been acknowledged that maintenance is dynamic – a continuation, not an absence, of change. People in maintenance may feel that they need occasional support to stop them from relapsing. Stabilising behaviour change and avoiding relapse are the characteristics of the maintenance stage.

Termination

The termination stage is achieved when there is no danger that an individual will revert to the original problematic behaviour, but, as has already been stated, for some behaviours it is impossible to be confident that this stage can ever be realised.

As most of us who have tried to change any behaviour know only too well, we seldom succeed first time! Research has shown that smokers make an average of three to four attempts at giving up before they are successful (Schachter, 1982); people relapse, or recycle, through the stages several times, modifying their behaviour and their approach to changing it on each occasion, learning from past mistakes. Fortunately, however, the majority of relapsers do not give up entirely but have another go at achieving the change, often re-entering the process at the stages of contemplation or pre-contemplation. It was this evidence that changed the conceptualisation of the change process from a linear progression to a dynamic spiral.

> In this spiral pattern, people can progress from contemplation to preparation to action to maintenance, but most individuals will relapse. During relapse, individuals regress to an earlier stage. Some relapsers feel like failures – embarrassed, ashamed, and guilty. These individuals become demoralized and resist thinking about behavior change. As a result they return to the pre-contemplation stage and can remain there for various periods of time. . . . Fortunately, this research indicates that the vast majority of relapsers – 85% of smokers, for example – recycle back to the contemplation or preparation stages. They begin to consider plans for their next action attempt while trying to learn from their recent efforts (Prochaska et al., 1992, pp 1104–1105).

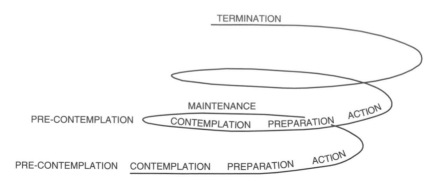

Figure 4.1.1 Spiral pattern of change. From *Systems of Psychotherapy: A Transtheoretical Analysis*, by J.O. Prochaska and J.C. Norcross. Copyright © 1994, 1984, 1979 Brooks/Cole Publishing Company, Pacific Grove, CA 93950, a division of International Thompson Publishing Inc. By permission of the publishers.

Although it might seem obvious, the idea that change is a dynamic process was in itself a breakthrough in understanding and supporting people to make required changes. Traditionally we have tended to respond as if change occurs 'out of the blue', and to interact with people as if they were ready for action, simply because there is sufficient evidence of directly attributable morbidity associated with the problematic health behaviour. Major mass media campaigns have targeted whole populations as if they were in the action stage, health professionals' advice assumes, based on the theory of reasoned action (Fishbein & Ajzen, 1985) that giving people convincing health information is sufficient persuasion for them to make significant behaviour changes. However, research from the USA indicates that only a small minority of people, between 10% and 15% are in the action stage, approximately 30%–40% are in the contemplation stage and 50%–60% are in the pre-contemplation stage (Abrams et al., 1988; Gottleib et al., 1990). Thus, by aiming interventions at action-oriented people alone, we are missing the opportunity of engaging with around 80% of the target population. To be effective, interventions must be tailored, stage-specific and where possible, personalised.

PROCESSES OF CHANGE

The model which underpins the analysis of behaviour change developed by Prochaska et al. is referred to as the transtheoretical model. This term, in effect, means that the model is eclectic, drawing on elements from a number of different psychological, psychotherapeutic and sociological theories to describe and explain the change process. Individuals use a variety of psycho-social techniques to support their behaviour change, and research has shown that it is possible to identify specific processes with the different stages of change. The transtheoretical model incorporates ten key processes or techniques of change. These were first identified in empirical research on smoking, obesity and with people experiencing psychological distress, and have since been substantiated across a range of behaviours.

TEN KEY PROCESSES OF CHANGE

Consciousness raising	or	Raising awareness or gaining insight by increasing information about oneself and the behaviour to be changed, using techniques such as reading (or bibliotherapy), and confrontation.
Self-re-evaluation	or	Assessing feelings and emotions about oneself and the problem to be changed; using techniques such as visualisation, value clarification, imagery, corrective emotional experience.
Self-liberation	or	Choosing and committing oneself to take action to change the problem behaviour or believing that you can do it. Techniques include making New Year's resolutions, decision-making therapy and commitment enhancing techniques.
Counter-conditioning	or	Substituting alternatives for problem behaviours: relaxation, desensitisation, assertion, positive self-statements.
Stimulus control	or	Avoiding or countering stimuli that elicit problem behaviours: restructuring one's environment (e.g. moving alcohol or fattening foods), avoiding risk cues, fading techniques.
Reinforcement management	or	Rewarding oneself or being rewarded by others for making changes. This may involve making contracts, overt and covert reinforcement, rewarding oneself.
Helping relationships	or	Being open and trusting about problems with someone who cares by joining self-help groups or asking for the support of significant others.
Dramatic relief	or	Experiencing and expressing feelings about one's problems and solutions by using techniques such as psychodrama and role play or grieving losses.
Environmental re-evaluation	or	Assessing how one's problem affects the physical environment. Typical techniques include the influence of documentaries or empathy training.
Social liberation	or	Self-empowerment. Increasing alternatives for non-problem behaviours available in society, for example by advocating for rights of repressed and attempting to influence social policy.

(adapted from Prochaska et al., 1994, p 33).

Table 4.1.1 Stages of change in which change processes are most emphasised. From *Systems of Psychotherapy: A Transtheoretical Analysis*, by J.O. Prochaska and J.C. Norcross. Copyright © 1994, 1984, 1979 Brooks/Cole Publishing Company, Pacific Grove, CA 93950, a division of International Thompson Publishing Inc. By permission of the publisher.

	Stages of change				
	Pre-contemplation	Contemplation	Preparation	Action	Maintenance
Processes	Consciousness raising Dramatic relief Environmental re-evaluation Self-re-evaluation				
			Self-liberation		
				Contingency management Helping relationship Counter-conditioning Stimulus control	

FITTING PROCESSES TO STAGES OF CHANGE

There is integration between the stages of change and the processes predominantly used in each stage.

In the pre-contemplation stage people tend to use the processes of consciousness raising, dramatic relief and environmental re-evaluation, the remaining eight processes being used in smoking cessation and weight loss indicated that 'pre-contemplators process less information about their problems, spent less time and energy on re-evaluating themselves, experienced fewer emotional reactions to the negative aspects of their problems; and are less open with significant others about their problems' (Prochaska et al., 1992, p 1109).

Focusing on raising pre-contemplators' awareness or increasing their understanding, can help the shift into contemplation. To move into contemplation a pre-contemplator needs to recognise the negative consequences of a behaviour, and perhaps to acknowledge the defensiveness – rationalisation, denial, defiance and so on – which they might be using to support the behaviour. The process of dramatic relief, with its powerful emotional impact, can help release emotions related to problem behaviours, and sometimes real-life events, such as the death of a friend or relative from an illness associated with the problematic health behaviour; or punishment, legally imposed, can have a powerful influence.

Contemplators are most likely to use bibliotherapy – reading about the problem behaviour and its consequences – to increase their awareness. They will often appear immensely knowledgeable about the problem behaviour and discuss it and its implications endlessly, as anyone who has worked with drug addicts and alcoholics will know. As people become increasingly aware of themselves and the nature of their problems, they can be more objective about how they think and feel about the problem relative to themselves. This self-re-evaluation process is in effect a personal assessment of the pros and cons of the behaviour – a decision about which aspects of the behaviour are important and which can more easily be abandoned. Contemplators also re-evaluate the effects of their behaviour on their environment, especially the people they care about most.

The move into preparation indicates an intention or readiness to change in the near future and draws on all the learning and understanding gained in the stages of pre-contemplation and contemplation. In making action plans, a person is preparing to control the change process in a way which is personally relevant. For example, one dieter may find the technique of substituting a healthier behaviour, such as eating fruit or taking exercise, an appropriate alternative response to the trigger to binge on chocolate, whereas another dieter may prefer to rigidly resist the temptation to binge, and yet another may decide to reduce the amount of chocolate they allow themselves to eat, or restrict it to certain situations and change its symbolism to that of a 'reward'. Each of these techniques is used as a process of counter-conditioning in the preparation stage. Another process or technique often used is that of stimulus control – or changing the routines which trigger the problem behaviour. For our dieter this might mean not pulling into the garage for a newspaper (and the bar of chocolate) on the way home from work. For a smoker, or someone with an alcohol problem, it might mean gradually cutting out, one by one, the times you respond to the trigger or stimulus to have a cigarette or drink.

In the action stage there is an increased feeling of self-worth or self-efficacy. The process identified with this feeling is self liberation – the belief that success is achieved by one's own efforts, even in difficult situations. Self-liberation, however, requires more than just an affective and cognitive belief in one's ability to control or change a behaviour, it also requires active effort to sustain the changed behaviour and techniques used in previous stages, such as counter-conditioning, stimulus control and contingency management. Many people actively sustaining a behaviour change also find the help and support of others useful. There is ample testimony to the supportive group from organisations such as Weight Watchers, Alcoholics Anonymous, Gamblers Anonymous and many of the campaigning groups working to bring about changes in legislation and practice.

Just as preparation for action is essential for success, so too is preparation for the stage of maintenance – or sustaining the changed behaviour. Successful maintenance draws on all the techniques which a person has found useful in the earlier stages of change, and uses them to sustain action and prevent relapse or recycling. For example, the 'chocoholic' may still find it necessary to deliberately avoid going to the garage for a newspaper, even if he or she hasn't had a chocolate binge for a considerable time, and the ex-smoker of six months or so may continue to need to resist the temptation to weaken and have 'just one cigarette' at a party.

To bring about successful behaviour change, then, requires giving appropriate help, or supporting the use of appropriate techniques or processes of change at the appropriate time, or stage of change.

THE CONTRIBUTION TO HEALTH PROMOTION OF DIFFERENT MODELS AND THEORIES OF CHANGE

The main contribution of the transtheoretical model to health promotion and the understanding of behaviour change is perhaps in providing a framework in which a number of significant variables can link up in patterns which provide the key to the system of change itself. Many of the variables were well known before the work of Prochaska and DiClemente began to be recognised as significant. For example, the work of Rosenstock (1966) and Becker (1974) had contributed the idea that a person considering changing their behaviour engages in a cost/benefit or utility analysis with themselves. They may consider the relative likelihood of contracting a disease or disability by continuing to engage in the behaviour, and weigh up a feasibility balance of the pros and cons of the behaviour. This model has come to be well known as the Health Belief Model, and has been expanded to include Bandura's concept of self-efficacy (Bandura, 1977; 1982) which suggests that individuals must have a belief in their ability to carry out and sustain a particular behaviour change. For the required behaviour change to occur they must have the incentive or motivation to change; feel a negative imbalance in their behaviour (the cons of current behaviour outweigh the pros); believe the changed behaviour would have advantages which outweigh the perceived benefits of the current behaviour (the pros of the changed behaviour outweigh the cons); and feel confidence in their ability to make and sustain the change. Identification of the stages of contemplation and preparation are influenced by Fishbein and Ajzen's Theory of Reasoned Action (Fishbein & Ajzen, 1985). This theory develops the Health Belief Model still further by separating people's beliefs from their attitudes in the context of health behaviour, and highlighting the interconnectedness of beliefs, attitudes, intention and practice with opinions and influences of significant others in health related decision making.

Subsequently, Ajzen (1985) added further to the Theory of Reasoned Action by incorporating Bandura's notion of a person's perceived ability to control their behaviour. The revised model, or Theory of Planned Behaviour, asserts that actions depend not only on beliefs and attitudes about the likely consequences of a particular health behaviour, but also on the extent to which people believe it is actually within their power to make and sustain the necessary changes. This gives implicit acknowledgement to the possibility that individuals cannot always influence or change some of the societal structures and systems which may provoke their problematic behaviour.

The decisional balance inventory (pros and cons) is clearly influenced by Janis and Mann's work on decision making in the 1970s (Janis & Mann, 1977). Their strategy of 'vigilant' decision making postulates that people do not always make decisions in the same way, but the process and outcome of decision making will vary according to a number of factors – for example, the situation, range of choices or alternatives, competency of the decision maker, information available and knowledge (both normative and objective). According to Janis and Mann much decision-making education is directed towards the development of rational choices, although real life seldom reflects these situations and normative and affective factors have to be given due weight, particularly in decisions relating to health. A person may be able to make the rational health decision not to have unprotected sex, or 'just to say no' to drugs for example, in abstract, but may be more vulnerable when faced with other influences in real life situations.

So how useful is the transtheoretical model as a framework for effective health promotion? Purists would argue that it is not a true model, but a useful eclectic tool for understanding behaviour change and matching the most receptive intervention points with the most appropriate interventions. No mean accomplishment in itself. The most frequently vaunted criticism is that the transtheoretical model advocates a prescriptive and individualistic approach to behaviour change, an approach, akin to the medical model, which assumes compliance based on reasoned action. Human behaviour is clearly not so logical, otherwise the vast majority of people would adopt healthy behaviours out of nothing more than rational choice. We know, from the outcome of health promotion campaigns that knowledge is not the only key to rational choice where health behaviour is concerned, but that a range of factors, such as social influence, disenfranchisement, economic power, emotional belief, media persuasion and normative influence are all strongly associated with behaviour outcome. Epidemiologists have been telling us for a considerable amount of time that morbidity and mortality which are directly attributable to unhealthy behaviour, such as smoking, high-fat diet, insufficient exercise and so on, can be mapped in terms of socio-economic and demographic characteristics. Similarly, variations in health can be attributed to different populations for different reasons. Many argue that these reasons are to do with social influence, apathy or alienation born of the belief that it is impossible to change your lot, poor educational attainment and economic circumstances, lack of skills, competence and self-esteem. But this does not explain why, in populations matched for social, economic and demographic characteristics, some people can, and do, change their behaviour.

Indeed, assessment of the population in relation to a variety of health behaviours seems to indicate quite consistently that around 40% are in the pre-contemplation stage, 40% are contemplators and 20% are preparing to take action. Furthermore, regardless of socio-economic characteristics, research indicates that the amount of progress people make following appropriately targeted stage-based interventions is a function of their pre-treatment stage of change (Prochaska & DiClemente, 1992). It seems that the earlier people can be helped to move from one stage to the next the better the chances of achieving a positive outcome. Prochaska and DiClemente in their research with smokers found that if a person can be helped to move from one stage to the next within a month, their chances of taking action to change the problematic behaviour is roughly doubled after six months. This fact challenges another of the criticisms sometimes made that the model disadvantages pre-contemplators. In a context which demands that scarce resources are targeted where they are likely to maximise effectiveness and efficiency, it is sometimes argued that pre-contemplators, who absorb a great deal of resource for little evidence of successful outcome, are likely to be excluded from targeted interventions. The fact that pre-contemplators and contemplators alike double their chances of successful outcome if they can move across a stage in the first month of an intervention, negates the argument. Evaluation of the effectiveness of interventions based on the model, and of their application in the real life systems and structures of service delivery, can, however, only be assessed by carrying out scientific randomised controlled trials. There is an urgent need for this research.

Finally, the model offers health professionals measurable feedback on progress relative to the stages and processes of change. As change agents it is important that they not only assess precisely where and how to target their intervention, but also that they are able to monitor progress from one intervention contact to the next. It is, after all, not just the client who needs the confirmation and reassurance that progress is being made!

REFERENCES

Abrams D B, Follick M J & Biener L (1988) Individual versus group self-help smoking cessation at the workplace: initial impact and 12 month outcomes. In: T Glynn (chair), Four National Cancer Institute funded self-help smoking cessation trials: Interim results and emerging patterns. Symposium conducted at the annual meeting of the Association for the Advancement of Behaviour Therapy, New York.

Ajzen I (1985) From intention to actions: a theory of planned behaviour. In: J Kuhl & J Beckman (Eds), Action control: from cognition to behavior. New Jersey: Prentice Hall.

Bandura A (1977) Self-efficacy: toward a unifying theory of behaviour change. *Psychological Review*, 84, 191–215.

Bandura A (1982) Self-efficacy mechanism in human agency. *American Psychologist*, 37, 122–147.

Becker M H (Ed) (1974) The belief model and personal health behaviour. Thorofare, New Jersey: Slack.

Cashdan S (1973) Interactional psychotherapy: stages and strategies in behavioural change. New York: Grune & Stratton.

DiClemente C C, Prochaska J O, Fairhurst K S, Velicer W F, Velasquez M M & Rossi J S (1991) The process of smoking cessation: an analysis of pre-contemplation, contemplation and preparation stages of change. *Journal of Consulting and Clinical Psychology*, 59, 295–304.

Egan G (1975) The skilled helper: a model for systematic helping and interpersonal relating. Monterey, CA: Brooks/Cole.

Fishbein M & Ajzen I (1985) Belief, attitude, intention and behaviour: an introduction to theory and research. Reading Massachusetts: Addison-Wesley.

Gottleib N H, Galavotti C, McCuan R S & McAlister A L (1990) Specification of a social cognitive model predicting smoking cessation in a Mexican-American population. A prospective study. *Cognitive Therapy and Research*, 14, 529–542.

Horn D & Waingrow S (1966) Some dimensions of a model for smoking behaviour change. *American Journal of Public Health*, 56, 21–26.

Janis I & Mann L (1977) Decision making. New York: Free Press.

Lambert M J, Shapiro D A & Bergin A E (1986) The effectiveness of psychotherapy. In: S L Garfield & A E Bergin (Eds), Handbook of psychotherapy and behaviour change. Third edition. New York: John Wiley.

Marlatt G A, Baer J S, Donovan D M & Divlahan D R (1988) Addictive behaviour: etiology and treatment. *Annual Review of Psychology*, 39, 223–252.

McBride C M & Pirie P L (1990) Post partum relapse. *Addictive Behaviour*, 15, 165–168.

Mullen P D, Quinn V P & Ershoff D H (1990) Maintenance of non-smoking post partum by women who stopped smoking during pregnancy. *American Journal of Public Health*, 80, 992–994.

Prochaska J O & DiClemente C C (1992) Stages of change in the modification of problem behaviours. In: M Hersen, R M Eisler & P M Miller (Eds), Progress in behaviour modification (pp 184–214). Sycamore, IL: Sycamore Press.

Prochaska J O & Norcross J C (1994) Systems of psychotherapy – a transtheoretical analysis. Third Edition. Monterey, CA: Brooks/Cole.

Prochaska J O, DiClemente C C & Norcross J C (1992) In search of how people change. Application to addictive behaviours. *American Psychologist*, 47 1102–1114.

Prochaska J O, Norcross J C & DiClemente C C (1994) Changing for good. New York: Morrow.

Rosenstock I (1966) Why people use health services. *Millbank Memorial Fund Quarterly*, 44, 91–121.

Schachter S (1982) Recidivism and self-cure of smoking and obesity. *American Psychologist*, 37, 436–444.

Shapiro S, Skinner E, Kessler L, Cottler L & Regier D (1984) Utilisation of health and mental health services. *Archives of General Psychiatry*, 41, 971–978.

Smith M L, Glass G V & Miller T L (1980) The benefits of psychotherapy. Baltimore: Johns Hopkins University.

Velicer W F, DiClemente C C, Prochaska J O & Brandenburg N (1985) A decisional balance measure for assessing and predicting smoking status. *Journal of Personality and Social Psychology*, 48, 1279–1289.

Section 4.2

The Transtheoretical Model: Profiling Smoking in Pregnancy

Liz Batten

THE HISTORY OF THE ADOPTION AND DIFFUSION OF THE TRANSTHEORETICAL MODEL IN THE UK

The publication of Prochaska and DiClemente's landmark paper in 1983 (Prochaska & DiClemente, 1983) caused a small ripple amongst those of us researching psychological approaches to smoking cessation in the UK at that time. I can remember a colleague sending a copy to me in 1984, who thought it might be of use in my work on community-based self-help approaches to stopping smoking (Batten & Taylor, 1982). Also in 1984, I later discovered, there was a conference in Scotland on alcohol and tobacco addiction, at which Professor Prochaska presented his ideas. Those who attended that conference were to be inspired by the potential transformation of their practice and possible improvement in outcomes, were they to adopt such an apparently simple model of how people naturally change their behaviour. There was at least one tobacco researcher present, a psychologist called Martin Raw, who had already been working on the idea of change as a cyclical process. Later in 1984 he was to present these ideas at a national conference on smoking cessation in Southampton (Batten, 1985). However, the majority of those present at the conference were drug and alcohol workers: practitioners who were there to focus on substance use and misuse, rather than on tobacco use. They took the conceptual framework into their everyday practice and began to transform their interventions. Researchers in the drug and alcohol field began to work with the model to develop different approaches to intervention.

Thus it was that the Stages of Change model, as it was then called, became a well-known and well-used concept within the drug and alcohol field in the UK long before it impacted on tobacco cessation research and practice. In 1986 I met Margaret Greaves, a member of the Standing Conference on Drug Abuse (SCODA), who had also attended the Scottish conference, and we began working together on the development of Smokestop training for health professionals.

Evidence-based Health Promotion. Edited by Elizabeth R. Perkins, Ina Simnett and Linda Wright.
© 1999 John Wiley & Sons Ltd.

Smokestop provided a range of in-service courses for those who wanted to become stop-smoking group leaders or smoking cessation counsellors. There were also courses for trainers and for workplace tutors. Most of the people who attended the courses were either practitioners in primary health care (health visitors, practice nurses, midwives, occupational health nurses) or health promotion officers. Margaret introduced me to the stages of change model in 1987 and it immediately became incorporated into the training programme. This was the first time that the model had been taught to primary health care practitioners, and it became an important feature of the distinctive Smokestop style of training. Smokestop also introduced the stages of change model to 'Look After Yourself' trainers during 1990 in a specially devised course on women and smoking. At around this time the smoking cessation literature produced by the Health Education Authority (and written by Martin Raw) began to introduce the idea of cessation as a 'revolving door', clearly related to the work of Prochaska and DiClemente, although not acknowledging this. Within a few years the HEA would commission training for practitioners called *Helping People Change*, and this, too, drew on the stages of change model (and was again written by Martin Raw).

During the 1980s, the Smokestop style of training had percolated widely throughout health promotion training, and with it the diffusion of the stages of change model. This process continued through *Helping People Change*, and through another training programme commissioned by the HEA called *Helping pregnant smokers quit* and continues today via the many publications on smoking cessation produced by the HEA.

PROS AND CONS OF ADOPTING THE STAGES OF CHANGE MODEL IN THE UK

The value of the stages of change model as a tool in experiential teaching and learning is beyond doubt. It gives credence and structure to the experience of trainers, trainees, practitioners and clients alike. As a trainer I find it delightful to introduce this model of behaviour change to a group of trainees. Within minutes, the impact of beginning to see smoking cessation as a process, something which has to be learned, is apparent to the trainees. They can relate their own experience of behaviour change to the model, can stage themselves in relation to any behaviour they might like to change, and can begin to identify the differences in language a person might use to talk about their experience, depending on which stage of change they are in. The model encourages practitioners to adopt an attitude towards smoking cessation, or any kind of behaviour change, which is supportive, encouraging and helpful; it helps them to become more aware of what kind of intervention will be most helpful for each individual; and helps them to learn to treat all experience as an opportunity for each individual to glean information about what works for them, and what does not, in their progress towards creating and maintaining change.

Importantly, the stages of change model removes the concept of 'success' and 'failure', both for the practitioner and client; it removes the idea that stopping smoking is an event and replaces it with the concept of change as a process, the techniques of which can be learned; it introduces the concept of change as a cyclical or dynamic process, where several attempts at change may be appropriate, in order to learn and practise new behaviour, before eventually achieving a goal of maintenance of a new behaviour.

More important still, when taking an evidence-based approach to smoking cessation intervention, the model helps the practitioner in two ways. Firstly, the battery of measures which comprise what is nowadays called the transtheoretical model provides a comprehensive means of measuring both individuals and their smoking attitudes and behaviour, and whole populations. If we can measure a population in this sophisticated way, then we can profile the populations we work with as practitioners in much more detail, and can provide much more highly targeted and appropriate interventions. Using the data gathered with this battery of measures, we can create a baseline assessment and then measure progress in much finer detail than has previously been possible. Secondly, interventions with individuals can be recorded in much more detail using the stages and processes of change as a basis, and subsequent interventions can register movement through the stages and utilisation of the processes, rather than a simple measurement of current cigarette consumption or abstinence. This means that both practitioner and client can remain involved in the process of change, because both are working with *what is*, rather than solely focusing on the ultimate goal of abstinence, which may not yet be appropriate or attainable. In other words, the client is being encouraged to work towards his or her ultimate goal at his or her own pace and in his or her own way, supported by the practitioner.

Finally, the interventions based on the transtheoretical model can reach a much greater proportion of the target audience (all current and recent smokers), because pre-contemplators and contemplators can also be engaged with and offered concrete opportunities to learn how to change. With this increase in the reach of such interventions there is an accompanying claimed increase in efficacy (Prochaska et al., 1993), and this, too, will help practitioners and their clients to feel more optimistic about the possibility of change.

On the downside, there are several problems with the way the model has been introduced into the UK. The HEA's various programmes and documents do not use the original labels for each stage of change: pre-contemplation, contemplation, preparation, action and maintenance. It is understandably tempting to re-word these labels, but the meaning of each stage can become subtly altered in translation. An example of this is the general tendency to substitute 'not interested in quitting' or 'not ready to quit' for pre-contemplation. (The US research team's definition is: Not intending to change (a given behaviour) in the next six months.) This led to several years of advice from the HEA and others to not put pressure on smokers in this stage to quit smoking, because it would not be appropriate. As a consequence, most practitioners have avoided doing anything other than offer leaflets to pre-contemplators, and felt unable to intervene. This in turn has led to another change in the use of the model within interventions by practitioners. The model has become a diagnostic tool for some, in order to locate those in the preparation stage who will be more responsive to an intervention. This is an improvement over previous methods, which largely gave the same intervention to the whole population of smokers, but still avoids providing an intervention for the 80% of current smokers who are in pre-contemplation and contemplation stages. The reason for this modification of the original scope of the model is that the processes of change, an integral part of the whole model, have not been taught alongside the stages of change, until recently. These are described in the previous section. Without an understanding of these processes, and how the experiential processes feature more in the early stages of change, and how the behavioural processes feature more in the later stages of change, practitioners had only half of the picture of how to intervene effectively with the whole population of smokers.

Another difficulty has been the absence of stage-based materials to offer smokers, which would help them to understand both the stages of change and the processes of change and allow them to plan their own individual pathway to change. These are now available in the UK.

Finally, the model has been widely adopted throughout the UK without the benefit of any comprehensive research on a UK population. Until very recently we have had no data to describe whether the model, and interventions derived from it, would be culturally appropriate, nor any information on whether a UK population would have the same characteristics as the US populations on which the model was tested and refined. Alongside this absence of UK data on the transtheoretical model is the often raised question (see for example the debate in the *British Journal of Addiction*, 1992, 87) of whether the descriptive validity of the constructs within the model can be utilised in a prescriptive way, to shape and define the interventions we use, or in a predictive way, to target the populations and corresponding interventions used. In other words, can this valuable conceptual framework for describing how people naturally change their behaviour be successfully translated into an intervention programme? We have yet to conduct studies in the UK to test this, although randomised controlled trials are under way in the West Midlands.

Development of a UK Database on Smoking in Pregnancy and the Transtheoretical Model

In 1995, West Midlands Regional Health Authority (now West Midlands NHS Executive) was putting considerable effort into training midwives to intervene with pregnant smokers, using a modification of the HEA's *Helping pregnant smokers quit* training manual. There was also, and continues, a concurrent development in the systematic recording of smoking prevalence data on pregnant women at several points throughout pregnancy. What became apparent was that, despite the additional training and improvement in data collection, what remained to be tackled was how to help the large numbers of women on a low income who seemed more likely to smoke during pregnancy. More detailed information was needed on the social and economic circumstances of pregnant women, together with a picture of how these might relate to their smoking status and intentions.

At this point I was invited to design a population survey of smoking in pregnancy in the West Midlands, and this would be the first UK survey to collect such detailed information together with data on the stages and processes of change. It was envisaged that the findings of the survey could then be used as a planning tool for smoking cessation interventions with pregnant women. The task before us was to explore whether a psychological model of behaviour change would be a sufficient descriptor in itself of opportunities for intervention with this group of women. We wanted to know how the transtheoretical model would fit with women's social circumstances. We wanted to know whether this information could offer anything useful to professionals faced with the task of reducing smoking prevalence in pregnancy as part of the *Health of the Nation* strategy. Was quitting smoking during pregnancy, or not smoking at all, a function of better social and economic circumstances, which a smoking cessation intervention on its own could not attempt to provide?

The questionnaire therefore contained a wide range of questions in various sections: about being pregnant (health issues, social support, loneliness and depression, smoking in the household, being asked about smoking, number of weeks pregnant, number of children, intention to breastfeed, planned or unplanned pregnancy); about you and your family (access to car, tenure, relationship, income and assessment of financial management, benefits claimed, smoking status and partner's smoking status); tempting situations (the short form situational temptation inventory); pros and cons of smoking (the short form decisional balance inventory); impacts on smoking (the ten processes of change); smoking history; and socio-demographics (age, education, employment status, partner's employment status, ethnicity).

We aimed to collect a total of 2100 questionnaires (700 from each of three sites) from each woman who attended for ultrasound scan over a period of approximately ten weeks. The questionnaires were administered by midwives in the ante-natal clinics in Coventry and Stoke on Trent, and in women's own homes in Dudley, and a total of 2102 questionnaires were administered, of which 2030 were eligible (97%). Of these, 188 were removed because of refusals, spoiled or part-completion, or not returned to the midwife, leaving 1842 valid responses (91% of eligible responses); a very high response rate.

Analysing the Data Collected

We needed to ask three main questions of the data collected: how representative was the group of women on whom we had collected the data?; did the model have the same characteristics when tested on a UK population as on a US population?; and what could we say about a population of pregnant women in the West Midlands in relation to their smoking status and social circumstances?

How Representative was the Study Population?

Around 97% of all babies in their catchment area are delivered by the maternity hospitals in this study, so attendance bias is unlikely in the two hospital sites (97% and 98% valid response), although administration in the women's own homes resulted in a lower response (73%). The 1842 women are representative of women in these three locations in the West Midlands by own and partner's social class when compared with the 1991 Census for the West Midlands. The distribution of respondents by ethnic group also closely resembles that of the 1991 Census. Overall, the women in this sample are poorer than a representative sample of the UK population. This is probably because they are younger, i.e. at the lowest earning point of their working lives, have children, and are located in the mostly industrial parts of the West Midlands.

Fifty-three per cent of respondents had never smoked, 29 per cent were current smokers, and 10.4 per cent had quit since becoming pregnant; while only 7.5% were longer term ex-smokers. There were fewer current smokers in Dudley, which may be due to the different method of administering the questionnaire (by community midwife in the women's own homes), but this is not a significant difference (p = 0.148, df = 4, n = 1813). These data are consistent with previous studies of smoking prevalence during pregnancy by the Infant Feeding Survey and the HEA Tracking Studies (Campion et al., 1994; White et al., 1992).

CHARACTERISTICS OF THE MODEL

Stage of Change

Respondents' stage of change was ascertained by use of a standard set of questions which assess intention to quit smoking and actual quit attempts during the past year. The results are shown in Figure 4.2.1. The action stage has been separated into those women who quit in the six months prior to becoming pregnant, and those who quit following confirmation of pregnancy. This separation emphasises the amount of recent quitting activity there is for this group of women. There is also a different proportion of current smokers by stage than has been found amongst US adult smokers. In this sample there is a stage of change ratio of 42:24:34 (pre-contemplator:contemplator:preparation). In adult populations of smokers in the US, a ratio of 40:40:20 (PC:C:P) has commonly been found (Velicer et al., 1994). It could be expected that there would be more women in the preparation stage in early pregnancy, but not that the proportion in pre-contemplation, in a pregnant sample, would remain as high as might be found in the general population.

Processes of Change, Decisional Balance, Situational Temptation and Confidence

The short form inventories for the other constructs of the transtheoretical model were used (Fava et al., 1995), except for confidence which was measured by one item. Reliability tests of these constructs show good internal consistency, and the relationships between stages and processes of change and these are similar to those in the US data, and have been reported on in detail elsewhere (Batten et al., in preparation a). These tests of validity on the measures within the transtheoretical model indicate that they are robust and culturally appropriate for use with a UK pregnant population. When we examined non-response to items and sections within the questionnaire it became apparent that there is a slight trend towards women on a low income (less than £200 per week) and those who did not have any further education to be more likely to be missing from the stage and process measures.

Stage of Change, Parity and Social Circumstances

Given the unusual stage of change ratio amongst current smokers in this study (see Figure 4.2.1), the data were analysed by parity. Figures 4.2.2 and 4.2.3 show that, in first pregnancy, most women have moved into the action or preparation stages, suggesting that pregnancy has an intervention-like effect in itself. On the other hand, women in their second or subsequent pregnancy are polarised into pre-contemplation, with many fewer in the action stage, and the proportions in contemplation and preparation stages remaining virtually the same, for first and subsequent pregnancies. It suggests that the enormous shift of activity early in first pregnancy may be primarily from pre-contemplation to action. Those women who made attempts to change their smoking behaviour and relapsed during or after the first pregnancy may be remaining in pre-contemplation in second and subsequent pregnancies. This finding has implications for support and intervention strategies for pregnant smokers.

The next question to be asked of the data was: Do women in the most deprived circumstances have the same profile by stage of change as women in more comfortable circumstances? We created three groups for comparative purposes: those in receipt of income support; those women, not in receipt of means-tested benefits, with a household income of £200 per week or less after tax; and those women, not in receipt of means-tested benefit, with a household income in excess of £200 per week, after tax. Table 4.2.1 shows the profile which emerges.

Most pre-contemplators are to be found amongst those claiming income support, and those who quit smoking before pregnancy or more than six months previously are most likely to be in the higher income group. Nevertheless, it is clear that very low income is not a barrier to many women attempting to change their smoking behaviour during pregnancy.

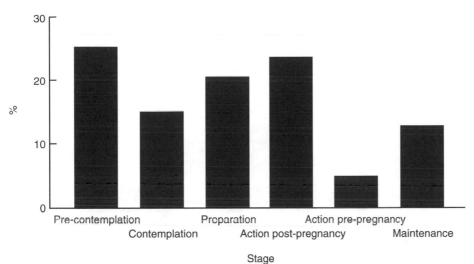

Figure 4.2.1   Respondents' stage of change

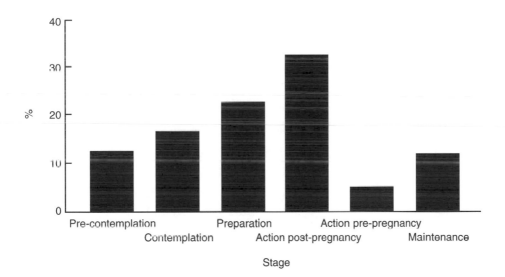

Figure 4.2.2   Stage of change by first pregnancy

Given that large differences by stage were found amongst women by parity, the analysis was repeated by income group (see Table 4.2.2).

Women expecting their first child, regardless of income or benefit status, were much more likely to be in action or preparation. Pre-contemplators were most likely to be in the group in receipt of income support and expecting their second or

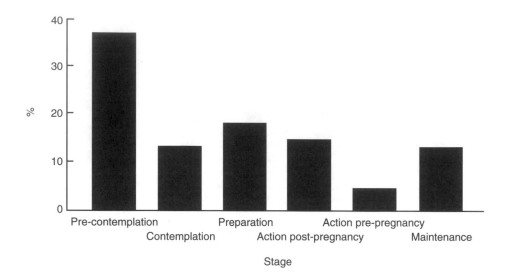

Figure 4.2.3   Stage of change by second or subsequent pregnancy

Table 4.2.1   Stage of change by income status

Stage	Income			Total
	Income support	Other low income	Over £200 pw	
Pre-contemplation				
n	107	26	49	182
%	45.0%	14.9%	15.5%	24.9%
Contemplation				
n	39	33	39	111
%	16.4%	18.9%	12.3%	15.2%
Ready for action				
n	43	45	63	151
%	18.1%	25.7%	19.9%	20.7%
Action after pregnant				
n	38	41	85	164
%	16.0%	23.4%	26.8%	22.5%
Action before pregnant				
n	3	8	21	32
%	1.3%	4.6%	6.6%	4.4%
Maintenance				
n	8	22	60	90
%	3.4%	12.6%	18.9%	12.3%
Total				
n	238	175	317	730
%	100.0%	100.0%	100.0%	100.0%

Table 4.2.2 Stage of change by parity by income status

| Parity | Stage | Income | | | |
		Income support	Other low income	Over £200 pw	Total
First child	Pre-contemplation				
	n	12	7	19	38
	%	20.7%	6.7%	11.2%	11.4%
	Contemplation				
	n	12	21	22	55
	%	20.7%	20.2%	12.9%	16.6%
	Ready for action				
	n	16	29	30	75
	%	27.6%	27.9%	17.6%	22.6%
	Action after pregnant				
	n	18	32	54	104
	%	31.0%	30.8%	31.8%	31.3%
	Action before pregnant				
	n		6	11	17
	%		5.8%	6.5%	5.1%
	Maintenance				
	n		9	34	43
	%		8.7%	20.0%	13.0%
Total	n	58	104	170	332
	%	100.0%	100.0%	100.0%	100.0%
Second+ child	Pre-contemplation				
	n	95	19	30	144
	%	52.8%	26.8%	20.4%	36.2%
	Contemplation				
	n	27	12	17	56
	%	15.0%	16.9%	11.6%	14.1%
	Ready for action				
	n	27	16	33	76
	%	15.0%	22.5%	22.4%	19.1%
	Action after pregnant				
	n	20	9	31	60
	%	11.1%	12.7%	21.1%	15.1%
	Action before pregnant				
	n	3	2	10	15
	%	1.7%	2.8%	6.8%	3.8%
	Maintenance				
	n	8	13	26	47
	%	4.4%	18.3%	17.7%	11.8%
Total	n	180	71	147	398
	%	100.0%	100.0%	100.0%	100.0%

subsequent child. Further statistical analysis (Batten et al., in preparation b) suggests that it is being in receipt of means-tested benefit rather than being on a low income that reduces the likelihood of intending to change smoking behaviour in pregnancy.

WHAT ARE THE IMPLICATIONS OF THIS BASELINE STUDY?

For the first time in the UK, we have a baseline assessment of smoking in early pregnancy by stage of change. Many practitioners will recognise their own experience in this dataset. It may provide confirmation of their observations in the course of their work about who is more likely to quit smoking during pregnancy. They may not, however, have seen before the large differences between first and second pregnancy in women's intentions to quit smoking. They will probably be very familiar with the impact of living on means-tested benefit on women's intentions to quit smoking.

There are several issues arising from this study:

1. It would be reasonable to hypothesise from this data that interventions based on the transtheoretical model will be appropriate for the majority of pregnant women who are not in receipt of means-tested benefit. Pregnant women have been targeted as a way in to smoking cessation in women more generally, and this study gives cause for hope that further reductions in smoking prevalence in this group can be achieved.
2. Measurements of smoking prevalence and of change, whether self-motivated or in response to an intervention, are strongly socio-economically related. If the stage-based interventions work as well as expected, might there then be an inadvertent increase in the already large divide between rich and poor and their ability to quit smoking? What kinds of intervention are likely to be most appropriate and acceptable to women living in the most deprived circumstances? This study suggests that tackling smoking cessation head on will not be the most fruitful approach. It is likely that being in receipt of means-tested benefit is a proxy for many facets of the experience of women in deprived circumstances. We need to pay attention to the detailed qualitative work by Graham (1996) and others which will help to guide our understanding of what needs to be done.
3. Utilising the transtheoretical model within a smoking cessation intervention is a sophisticated procedure, which requires intensive training and continuously supervised practice. This is, after all, a particularly focused form of counselling, and ethical standards dictate that appropriate training and supervised practice should be in place. This is not the norm in the UK, nor is there any official body which oversees the quality of training and practice and the ethical procedures associated with this. Maybe there should be one. In the US, the

interventions have been delivered only by qualified psychologists, so far, and with the benefit of the stage-based self-help manuals and the interactive computer system to support them. It seems advisable that such materials be made available to practitioners in the UK.

4. Another ethical issue to arise from the use of the transtheoretical model in the UK to date has been its use as a diagnostic tool to identify and target interventions at those who will be more likely to want to change in the near future. This has been raised by others (Whitehead, 1997). This is not the intention of the creators of the transtheoretical model and, if used correctly, the stages and processes of change will provide an appropriate intervention for each person, according to stage of change, and does not eliminate anyone from the opportunity of receiving an intervention.

It is intended that the existing dataset will be explored to examine whether being on means-tested benefit is a proxy for other important issues in the lives of women in the most deprived circumstances. These may be social issues, such as the stress and distress caused by poor housing, poverty and inadequate education. We clearly also need a policy-led approach to eliminating poverty and improving education for all in order to make further inroads into the association between smoking and deprivation.

REFERENCES

Batten E (1985) Smokestop National Conference Proceedings. Health Education Council/ University of Southampton.

Batten E & Taylor D H (1982) Operation Smokestop: smoking cessation self-help groups in Wessex. Lifeline Report no. 5, Wessex Regional Health Authority.

Batten E, High S, Graham H, Rossi J & Ruggiero L (in preparation a) Applying the transtheoretical model to a West Midlands pregnant population: 1. Reliability and validity of the model.

Batten E, High S, Graham H, Rossi J & Ruggiero L (in preparation b) Profiling smoking in early pregnancy: integrating the stages and processes of change with social and economic circumstances.

Campion P, Owen L & McNeill A (1994) Smoking before, during and after pregnancy in England. *Health Education Journal*, 53(2), 163–173.

Fava J L, Velicer W F & Prochaska J O (1995) Applying the transtheoretical model to a representative sample of smokers. *Addictive Behaviors*, 20(2), 189–203.

Graham H (1996) Researching women's health work: a study of the lifestyles of mothers on income support. In: P Bywaters & E McLeod (Eds), Working for equality in health (pp 161–178). London: Routledge.

Prochaska J O & DiClemente C C (1983) Stages and processes of self-change of smoking: toward an integrative model of change. *Journal of Consulting and Clinical Psychology*, 51(3), 390–395.

Prochaska J O, DiClemente C C, Velicer W F & Rossi J S (1993) Standardized, individualized, interactive, and personalized self-help programs for smoking cessation. *Health Psychology*, 12, 399–405.

Velicer W F, Rossi J S, Ruggiero L & Prochaska J O (1994) Minimal interventions appropriate for an entire population of smokers. In: R Richmond (Ed), Interventions for smokers: an international perspective (pp 69–92). Baltimore: Williams and Wilkins.
White A, Freeth S & O'Brien M (1992) Infant feeding 1990. London: HMSO.
Whitehead M (1997) Editorial: How useful is the 'stages of change' model? *Health Education Journal*, 56, 111–112.

Chapter 5

Training and Education

Elizabeth R. Perkins

INTRODUCTION

Health promotion often involves an extension of skills or knowledge acquired in initial training, and health promotion departments have traditionally been seen as one possible local source for this extra help. It is in the nature of the need for extra training that potential trainees do not know enough about the problem to be able to identify clearly what they need to know. This presents problems for individuals trying to access help, for managers trying to assess the right kind of course to support their staff, and for those who run courses trying to work out what to provide. Many courses put on by health promotion departments have been based on informed guesses about what was needed, and the role of evidence has often been limited. The same can be said for courses provided from within higher education, where the scope for the academic discipline, rather than the demands of practice, to determine the curriculum is considerable.

An evidence-based training and education process would use evidence both in the design of the programme and in the evaluation of its effects. Evaluation is discussed in Chapter 16. This chapter considers two systematic approaches to programme design, training needs analysis (TNA) and professional competencies.

The first section, *Training needs analysis*, explains this approach in general terms.

The second section, *Primary care nursing: a TNA case study*, is an account of one health promotion department's application of this process to health visitors' training needs. It illustrates both the advantages of undertaking a TNA and the lessons which can be passed on to others undertaking one for the first time.

The third section, *National occupational standards for health promotion and care*, describes the recently developed framework of competencies deisgned specifically for health promotion and discusses the scope for using them in relation to evidence-based practice.

Evidence-based Health Promotion. Edited by Elizabeth R. Perkins, Ina Simnett and Linda Wright.
© 1999 John Wiley & Sons Ltd.

The fourth section, *Making use of competencies*, draws on experience in using the more established sets of competencies available for management, and training and development, to show the practical possibilities of this approach.

Section 5.1

Training Needs Analysis (TNA)

Linda Wright

WHY BOTHER WITH TRAINING NEEDS ANALYSIS?

Training is expensive. Within the prevailing culture of contracts and cash limits, health promotion training increasingly faces demands for evidence of both need and effectiveness. Scepticism is fuelled by the fact that training often fails to have an impact on practice; Georgensen and Del-Gaizo (1984) estimate that only 10% of training makes a difference to how people behave at work. Health promotion training will usually be only one of many competing demands made on an organisation's limited training budget. Providers of health promotion training, e.g. the specialist NHS health promotion services, are also often seeking to influence training practice in institutions outside of their own, e.g. education authorities and social services departments, and therefore need to convince managers that such training is needed.

Some providers of health promotion training continue to circulate a menu of training courses to managers, for them to decide which ones to send their staff on. This has been dubbed *'the scattergun approach to training – firing off a hail of pellets [courses] in the hope that one might find the mark i.e. meet the need – whatever it is!'* (Bee & Bee, 1994, p 3).

Basing your training mainly on what you think is important or useful may fail to take into account the needs and goals of the organisation or the needs of individual work roles within it. Such provision may not be considered a good return on investment. Training needs analysis (TNA) and training evaluation are therefore vital tools in ensuring that heath promotion training is properly focused. Attention paid to TNA will provide evidence to justify investment in health promotion training and will also inform decisions about whether training is the most appropriate response to the needs identified.

Evidence-based Health Promotion. Edited by Elizabeth R. Perkins, Ina Simnett and Linda Wright.
© 1999 John Wiley & Sons Ltd.

TNA IN HEALTH PROMOTION

Originating in business training practice, TNA's adoption by health and social care training agencies has been slow and sporadic. A feasibility study of methods to assess training needs of health promoters in Scotland (Inglis et al., 1996) found that TNA was not widely understood by either health promotion specialists or health promoters. A limited range of approaches to TNA were used, focusing on the felt needs of potential trainees (mainly nurses) and tending to overlook the needs of their managers and organisations. This study also acknowledged some of the difficulties of using TNA in health promotion: the diversity of disciplines with a health promotion role, the range of contexts in which health promotion is practised and the contested nature of health promotion itself. To this list we can add the more mundane problem of finding sufficient time and money to do a TNA!

Essential Elements of TNA

TNA involves more than the identification of training needs; it is the whole process of:

- training needs identification
- training needs specification
- translating training needs into action.

Each of these three elements is essential: there is little point spending time identifying training needs if you don't then pull them together into a coherent needs specification. Equally, deciding whether training *is* the most appropriate way of meeting the needs identified (rather than other strategies such as changes in working practices or organisational change) will be important in ensuring that investment in human resources development is properly managed.

Identifying Training Needs

Business models of TNA usually incorporate three levels at which training needs should be identified:

- the organisation
- the job or occupation
- the individual.

To which, in health promotion, we should add a fourth level:

- the client, patient or service user.

Asking Questions about Health Promotion Training Needs

In deciding how you might identify training needs, start by setting some bound-aries to your enquiry. Define the group to be trained, the subject area and the time and resources you have available. It is unlikely that health promoters and their managers will share your understanding of the philosophy and practice of health promotion (Inglis et al., 1996; Nettleton & Burrows, 1997) and you will almost certainly need to take this into account in framing your questions and negotiating a TNA methodology.

The operational needs of the organisation (i.e. what it needs to do to achieve its goals) is the starting point for TNA. You should be able to clearly demonstrate how the training that you propose is relevant to organisational goals. For example, an operational goal of the Probation Service is offender rehabilitation. Drugs training for probation officers will therefore be centrally concerned with enabling them to address drug-related offending behaviour in their service users; training for a broader role in drug misuse prevention, however important this might be to you, is unlikely to be supported by the organisation.

The question most usually asked to identify health promotion training needs is:

In what skills/knowledge/personal attributes are you in need of training?

From the learning standpoint, this is a very good question, providing information about salient felt needs and learner motivation. Where people say they do not need training (even if their managers think otherwise) they will be very resistant to it. However, asking three more questions would provide a more complete picture:

What skills/knowledge/personal attributes are important in your job?

This provides information about importance of your subject in the job, its relevance and the possibilities for linking training with the intrinsic rewards of the job itself. If it is not considered to be important in the job, motivation to learn will be low.

What skills/knowledge/personal characteristics are likely to be encouraged, recognised or rewarded by your manager/organisation?

Responses relate the value of the training to the individual's organisation, includ-ing the rewards (financial, bonuses, promotions) and the realities of line manage-ment. If your subject is unlikely to be recognised or rewarded by the organisation, then even if motivation is high and the individual learns a lot, change is likely to be undermined as soon as the learner returns to work. If you encounter this, you might consider the following strategies:

- asking managers to look to the system for blocks to change
- including managers in the training strategy

- making time for action planning within the training
- negotiating follow-up and after care support for learners.

What skills/knowledge/personal characteristics will result in better health for your clients/patients/service users?

This final question, not usually incorporated in business models of TNA (e.g. Fairbairns, 1991) would seem to be central to an ethical approach to health promotion training.

The area of overlap between all four questions (see Figure 5.1.1) represents the best focus for your training efforts. It is the point where strategic, operational, individual and ethical priorities for learning converge.

Methods of Gathering Evidence about Training Needs

Many of the recommended methods for identifying training needs, particularly at the organisational level, are only available to a dedicated training department located within the organisation. The business plan, plans for human resource management, or a full analysis of internal and external environmental factors affecting the organisation may simply not be available to you, particularly in contexts where business competition exists. However, it should always be possible to ask managers the questions *'What are the goals of your organisation?'* and *'How will this training benefit the organisation?'* This will usually enable you to identify how the TNA fits into the organisation's plans and priorities. It is also important to check out your assumptions about the organisation, its mission and its culture, if the proposed training initiative is to have any chance of having lasting impact on the work practices of the trainees.

Essentially, identifying training needs involves identifying the 'performance gap', the gap between what people know and do and what they should know and do in order to achieve the organisation's goals and maximise individual job performance. The mechanistic model of training requires that job specifications should be broken down into key tasks and those tasks into specific competencies. This competency-based approach to training has been enabled by the training and development lead bodies' efforts to define the competencies required for work roles, including those of health promotion (see Section 5.3). Unless your training relates to a very specific set of skills (e.g. how to use an overhead projector) or an extremely prescribed role, it is usually not feasible for a health promotion trainer to start from scratch in defining key tasks and competencies. You will usually need to focus your attention on asking managers: *'What do you want trainees to be able to do differently as a result of their training?'* and in identifying the shortfall between what is desired and current practice.

The feasibility of using any or all of the methods of training needs identification listed below will depend on your role as a trainer and on the resources you have

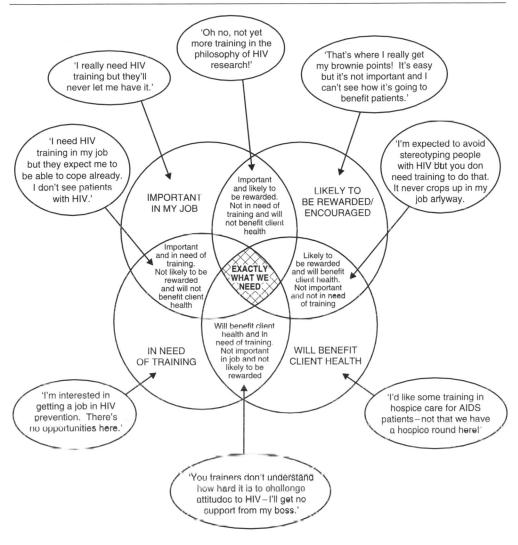

Figure 5.1.1 A four-question approach to training needs analysis in health promotion: examples from HIV prevention (Reproduced by permission of *Personnel Management*)

available. Whatever methods you use, make sure that you have taken the four levels of training need into account before you develop the specification.

Specification of Training Needs and Translating Them into Action

This is the stage where you assemble all of your evidence on training needs, identify where evidence from the four levels of needs assessment overlaps (and where it does not), write a detailed specification of the knowledge and skill levels to be achieved and develop a detailed training plan. Part of this process will be deciding whether training *is* the best solution. Non-training solutions could include:

- developing policies and management structures
- tackling problems with materials, equipment or the work environment
- increasing money or staff
- reorganising work methods
- improving communication practices and systems
- redesigning jobs
- changing personnel
- increasing motivation
- or even . . . doing nothing.

The key questions to ask are:

Will the chosen solution effectively meet the needs? and

Will it do so at the lowest cost?

A MENU OF METHODS

- asking them (perceived/felt needs) – individually/groups
- asking their managers
- asking their employer/organisation
- asking their clients – individually/groups
- reading:
  - publishing literature/research reports
  - training standards, TDLB core competencies
  - professional associations' guidelines, government reports
  - operational and strategic plans, annual reports, business plans
- direct observation of practice (shadowing, non-participant observation)
- critical incident analysis
- performance review
- staff appraisal
- organisational review
- community analysis
- job specifications, job descriptions and task analysis
- practice audit
- current training provision, demand and uptake

Training Needs Specification

As with needs identification, many of the techniques for specifying training needs are simply beyond the resources of most health promotion trainers. They all involve gathering data about the performance gap so that training requirements can be precisely specified as learning outcomes:

- key person consultation
- self-completed questionnaires/reports/diaries
- document/record analysis
- observing practice
- individual and group interviews (including appraisal)
- examining competencies (see above).

The first two techniques are commonly used in health promotion TNA, but work usually stops short of a detailed specification of the actual performance gap. The more detail you can give about the amount of knowledge and skill improvement that learners need to achieve to do a particular health promotion task, the better the training will be tailored to their needs.

USING EVIDENCE FROM TRAINING NEEDS ASSESSMENT TO INFORM A PROFESSIONAL DEVELOPMENT AND TRAINING STRATEGY

Having invested time and effort in the first two stages of TNA, you will now be ready to translate your evidence into a training specification, your blueprint for how the training is to be carried out and assessed. This should detail the:

- goals of the organisation
- training needs and gaps in performance
- target population
- aims
- objectives
- methods
- trainer(s)
- evaluation
- time-scale
- constraints.

It is beyond the scope of this chapter to discuss each of these elements fully. In my experience, health promotion trainers are much more confident in specifying training than they are in gathering the evidence that precedes it – hence this focus on TNA.

REFERENCES

Bee F & Bee R (1994) Training needs analysis and evaluation. London: Institute of Personnel and Development.

Fairbairns J (1991) Plugging the gap in training needs analysis. *Personnel Management*, February, 43–45.

Georgensen D & Del-Gaizo E (1984) Maximise the return on your training investment through needs analysis. *Training and Development Journal*, 38(8), 42–47.

Inglis B, Duffield J, Low L & Morris B (1996) Devising methods to assess training needs of health promoters in Scottish Area Health Boards. Final report for the Health Education Board for Scotland. Stirling: University of Stirling, Department of Education.

Nettleton S & Burrows R (1997) If health promotion is everybody's business what is the fate of the health promotion specialist? *Sociology of Health and Illness*, 19(1), 23–47.

FURTHER READING

Boydell T & Leary M (1996) Identifying training needs. London: Institute of Personnel and Development.

Section 5.2

Primary Care Nursing:
A TNA Case Study

Kenny Richardson and Sandy Burnham

BACKGROUND

The Borders Health Board area has a population of around 106 000, which is spread over a large area in small towns and villages. The population has the largest percentage of elderly population in Scotland and also one of the lowest average incomes. While there are concentrated areas of relative deprivation, there are also problems caused by rural isolation and access to services. In 1995, health service delivery was re organised and split into a health board, an acute trust and a community trust. The acute trust comprised the Borders General Hospital, while the community was responsible for health centres, community hospitals, mental health services, learning difficulties and community PAMS (Professions Allied to Medicine).

Historically, the Health Promotion Department (HPD) has maintained positive links with most NHS staff since its early days as a provider of leaflets, posters and videos. However, as the role and aspirations of the HPD advanced we recognised a need to increase our influence over the development of nurses' health promotion practice, but found some resistance by them to attending courses. We decided to undertake a training needs assessment exercise with nursing staff in the Community Health Services Trust. Informal feedback gave us an impression that nurses were generally confident about their health promotion practice with their clients and did not feel the need to develop their skills and understanding in this area. This did not match our perception of local practice or the overall findings of research into nurses' health promotion practice (Atkins et al., 1994; Gott & O'Brien, 1990).

Galli (1978) described health promotion as 'an essentially contested concept'. Recent research by Stirling University (Inglis et al., 1996) investigated the training needs of health promoters in Scottish Area Health Boards and a key finding was that 'the most important area of unmet training need is that of appreciating the concept of health

Evidence-based Health Promotion. Edited by Elizabeth R. Perkins, Ina Simnett and Linda Wright.
© 1999 John Wiley & Sons Ltd.

promotion'. Our own experience in an earlier training needs exercise through questionnaire was that when invited to express their training needs, nurses tended to concentrate on ways of getting the message across or learning how to persuade patients to change their behaviour. We found that staff were happy to attend topic- or skill-based courses but were not enthused by the prospect of spending a day attending a foundation course on Health Promotion Principles and Practice.

In the course of discussions with nursing staff in the context of other work, it seemed that there was scope for increasing interest in our foundation courses. There was a sense that there were inconsistencies in the extent to which health promotion work being carried out by nurses employed theories such as Social Learning Theory (Bandura, 1977) and Prochaska and DiClemente's Model of Behaviour Change (Prochaska & DiClemente, 1984), in which health promoters could look for indicators other than behaviour change as measures of success.

It became clear to us that if we were to overcome the barriers to training we should apply both health promotion and organisational development theory to this problem and adopt a client-centred approach to finding out nurses' views of health promotion. It is important to identify the need for and benefits of change and to share joint goals. It was decided to carry out a focus group discussion with a group of nurses and to use the findings to construct a questionnaire to circulate to all nursing staff in primary care.

It was important at this stage to get the support of senior management to ensure continuing commitment to health promotion training for nursing staff. It was also important to clarify that we did not wish to interfere with the clinical expertise of staff, but were concerned with appropriate and effective educational methods. We met with the Director of Nursing and Quality in the Trust, gained his support for the project and were able to move on to the research itself.

METHODS USED

Focus Group Discussion

As health visitors see health promotion as a key area of their work it was decided to approach a small group in Hawick, a town in the Scottish Borders with a population of nearly 16 000. Some parts of this town suffer many of the problems associated with low income and deprivation. Two health promotion specialists carrying out the research met with five health visitors, one of whom was also the local line manager. The session aimed to find out the group's views on promoting the health of their clients, what they felt was successful, what was challenging and what they felt their training needs were in order to enhance their health promoting skills. The format used was a semi-structured interview developed from a previous needs assessment questionnaire (carried out with community nurses two years earlier) and drawing on the principles of health promotion, particularly focusing on a client-centred approach. The group did not want the session recorded on tape so the researchers made manual notes of the session. These were subsequently analysed to draw out the main themes. Much of the work at this stage involved finding phrases and concepts which clearly resonated with the health visitors which could be translated into useful statements for the questionnaire.

The Questionnaire

The questionnaire was aimed at all nursing staff working in primary health care teams in the community. It was decided to use the first few questions to gauge the level and type of health promotion activity being undertaken by nurses in the Borders. The next section was designed to establish nurses' perspectives on priorities in promoting health and to identify their own health promotion training needs. It was here that the discussion with the health visitors was most useful in encapsulating the health promotion principles in phrases which derived from their own perceptions as relayed to the researchers. Also included in this section was a question which broke down the elements of a training course in health promotion and asked respondents to prioritise their needs. Other areas included in the questionnaire related to interest in accredited training and training which was linked to topics such as diet or stress.

Refining the Questionnaire

Once the final text had been agreed with colleagues, a pilot questionnaire was sent to the health visitors who had taken part in the focus group for completion and comment. It was then revised and after a final check with the director of nursing was distributed through line managers to all community trust nursing staff working in primary care.

RESULTS

One-hundred-and-eighty-nine questionnaires were distributed. Forty-eight (25%) were returned; a disappointingly low level of response. Of these, health visitors were the largest group responding, with others ranging from nurse co-ordinators, district nurses, school nurses, midwives and treatment room nurses. The results gave a helpful picture of the range of client groups worked with, methods used and the types of health promotion activity staff were involved in.

In response to the question on priorities in health promotion, 78% of respondents selected 'Identifying health promotion needs in your client group and applying an appropriate strategy' as a high priority and it was encouraging that developing a dialogue with patients and understanding the influences on their health were a considerably higher priority for nurses than giving patients leaflets. However, only 55% rated 'working with other agencies to promote health' and 39% felt 'Evaluation' as high priorities, which suggested the need for training to explore the benefits of collaborative working and evaluating health promotion activities.

Having a dialogue with patients and making them partners in promoting their own health is fundamental to health promotion for staff working on a one-to-one basis with clients. In response to the question: 'To what extent do you base your work on issues raised by your clients?', Figures 5.2.1 and 5.2.2 below showed that there was a bias towards a client-centred approach but that the nurses themselves saw a need for further training in this area.

The key question in the survey related to health promotion training needs and there was a surprisingly good response to the listed elements of a training programme. This suggests that the focus group discussion had been successful in breaking through the previously held barriers in nurses' perceptions about their need for training in health promotion (Table 5.2.1 below).

Although the response rate was poor, it was encouraging that the questionnaire did achieve a clearer indication of these community nurse practitioners' real as opposed to perceived training needs. It was later possible to build a foundation course in health promotion based on the findings.

One-day courses were subsequently offered using a programme which was more 'user-friendly' and there was an increasing interest in these. Since then, discussions have been held with Napier University to accredit a course developed by HEBS called 'Promoting Health: a short course in developing effective practice'. There has been enthusiasm for this course stimulated we believe by the fact that it is to be accredited, a factor which got a high rate of approval in the responses to the questionnaire.

REFLECTIONS ON THE PROCESS AND OUTCOME OF THE RESEARCH

As a marketing exercise this project proved invaluable not only in gathering information about our clients, but also in clarifying our relationship with other health promoters, specifically nurses in the Trust. Although the low response rate meant we could not claim we had an exact picture of training needs, we believe we gained a strong flavour of current practice and that this was a reasonable basis for creating a coherent structure for a health promotion training programme.

Informal feedback from the project has reported that our meeting with the focus group showed a 'sense of commitment' on our part to listen to the views, feelings and frustrations of the group. It gave us more of an insight into the day-to-day problems of community nurses. Since the needs assessment, we have shadowed community nurses to keep abreast of the context in which health promotion takes place.

This was the first major exercise of its kind carried out in the Borders and we have gained valuable lessons from both the qualitative and quantitative elements of the research. As well as the benefits outlined previously, the focus groups gave us a

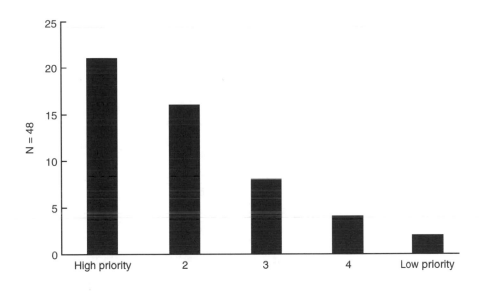

Figure 5.2.1 How much of your health promotion work is based on your clients' issues?

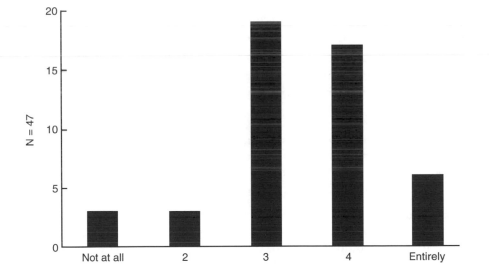

Figure 5.2.2 How important is your need for training in a client-centred approach?

Table 5.2.1   The ranking of training needs in eight selected areas

Training needs	Staff stating 'High priority' (%)
1. Helping a patient who has multiple needs in terms of lifestyle change (knowing where to start)	79
2. Health promotion. What can be achieved	78
3. Valuing your own work – recognising success	76
4. Understanding how people learn and change behaviour	75
5. A client-centred approach (promoting health by starting with the patient's agenda)	75
6. Encouraging a reluctant patient towards a change to a healthier behaviour	72
7. New ideas for getting a group talking and working	60
8. Working with other agencies to promote health	58

sound basis on which to develop our questionnaire helping us to hone in on areas we needed to explore further. For example, there was a sense from those interviewed that they were doing health promotion well. This was borne out by the questionnaire. We know we now need to explore with health promoters if 'well' means effectively and efficiently in relation to agreed criteria.

There was a general consensus that health promotion was a major part of the health visitors' role. It was highly rated as a training need, though not necessarily in the areas of methodology, theory and skills. We aim to address this with senior management and through a 'Developing Effective Practice in Health Promotion' course which we believe will meet the needs of health promotion specialists and health promoters.

There are many aspects which we would change in the questionnaire design and delivery. A major source of disappointment was the low response rate of around 25%. This made the drawing of precise conclusions difficult. While there are inevitably some communication problems within a large organisation, we should have followed-up non-respondents to find out specific reasons for the failure to return their questionnaires. We also speculated that by using examples of health promotion in the letter accompanying the questionnaire we were viewed as patronising. This was reinforced by verbal feedback.

Designing a questionnaire by committee was problematic. Unlike larger health board areas, we do not have access to a research specialist. This exercise has shown the need for collaboration between practitioner and researcher in the design process. We feel investment at this stage would have been more cost-effective. The exercise would have benefited if focus groups had been held in different localities throughout the Borders; this may have raised more awareness and created a sense of ownership. Had this taken place we would have piloted the questionnaire with people who had not been in the focus groups. Focus group participants had experienced the discussion and the process had clarified differences in terminology.

Certain answers highlighted ambiguities in questions which we could have identified earlier.

While there was some retrospective disappointment, we feel we have gained greatly from this project and view it as an important learning experience. The discussions held with senior management certainly brought us closer to a common agenda, clarified our role and increased our credibility in the Trust. We are now contributing a health promotion perspective to an ever increasing range of organisational development projects. Looming before us however are further questions concerning the impact of our project; a measure of our success will be attendance at future training events and their evaluation, changes in health promotion practice in our target group and whether this impacts ultimately on the lives of their clients. We know we need to design appropriate and meaningful research to demonstrate this.

REFERENCES

Atkins K, Hirst N, Lunt N & Parker G (1994) The role and self-perceived training needs of nurses employed in general practice: observation from a national census of practice nurses in England and Wales. *Journal of Advanced Nursing*, 20(1), 46–52.

Bandura A (1977) Social learning theory. Englewood Cliffs, NJ: Prentice Hall.

Galli N (1978) Foundations and principles of health promotion. Chichester: John Wiley.

Gott M & O'Brien M (1990) The role of the nurse in health promotion. *Health Promotion International*, 5, 2.

Inglis B, Duffield J, Low L & Morris B (1996) Devising methods to assess training needs of health promoters in Scottish Area Health Boards. University of Stirling.

Prochaska J O & DiClemente C C (1984) The transtheoretical approach: crossing traditional boundaries of change. Homewood, IL: Dorsey Press.

National Occupational Standards for Health Promotion and Care

Liz Rolls

In Section 3.2 we looked at the challenge of evidence-based practice for health promotion and identified the need to derive *appropriate* evidence on which to base health promotion activities and practice and on which to determine the effectiveness of health promotion activities, practices and services. One way of meeting this challenge is to provide *evidence of the quality of the human resources* assessed against a set of agreed criteria for the best practice of health promotion; that is, evidence of the competence of the practitioners engaged in promoting health.

National Occupational Standards for Professional Activity in Health Promotion and Care provide, for the first time, criteria of what constitutes good health promotion practice. What the standards represent is a set of nationally agreed, publicly available, consistent descriptions of expected performance for health promotion practice based on:

- what is happening now
- what is considered good practice
- what is not happening now – but should be happening
- what can be anticipated about the future and so what might need to happen (Care Sector Consortium, 1997, p 10).

They provide a way of determining competent performance for all health promotion roles and functions and make explicit the knowledge and understanding required to undertake health promotion competently.

In this way, national occupational standards for health promotion and care contribute to evidence-based practice by providing a framework against which to:

- assess evidence of competence
- determine the need for education and training of health promoters
- plan professional development and training activities for health promoters
- provide evidence of the relevance and quality of these activities.

Evidence-based Health Promotion. Edited by Elizabeth R. Perkins, Ina Simnett and Linda Wright.
© 1999 John Wiley & Sons Ltd.

This chapter will outline national occupational standards for health promotion and care and describe:

- how they can make this contribution to evidence-based health promotion professional practice
- the implications for professional development and training activities to support that practice.

WHAT ARE NATIONAL OCCUPATIONAL STANDARDS AND HOW CAN THEY BE USED?

What are National Occupational Standards?

A national occupational standard is a specification 'from the perspective of service users [of] what needs to be achieved in the delivery of high quality services no matter who is involved in whatever employment setting' (Care Sector Consortium, 1997, p 7). They describe the key roles and functions undertaken by any particular sector and indicate the performance outcomes needed to achieve them. Nationally agreed standards of good practice provide both a benchmark for quality activity and a set of criteria against which evidence of competent practice can be assessed.

National occupational standards consist of a number of features:

- the outcome (or title of the standard)
- performance criteria against which quality can be judged
- range statements, which outline the contexts and situations in which the standards apply
- knowledge, understanding and skills which the individual needs to have acquired

The component parts of national occupational standards are shown in Figure 5.3.1.

What are the Uses of National Occupational Standards?

Broadly speaking, national occupational standards provide protection for service users and assure quality within an organisation. Specific uses for national occupational standards can be grouped under one of three headings:

- *The organisational focus* – for high quality service delivery
- *The common focus* – for the development of individual competence to deliver high quality services
- *The individual focus* – for the development of individual competence.

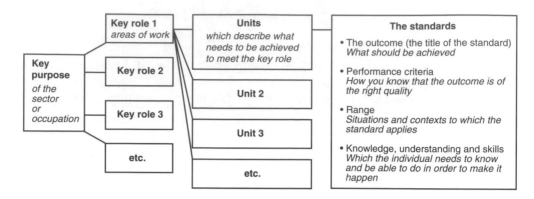

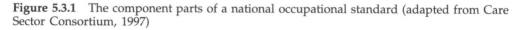

Figure 5.3.1 The component parts of a national occupational standard (adapted from Care Sector Consortium, 1997)

These include:

- linking individual and organisational development and the management of performance in the workplace
- assisting the development of work roles to meet the needs of user-centred services
- providing a common language about professional activity in health promotion and care to support more effective dialogue between commissioners, providers of services, providers of education and training, and users of services
- establishing quality standards
- facilitating the development of clearer links and relationships between academic, professional and vocational qualifications (Care Sector Consortium, 1997, p 8).

Figure 5.3.2 links these together diagrammatically.

How were National Occupational Standards for Health Promotion and Care Generated?

National occupational standards are derived through an 'interactive and iterative process of analysis based on consensus forming with practitioners' (Care Sector Consortium, 1997, p 14). An iterative research process is one in which people are seen as partners in the research process rather than the objects of it and as such are actively involved in the formation of the data (Mikkelsen, 1995).

Three major groups of practitioners were involved in the generation of national occupational standards for health promotion and care:

ORGANISATIONAL FOCUS	COMMON FOCUS	INDIVIDUAL FOCUS
STRATEGIC: • Organisational mapping • Decision making • Defining education and training needs	←——————→	• Identifying initial and continuing learning needs
OPERATIONAL: • Job descriptions • Recruitment specification • Appraisal and performance review	←——————→	• Define the learning outcomes • Plan education and training

Figure 5.3.2 Broad uses of national occupational standards (adapted from Care Sector Consortium, 1997)

- *Health promotion practitioners* (those for whom it is their whole role as well as for those for whom health promotion is part of their role).
- Six *professions allied to medicine* focusing on the 'standards in common' in post-qualifying practice. The practitioner groups included dietitians, occupational therapists, physiotherapists, podiatrists, radiographers and speech and language therapists.
- *Complementary medicine* particularly aromatherapy, homeopathy, hypnotherapy and reflexology.

Participants in the development project were actively engaged in informing the ideas and articulating the concepts which formed the basis of the standards in three ways. Firstly, a series of 35 workshops were held across the UK to provide the primary data on which to frame the draft standards. These workshops involved over 160 practitioners drawn from the statutory and voluntary sectors, from across the breadth of practitioners within the health and social care sector and from the different levels of service (for example from professional bodies and from those working at national, regional and local levels). Secondly, a wider consultation process across the UK resulted in amendments to the draft standards. Thirdly, the original workshop practitioners were invited to comment on and further contribute to the analysis of the data as well as support further conceptualisation of the standards framework.

This iterative analysis included the following stages:

- the development of a broad statement to describe the overall purpose of the area or sector of work – *the key purpose*

- the key purpose is broken down into a number of areas of work – *key roles*
- the key roles are explored to determine the range of different things which have to be achieved to meet each of the key roles – *units*
- from the units, the national occupational *standards* related to each are developed (Care Sector Consortium, 1997, p 15, my emphasis).

What are the National Occupational Standards for Health Promotion and Care?

National occupational standards for health promotion and care cover 12 key roles grouped into three broad areas:

- *Foundations for professional activity.* These key roles describe the activities with which *all* practitioner groups, to a greater or lesser degree depending on their specific role and function, need to engage.
- *Context of professional activity.* These key roles describe the areas of context in which practitioner activity takes place.
- *Range of professional activity.* These key roles describe a range of strategies which may be undertaken by practitioners to optimise health and social well-being.

These broad headings and the key roles are outlined in Figure 5.3.3.

The Informing Principles

As with all standards, national occupational standards for health promotion and care are built on a number of principles. In this instance, the principles include:

- Balancing people's rights with their responsibilities to others and wider society and challenging those who affect the rights of others.
- Promoting the values of equality and diversity, acknowledging the personal beliefs and preferences of others and promoting anti-discriminatory practice.
- Recognising and promoting health and social well-being as a positive concept.
- Enabling people to develop to their full potential, to be as autonomous and self-managing as possible and to have a voice and be heard.

NATIONAL OCCUPATIONAL STANDARDS AND EVIDENCE-BASED PRACTICE

National occupational standards for health promotion and care make a significant contribution to evidence-based practice in two ways; firstly, by providing evidence of best practice against an agreed framework and secondly, by indicating areas for professional development.

A. FOUNDATIONS OF PROFESSIONAL ACTIVITY			
BROAD AREA	*0* *(First principles/ values)* *(3 units)*	*1* *Developing own knowledge and others' practice* *(2 units)*	*2* *Promoting effective communication* *(8 units)*	*3* *Building and sustaining relationships* *(2 units)*
KEY ROLE	0 Promote and value the rights, responsibilities and diversity of people	1 Develop own and others' knowledge and practice to optimise the health and social well-being of people	2 Promote effective communication with people	3 Build and sustain relationships with and between practitioners and agencies
B. CONTEXT OF PROFESSIONAL ACTIVITY			
BROAD AREA	*4* *Influencing and developing policies* *(3 units)*	*5* *Commissioning research* *(5 units)*	*6* *Commissioning different means for optimising health* *(4 units)*	*7* *Manage processes* *(11 units)*
KEY ROLE	4 Influence and develop policies to promote health and social well-being	5 Commission research to develop knowledge and practice about health and social well-being	6 Commission a range of different means to optimise health and social well-being	7 Manage processes to optimise health and social well-being
C. RANGE OF PROFESSIONAL ACTIVITIES			
BROAD AREA	*8* *Create and maintain environments and practices* *(6 units)*	*9* *Enable people to address issues which affect health and social well-being* *(9 units)*	*10* *Enable people to manage disability and change* *(10 units)*	*11* *Assess individuals' needs and develop, implement, monitor and review programmes of care* *(7 units)*
KEY ROLE	8 Create and maintain environments and practices in which to promote people's health and social well-being	9 Work in partnership with individuals, families, groups, communities and organisations to enable them to address issues which affect health and social well-being	10 Enable people to manage disability and change	11 Assess individuals' needs and develop, implement, monitor and review programmes of care to meet them

Figure 5.3.3 Broad areas and key roles of health promotion and care (adapted from Care Sector Consortium, 1997)

Providing Evidence

National occupational standards provide an agreed and visible best practice framework against which to assess evidence of:

- *Practitioners' competence.* As a result of this nationally agreed framework, national occupational standards for health promotion and care provide a set of performance criteria against which individuals can generate evidence of their competence as health promotion practitioners.
- *The relevance and quality of professional development activities.* Because of their visibility (including the criteria for performance and underpinning knowledge and skills), national occupational standards for health promotion and care provide evidence for assessing and reviewing the quality and relevance of professional development activities and their effectiveness in contributing to the development of the competence of the practitioner.

Particular Ways this Evidence Contributes to Professional Development and Training

This evidence contributes to professional development and training in two ways. Firstly, whilst practitioners and their managers are assessing competence against the criteria for performance, they can use the national occupational standards as an invaluable tool for determining and reviewing individual and organisational professional development needs. Secondly, because national occupational standards describe the required performance criteria and underpinning knowledge and skills, they provide a framework for determining the content and desired outcomes of professional development activities, whether it is through a formal curriculum or more informal 'on the job' learning activities.

The particular benefits for professional development and training, therefore, include:

- Raising the 'quality' of occupational training
- Fitting occupational training to operational requirements
- Providing goals for learners
- Evaluating learning programmes
- Planning careers
- Giving credibility to learning programmes/training schemes
- Enabling progression for individuals.

Using Standards in Practice

National occupational standards can be used for professional development and training activities in four ways:

Using Standards to Assess Evidence of Practitioners' Competence

Using standards to assess evidence of practitioners' competence is a two-stage process.

Being Clear about the Practitioner's Role Description

It is important to be clear about the roles and functions which the particular post demands. By using, in turn, the headings of the broad areas, the key roles and unit headings, a practitioner or their manager can outline a particular role description.

Unit summaries provide information about the elements contained within the unit and describe for whom the unit is aimed, the principles of good practice which underpin the unit and its relationship to other units. Working with each of the key roles and units in this way, a full role description can be mapped.

Assessing Competence Against the Relevant Standards

Having determined which of the units within each of the key roles are relevant to the particular circumstances of the practitioner's post, the standards can be used to assess current levels of performance (competence). This is done by studying each unit in greater depth and assessing competence against the performance criteria and range and the underpinning knowledge and understanding outlined in the unit and elements which are required to perform competently.

Using Standards to Identify One's Own or Others' Learning Needs

Once a practitioner has mapped their role description and has assessed their competence against the relevant standards, they can then identify their learning needs, related to deficits in performance, range and/or underpinning knowledge. How these needs are met will depend on whether it is the need for practical or theoretical development. In either case, a plan of action to meet these needs can be devised.

Using Standards to Plan Professional Development and Training Activities

National occupational standards can be used to plan professional development and training activities in four ways.

To Identify Learning Outcomes

Providers of professional development and training activities can use the standards to identify the learning outcomes of their programmes by using the performance criteria and broad range indicators associated with the unit and element which they are trying to develop. As these define what is required in practice they indicate the necessary learning outcomes.

As a Basis for the Design of Programmes/Curriculum

National occupational standards provide the template for curriculum/programme design. For the provider of professional development and training activities, a process of checking and matching the performance criteria and underpinning knowledge requirements and a full consideration of what evidence of performance can be generated within the course work of the learning programme will provide both a starting point and parameters for the design of the learning experience.

To Identify Underpinning Knowledge and Understanding

Underpinning knowledge and understanding is particularly important in the higher level occupations, including health promotion. Academic programmes of study can offer the opportunity for both learning and for generating evidence of knowledge and understanding.

To Assess Learning and Generate Evidence

The performance criteria, range statements and underpinning knowledge and skills can be used to assess learning. Equally, professional development and training activities provide ideal opportunities for participants *to generate and collect evidence* of performance matched against the specific standards. These can take the form of products such as video and audio taped activities and completed paper exercises such as essays and other course work. Peer assessment is another welcomed source of evidence of competence.

Using Standards to Provide Evidence of the Relevance and Quality of these Professional Development Activities

For professional development and training programmes based on national occupational standards, providers will be able to make visible the intended learning outcomes, the performance evidence which will be generated and the relationship of these to the relevant standards. In this way, individuals, managers and commissioners can assess the appropriateness and the quality of particular learning programmes.

The inter-relationship, outlined above, between assessing competence, identifying learning needs and assessing the quality of provision is demonstrated in Figure 5.3.4.

THE IMPLICATIONS FOR COMPETENCE-BASED PROFESSIONAL DEVELOPMENT AND TRAINING

Competence-based professional development and training differs from other activities in three ways.

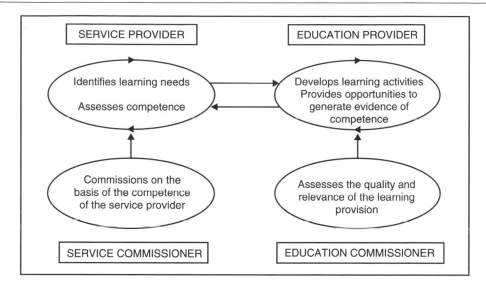

Figure 5.3.4 The relationship between assessing competence, identifying learning needs and assessing the quality of provision

Change in Emphasis

Because a key feature of the standards is the emphasis on the ability of a practitioner to perform competently, this shifts the emphasis in any learning programme from content and syllabus (input) to the assessment of a practitioner's competence (output). Thus, in designing education and training programmes, as well as being concerned with developing underpinning knowledge and understanding, emphasis needs to be on the design of activities which will create opportunities to generate performance evidence for assessment. As a result, the facilitative rather than teaching role of the educator and trainer is emphasised and the development of a portfolio is encouraged. However, this does not mean that the training method or the process of learning is not important; some of the standards are best learnt and understood through experiential learning.

The Programme Design

As well as the usual steps in programme design, Fletcher (1991) sets out a series of questions which designers of competence-based professional development and training activities need to take into account. These are outlined in Figure 5.3.5.

Issues for Assessment and Evaluation

Performance criteria provide clear indications of the evidence required to demonstrate that a standard is met. Assessment methods must, therefore, relate

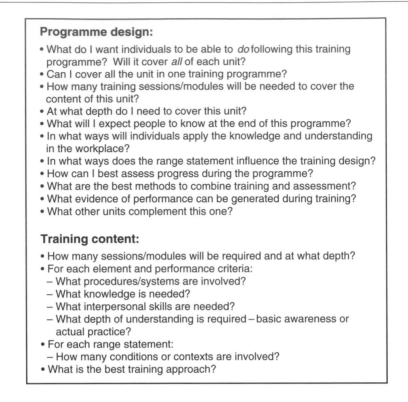

Programme design:

- What do I want individuals to be able to *do* following this training programme? Will it cover *all* of each unit?
- Can I cover all the unit in one training programme?
- How many training sessions/modules will be needed to cover the content of this unit?
- At what depth do I need to cover this unit?
- What will I expect people to know at the end of this programme?
- In what ways will individuals apply the knowledge and understanding in the workplace?
- In what ways does the range statement influence the training design?
- How can I best assess progress during the programme?
- What are the best methods to combine training and assessment?
- What evidence of performance can be generated during training?
- What other units complement this one?

Training content:

- How many sessions/modules will be required and at what depth?
- For each element and performance criteria:
  - What procedures/systems are involved?
  - What knowledge is needed?
  - What interpersonal skills are needed?
  - What depth of understanding is required – basic awareness or actual practice?
- For each range statement:
  - How many conditions or contexts are involved?
- What is the best training approach?

Figure 5.3.5   Programme and training design checklist (adapted from Fletcher, 1991)

directly to the standard and be based on the performance criteria. Evidence should be current, up-to-date and authentic, but it is worth remembering that not all evidence for a unit will necessarily come from one training programme.

When designing teaching and learning activities it is worth considering how best to assist the generation of high-quality evidence of performance or underpinning knowledge and understanding. There is also a need in planning activities to include practical and applied work as well as assessment of progress and to consider what forms of evidence these activities will generate.

THE WAY FORWARD: USING NATIONAL OCCUPATIONAL STANDARDS IN PRACTICE

This chapter has looked at the contribution that national occupational standards for health promotion and care can make to evidence-based health promotion. The standards, which are available from the Local Government Management Board (see Useful Addresses at the end of this section), provide a unique opportunity for collaboration and partnership between practitioners, their managers, educators and commissioners by providing a common language with which to 'unpack' and discuss the role and performance requirements of health promoters. The particular value of the standards is that they were generated by this constituency through a consensus process which accommodated the variety of roles and functions of the diverse range of practitioners within health promotion. The impact on professional development and training activities will be as great as the imaginations of all those involved.

Since they were developed the standards have been subjected to further scrutiny. During the period of November 1997 to March 1998, the Health Education Authority supported a project to pilot the standards in a number of sites for two different uses: curriculum mapping and health promotion role mapping. The project was designed to determine the quality and coverage of the standards in practice, with particular reference to the content, accessibility of the language of the standards and the ease of use. It specifically asked pilot sites to identify areas of practice which the standards did not address. The project produced a 'User's Guide' and a set of 'Case Studies'. These are available from the Professional Development Account at the Health Education Authority.

In addition, the National Health Service Executive set up a pilot project drawing on the experiences of a number of sites with the NHS. This project, which began in January 1998, was due for completion in March 1999. Further details are available through the NHSE.

REFERENCES

Care Sector Consortium (1997) National occupational standards for professional activity in health promotion and care: introductory guide. London: HMSO.
Fletcher S (1991) Designing competence-based training. London: Kogan Page.
Mikkelsen B (1995) Methods for development work and research. London: Sage.

USEFUL ADDRESSES

National occupational standards for health promotion and care can be obtained from:

The Publications Department
The Local Government Management Board
Layden House
76–86 Turnmill Street
London EC1M 5QU
Tel: 0171 296 6600
Fax: 0171 296 6523

The address for details of the Health Education Authority pilot project is as follows:

Professional Development Account
Health Education Authority
Trevelyan House
30 Great Peter Street
London SW1P 2HW
Tel: 0171 413 1945

The address for details of the NHSE pilot project is:

NHS Executive
Quarry House
Leeds LS2 7UE

Section 5.4

Making Use of Competencies

Lesley Jones

Back in the early 1980s I was asked by the then Health Education Council to design and run a workshop on management for Health Education Unit managers. Looking back, although it was well attended and repeated, I cringe at the way we decided what material, information and exercises should go in the workshop. It was a mixture of the pragmatic, 'What works for me in my own District with my own staff', and ideas and exercises I had found useful on workshops I had attended.

The pity of it is that some short courses and workshops are still being designed in this fashion. True, the facilitators might also read up on it in the journals or chosen books, but where is the proof that they cover all that the learner needs? What is the material based on, is it transferable to other Districts, how do I know what a person has learnt on such a course if they apply to me for a job? The facilitator who runs the course will have a level of competency which is difficult to find out about without reviewing their CV and getting independent references. This is a lot of work when you are trying to assess whether this is the course for you.

These days I would turn to the National Management Standards (MCI, 1997). There is evidence that about one in ten UK businesses use these standards in some way. They cover the four key roles of managers: to manage activities, to manage resources, to manage people and to manage information. There are also three additional units which cover: to manage energy, to manage quality and to manage projects. They are well laid out, with information on what is involved in these roles, what performance standards are required, what range of circumstances they apply to and what background knowledge is required to carry out these roles. These are available at three levels corresponding to supervisor, middle manager and senior manager.

The key roles listed above are comprehensive in what they cover. For example, the key role 'Manage People' includes units on:

Evidence-based Health Promotion. Edited by Elizabeth R. Perkins, Ina Simnett and Linda Wright.
© 1999 John Wiley & Sons Ltd.

- develop your own resources
- develop productive working relationships
- select personnel for activities
- develop teams and motivate to enhance performance
- manage the performance of teams and individuals
- respond to poor performance in teams.

The following is an example to give an idea of what one of these units would contain. The unit 'Develop Productive Working Relationships' includes performance indicators on:

- develop the trust and support of colleagues and team members
- develop the trust and support of your own manager
- minimise interpersonal conflict.

These management standards and their competence base are particularly relevant to health educators, since a large part of what they are attempting to achieve involves managing people. They may not be directly accountable for these people but nonetheless must influence them.

Courses on how to train and develop in adult education can also benefit from a competence-based approach. The practical nature of the planning and execution of training means that it cannot all be taught in the classroom. The National Standards for Training and Development (TDLB, 1995) are helpful with the following functional breakdown of the training role. To develop human potential to assist organisations and individuals to achieve their objectives:

- identify training and development needs
- plan and design training and development
- deliver training and development
- review progress and assess achievement
- continuously improve the effectiveness of training and development.

The TDLB competencies can be used as a checklist for anyone looking for an effective course on training and adult education.

The process of creating a national standard set of competencies for a job or role is carefully and painstakingly worked through with representatives of that profession or occupation and other stakeholders. It requires consultation and testing and is overseen by a lead body made up of representatives of the profession involved. Once written, the competencies can then be best tested by being used in a variety of ways, including using them as a basis for those wishing to obtain a qualification by proving current competence. Inevitably refinements will be needed and the two I mention, 'Training and Development' and 'Management Standards' have been altered quite considerably over the last two years, as those using them found their weaknesses and hit problems. The strength of what we now have is national agreement on what it is to carry out the training and development function and what a manager actually does. There is no excuse for anyone reinventing the wheel on either of these.

However, people will try! A colleague attended a recent meeting of senior college staff and sat through an interminable discussion on what skills they needed for managers in colleges of higher education. When she pointed out that management standards already exist and what about starting from them, some of those present opined the view that their situation was 'different'. Her response was to ask how it was different, which they could not respond to since they were not familiar with these standards. Many work groups feel their situation is special in some way. Using standards as a starting point can identify both common features with other groups and those areas where they genuinely are different.

The problem with competencies as a description of what skills, knowledge and abilities are needed to do a particular job is the very way they are written. They are precise, pedantic and repetitive and often use jargon unfamiliar to the reader. This is a turn off, but once you get used to it this very pithy precise competence style is useful because it keeps you on track and will not allow you to miss bits out. However those who prefer to gain their knowledge from books with interesting illustrative case studies will find this dry stuff. They are not meant to be used as resources from which to learn directly. Materials should be based on them using the competencies as a framework and so designed as to bring them alive and respond to the range of ways people like to learn.

The training and development and management standards are just two which are relevant to health promotion. Others include Advice, Guidance and Counselling, Project Management, and Customer Care. It should be stressed that these competencies are to be used as a framework for a number of activities including:

- training needs analysis
- writing and updating job descriptions
- criteria for performance
- understanding of organisational objectives and individual responsibilities
- a methodical approach to developing others
- benchmarking best practice
- new ways of conceptualising work tasks
- looking at quality of service
- better procedures and monitoring of actions
- more strategic behaviour
- curriculum development
- appraisal.

Competencies are the beginning, to be used in many different ways, not the end result.

When the health promotion competencies have 'come of age' and been tested to iron out some of the problems which you only find when you try to use them, they will be ideal to use as a basis of identifying training needs. Training needs analysis

(TNA) is always related to role and expectations within this role. Using these competencies in conjunction with an up-to-date job description will shortcut the need for an in-depth analysis before the TNA can be carried out. They will also be useful for those who wish to gain a qualification by proving current competence rather than following a course of academic study away from the workplace. Taking time out is not always an option and can also be frustrating when you feel that you have the knowledge and skills anyway and just require the proof of this knowledge in the form of a qualification. Evidence of such competence can be proven by collecting a portfolio of information, being assessed in the workplace, or by guided discussion with an assessor. The existence of nationally agreed competencies means that you no longer have to re-invent the wheel – you can gild it instead.

REFERENCES

Management Charter Initiative (1997) Management standards. London: Management Charter Initiative.
Training and Development Lead Body (1995) N/SVQ Level 4: Learning development. Rotherham: Cambertown Ltd.

Chapter 6

Organisations and Social Systems

Elizabeth R. Perkins

INTRODUCTION

Most people involved in health promotion work in organisations. Even those who occupy a more detached position have to relate to them at some point. In addition, many of the people whom health promoters wish to influence are involved with organisations, for example as school children or patients, and this provides a point of contact where health promotion can take effect. Organisations are therefore very important to health promoters. Health promotion has also been concerned with communities, as an alternative contact point for clients and an alternative social setting with which people are likely to identify more fully than the organisation where it may be convenient for professionals to contact them.

Social systems, whether they are institutions or communities, can deliver messages to individuals which can reinforce or oppose explicit health promotion messages. They can also, in their effects on staff, make those messages easier or more difficult to deliver. Staff who find their own individual concerns are not respected may find it difficult to give individual attention to the needs of those they serve.

On a larger scale, organisations and communities can become the focus for health promotion planning, as in the encouragement of Health Promoting Schools and Health Promoting Hospitals, and in work with communities to determine their own health needs and their preferred methods of meeting them. Social systems, whether they are institutions or communities, can be treated as potential health promotion interventions in their own right. This chapter considers the broader theory and provides two more detailed case studies of work within workplaces. Other types of organisations are discussed in Part II; see Chapter 8 for schools, Chapter 10 for prisons and Chapter 11 for hospitals. Sections in other parts of this book are concerned with small-scale studies in a community (for example, Beth Lindley in Chapter 9 (Section 9.2), Kathy Brummell and Alison

Evidence-based Health Promotion. Edited by Elizabeth R. Perkins, Ina Simnett and Linda Wright.
© 1999 John Wiley & Sons Ltd.

Mitchell's sections (11.2 and 11.3, respectively) in Chapter 11, and the whole of Chapter 14 on needs assessment). These can be read as complementary to the organisational studies here.

The first section, *Social system intervention*, takes the most wide-ranging view of the possible relationships between health promotion and social structures, and considers the kind of evidence which is relevant to this approach to health promotion.

The second section, *Applying the evidence to workplace catering*, narrows the focus to a particular health issue and a particular field of practice and discusses research evidence on the scope for intervention within organisations to encourage healthy eating.

The third section, *A workplace stress survey*, is an example of an initiative taken in one organisation in response to concerns about stress at work. It provides a practical example of the problems inherent in this kind of work and the strengths and limitations of evidence collected in this way.

Section 6.1

Social System Intervention

Dominic Harrison

THE DETERMINANTS OF POPULATION HEALTH

It is not possible to consider what evidence-based health promotion might be without reviewing contemporary evidence on the determinants of population health. As Blane et al. (1996) argue, 'There is a growing recognition that the most powerful determinants of health in contemporary populations are to be found in social, economic and cultural circumstances.'

For many years traditional public health approaches have focused on analysis and prescription for effective action to improve health on disease-orientated risk-factor epidemiology. This sought to know about the social, behavioural and bio-medical causes of disease. Recent work over the past ten years (Brunner, 1993; 1996; Evans, 1994; Hertzman, 1996; Marmot, 1996; Syme, 1996; Wilkinson, 1996) has been highlighting the inadequacy of this foundation for policy and action in the promotion of health. Syme (1996) asks, 'How is it possible that after 50 years of massive effort, all of the risk factors we know about, combined, account for less than half of the disease that occurs? Is it possible that we have somehow missed one or two crucial risk factors?' (p 21). He suggests that about 60% of preventable morbidity and mortality are located neither within individual sovereignty nor the domains of individual behaviour, lifestyle or 'risk' but within social organisation. Marmot (1996) has shown how control and autonomy are crucial determinants of health often more powerful in explanatory value than smoking and Wilkinson (1996) has shown how inequality itself rather than poverty *per se* may be a major cause of preventable morbidity and mortality in most industrialised societies. Antonovsky (1996) has reminded us that disease-oriented risk-factor epidemiology is only half the story. We know the bio-medical causes of why 40% of people smoking 20 cigarettes a day may die early. We do not know the bio/psycho/social reasons why 60% do not. We have no real epidemiology of health (salutogenesis).

Even within a narrow bio-medical model we now have evidence to discredit the received wisdom on which most individual, behaviour change focused, health promotion/education has been undertaken. This is not to say it was not effective, just that it was largely irrelevant and certainly an inefficient use of very scarce specialist resources.

Syme (1996) and others suggest there is an urgent need for a paradigm shift in the conceptual framework and problem-solving strategies for public health. This must recognise that most health risk and most determinants of health are systemic, located within complex, dynamic and interactive social relationships which themselves are determined by social institutions and organisations including families, communities, workplaces – indeed the health care system itself. Such a change of paradigm requires population health to be seen not as the 'additive' outcome of the application of health care resources but as an integrative social product arising from the impact of social systems on individuals, communities and societies. Determinants of population health are mediated *through* social systems but are determined *by* social relationships within those systems. This understanding has enormous implications for the efficacy, effectiveness and efficiency of health investment and the search for an evidence-based health promotion within social systems.

HEALTH INVESTMENT STRATEGIES AND THE PURPOSES OF HEALTH CARE

'Humankind would not die out if formal healthcare systems did not exist – they are not biologically necessary for the survival of the species' (Vang, 1997). In fact the 7% of GDP spent on health care is not the total health care system. One recent analysis of UK health spending, for instance (NHS Executive North West, 1994), suggested that only about half of all UK health care is accounted for through the NHS. Much health care is undertaken in an unplanned and unsupported way outside the statutory health care system. The total cost of NHS spending in 1996 was approximately £42 billion, but the value of informal health care outside the NHS is over £39 billion (1994 prices), with £34 billion of this amount accounted for by carers, the balance being accounted for in large part by self-help, self-medication and alternative therapies.

It is salutary to reflect that in the UK, in the late eighteenth century, lay perspectives on medical care were an integral part of both medicine and hospitals. The clinical organisation of hospitals, including patient admission had, from inception, been dominated by non-qualified persons and it was not until the 1880s that consultants firmly gained control of medical appointments and teaching. A key determinant of this was that, in the domestic world which at that time remained the principal locus for healing, popular remedies and therapeutic systems could easily match the effectiveness of hospital-based clinical medical practice (Toth, 1996). The unifying goal of the NHS is to improve the health for all of the population (NHS Executive, 1996).

But in this task, Smee (1995) and Smith (1996) argue that evidence-based health investment needs to pay particular attention to increasing allocative efficiency in the

NHS. Smee defines technical efficiency as 'doing things right' and allocative efficiency as 'doing the right things'. The suggestion is that even if the NHS is achieving good health outcomes from health care there is still a need to review whether the same investment made elsewhere could bring increased benefit to population health. The World Bank has raised similar concerns at a global level. Reviewing the relationship between national health expenditures and population health outcomes in 1993, it stated: 'At any level of [population] income and education, higher health spending should yield better health, all else being equal, but there is no evidence of such a relation' (World Bank, 1993, p 53).

The fact that international health sector investment is unrelated to population health outcomes is not perhaps surprising. The US Surgeon General (May, 1996), addressing this issue, has listed the general causes of premature death and disability (and thus avoidable health sector cost which could be reinvested in promoting health) as:

- 10% due to inadequate access to medical care.
- 20% genetic.
- 70% due to environmental/behavioral/lifestyle factors.

Despite this and similar evidence on the poor population health outcomes of health sector spending from around the world, NHS activity is overwhelmingly dedicated to the treatment and care of prevalent disease in individuals. Resources are focused only on the small percentage of the population who are ill at any one time, to the exclusion of those who certainly will be ill if preventive action is not taken through the investment of those resources elsewhere. The first purpose of developing a body of knowledge about evidence-based health promotion must therefore be to assist the NHS, at a global whole system level, in 'doing the right things', thus increasing the allocative efficiency of its resource allocation.

IN SEARCH OF RELEVANT EVIDENCE

General practices, health authorities and trusts spend 7% of UK GDP on health, but their annual reports would not look any different were all the patients to have died. It sometimes seems that whilst everyone knows what they are busy *about* in the health care system, what they are busy *for* seems less important.

Ironically, the most frequently asked question of health promotion by all these agencies is – 'Does it improve health?' But planned health promotion interventions enjoy budgets of less than 1% of the UK total spend on health (Limb, 1996). With such levels of investment it is inconceivable that they could be anything other than largely irrelevant to population health, except perhaps on a political and symbolic level. Yet researchers undertaking so called 'effectiveness reviews' employed by the HEA, York University and the International Union of Health Promotion and Education (IUHPE) earnestly search for evidence of effectiveness solely within that 1%, as if it might make a difference whatever the answer was. Furthermore, it has been suggested that only about 1% of the evidence already available on effective health care interventions has ever been used as a basis for routinised health care practice or purchasing (ECHHO, 1997). Indeed Weiss (1991) convincingly demonstrates that there is evidence to show that research has 'very little' impact at all on *any* public policy (Alkin et al., 1979; Bulmer, 1978; Caplan, 1977; Deitchman, 1976; Dockrell, 1982; Knorr, 1977; Leff, 1985; Rich, 1977; Weiss & Bucuvalas, 1980). Weiss argues that research rarely determines policy; rather it tends to be used to illuminate the consequences or support the advocacy of decisions already made on the basis of custom and practice, values or interests.

In searching for an evidence base for the practice of health promotion that is relevant, it may be necessary to problematise some of the questions traditionally asked and to look at the cultural whole system context within which both questions and answers are being framed. Evidence-based health care, medicine and purchasing and evidence-based health promotion might then best be seen as distant subjects in search of separate objects. Evidence-based health care might ask, 'What is the most efficient and effective (least cost greatest outcome) intervention that can be undertaken with this group or to this patient, that will restore or maintain health?' Evidence-based health promotion should be asking, 'What are the determinants of this population's health status and what are the most effective and efficient interventions to protect and improve it?'

Evidence of effective health care is generally narrowly focused within the 7% of GDP spent on health and as Schwartz and Bitzer (1997) warn:

> There is no common understanding about what constitutes 'evaluation in health care'. Beginning with an acknowledgement of the essential judgmental nature of any evaluation activity, health care evaluation is defined in broad terms as a comprehensive scientific assessment of positive and negative effects of products, technologies, projects, models, institutions or programs in health care (p 2).

Evidence-based health promotion must look elsewhere, beyond health care and beyond the bounds of that which recognizes itself as health promotion.

That health promotion is evidence based may logically mean there is:

- *Evidence about*: appropriateness, efficiency (technical, allocative, clinical, social or institutional), efficacy, effectiveness, equity, equality, productivity, sustainability or ethical behaviour found in relation to a specific intervention in a specific context at a specific time.
- *Evidence in relation to*: input, process output, outcome or impact of a specific activity. (It can also mean the opposite of these things, but there are few databases of that sort of evidence even though it is half of the reality that may be found.)
- *Evidence for*: stakeholders with various interests and perspectives. Vang (1997) has characterized these as:
  - The perspective of the patient and their expectations on the outcomes of care

- The perspective of the professional of the quality and process of care
- The perspective of commissioners and managers on the productivity, efficiency and cash-flow of care
- The perspective of politicians about the social institutions of health care and its relationship to broader societal management and objectives
- The perspective of NHS staff and unions in their assessment of health care systems as workplaces.

All of these domains are valid and it should be noted that good practice in health promotion means involving the perspectives of all stakeholders. This is a very difficult process. As Smith and Cantley (1985) observe:

> There may well be disputes about which findings are relevant or significant. Success means different things to different groups of people who each have their own agendas or interests (p 37).

Evidence-based health promotion is of course not a science at all but an *applied* science. This means that it requires judgement in its application. Judgement depends on values and the privileging of one judgement or set of values against another requires power. The meaning and importance of evidence is thus really only amenable to political choice. Which choice is taken depends on whom amongst the stakeholders in a given situation has the greater positional power, which in turn is mediated through the nature of the micro-political system of the health care system itself. Echoing Weiss (1991), we must conclude that application of relevant health promotion knowledge depends on stakeholder democratisation in the social construction of meaning and significance – it is not so much that 'knowledge is power' but that 'power in knowledge' in the health care system.

SOCIAL SYSTEMS INTERVENTION

In a totalitarian state it would be possible to decree that all social systems and organisations would be health promoting. Even if health promoters had the power, the repression necessary to achieve such change would outweigh the benefits of the change itself. Change that is sustainable has to be owned, negotiated, mediated, lobbied and advocated for and consensually agreed.

Evidence in Theory

Durkheim's study of the 'causes' of suicide was perhaps the first seminal work that identified determinants of health-related behaviour as existing systemically at a population level beyond the sovereignty of individual choice alone (Rose, 1993). Medical and social anthropology have traced the social construction of disease and identified ways in which macro settings or 'environments' determine health behaviour and health risk at the macro, meso or micro (individual) level. In the late modern age most life experience and individual behaviour is mediated through social systems (families, religion, communities) or organisational systems (workplaces, schools, health care, etc.) (Grossmann & Scala, 1994).

As long ago as 1984, WHO stated:

> Health Promotion has come to represent a unifying concept for those who recognise the need for change in the ways and conditions of living in order to promote health. Health Promotion represents a mediating strategy between people and their environments, synthesising personal choice and social responsibility in health . . . (p 1).

Evidence-based intervention within social and organisational systems is a shift away from a direct focus on intervention in the ways of personal living to a focus on the *conditions* of that living – conditions that are generally governed by management and organisational dynamics within a whole system.

In their early study of 'Some conditions of obedience and disobedience to authority', Stanley Milgram (1965) and colleagues demonstrated the power of social systems on individual behaviour choosing a discourse of 'obedience to authority' to explain its influence. They concluded:

> . . . are these forces to be conceptualised as individual motives and expressed in the language of personality dynamics or are they to be seen as the effects of social structure and pressures arising from the situational field?

The opening of such perspectives on the determinants of human behaviour found their way into the field of management science in the 1960s and 1970s as the systems approach to organisational change. It applied insights from systems theory to the improvement of organisational effectiveness.

Grossmann and Scala (1994) use systems theory to define the key challenge of contemporary health promotion as intervention in social and organisational systems to develop health. They describe the current health care system as an illness system. Its characteristics are that it has 7% of GDP (in the UK), recognised and regulated professions such as doctors and nurses and social roles such as the sick role (i.e. if you are off work 'sick' it is not socially acceptable to be seen smiling and shopping!). For health there is no such social system as that for managing illness. Health is an unincorporated cloud that hovers amorphously, part of all other social systems – education, agriculture, politics, etc. There is no percentage of GDP to pursue it, and no professional or social roles for its development and integration.

They suggest that if it is everything else other than the health care system that creates population health, then the main function of health promotion is to develop social system interventions that build systems for health (organisational competencies) into other established social structures. Their argument is that this method is sustainable in that it 'builds in the intervention into the permanent context of everyday social systems (workplace, school, etc.)' rather than it being constantly dependent on continued practitioner/specialist intervention. Health becomes an integrative goal of the organisation. They argue that this has specific implications for the skills base for health promotion. Health promotion specialists should be primarily skilled in organisational development and change management. Health is the goal but change management is the process. Knowledge about the aetiology of health and disease are important but their transmission is not the outcome measure of relevance in intervention. What is relevant is whether health investment has been made and whether an infrastructure for health promotion has been constructed within the formal or informal fabric of the organisation or social system. Indicators may include:

- written roles/job descriptions that include health responsibilities (not health care or disease treatment)
- evidence of health related infrastructures such as policy on health or environmental audits that are routinised/integrated into core business
- formal health committees adopted
- changes in values/policies within the organisation such as a shift to equal opportunities, job sharing employment practices or 'mental health days' as a right.

Evidence in Practice

Workplace

Oblique reviews of that which promotes the health of workforces (rather than just individuals at work) seem to demonstrate that managerial and organisational development strategies for health are surprisingly similar to those for increasing organisational efficiency as a whole (see for instance Newall, 1995). The general focus of many management writers unconcerned with health *per se* is now that organisations wishing to increase efficiency need to ensure that staff have their social, emotional, economic and other satisfactional needs met within the workplace if they are to function to their maximum capacity. Also, workplaces now seek to foster decentralisation, non-hierarchical social relationships and autonomy-promoting employment structures and technology use (Cooper & Payne, 1990; Handy, 1995; Kanter, 1993; Newall, 1995; Peters & Waterman, 1982; Ranade, 1995). This agenda overlaps considerably with the structural prerequisites of positive health at work. Much evidence for effectiveness in implementing social systems intervention for workforce health can thus be gleaned from an intertextual analysis of research on the effectiveness of management change. One can conclude that:

1. Initiatives aimed at improving the general health of workforces are inextricable from issues of general and human resource management. This is particularly

true in relation to areas of employment practice and reward strategies. It is also true for recruitment and retention of staff issues, employee motivation and satisfaction, quality development and in relation to the improvement of consumer relations.

2. Investment in improving the general and mental health of workforces, in the sense of constructing a working environment which seeks to meet their psychological, social and other satisfactional needs may well make economic and commercial sense. It is already a key organisational strategy for achieving economic efficiency in the commercial and industrial world.

3. Evidence relating to the nature of effective intervention for improving work-force efficiency suggests that management and organisational development are key tools. Interventions aimed at effecting structural change within working conditions and systems are a key focus of contemporary approaches. Much leverage will be gained by the overwhelming evidence that shows that organ-isations wishing to promote both health *and* efficiency within the workforce/workplace may well gain added value from integrative approaches to work-force health development.

Community

'Social capital' has been formally defined as 'those features of social organisation, such as networks, norms, and trust, that facilitate co-ordination and co-operation for mutual benefit' (Putnam, 1993, p 114). The development of 'social and organ-isational capital for health' is particularly important for the future health and social welfare of the whole population. Here, evidence of effective health promotion is actually evidence of community and institutional development which creates social capital facilitating infrastructures within civic society. As with the health care system, and workplaces, such evidence shows that increasing the accountability and democratisation of institutions is a key prerequisite for population health improvement. Crucially all activity here is also precisely aligned to the deter-minants of population health.

This concept is linked to that of 'civic society'. Civic societies are those 'which value solidarity, civic participation, and integrity; and where social and political networks are organised horizontally, not hierarchically' (Putnam et al., 1993, p 115). Social and organisational capital and the construction of civic society is seen as an area of social development widely neglected by monetarist approaches to economic and social development in the west and by state capitalist systems in the east. The consequence for both has been a rapid reduction in the quality of life, a decimation of the 'co-operative economy' (what we do for each other without the exchange of money such as childrearing, self-help, organising community events, etc.) and these factors in turn are major sources of loss of social cohesion, 'public life in public space'; crime and health status in communities (Real World Coalition, 1996).

Most importantly, Putnam et al. (1993), in a study of the impact of Italian Regional Government (introduced in 1970) has established a number of measurable constructs of civic society which show close correlation between infant and child mortality and social capital – the higher the indicators of social capital the lower the mortality. The relationship is striking but does seem to disappear by mid-life for reasons that are not as yet fully understood.

Evidence of the wealth and health creating power of community is well illustrated in Lima's largest squatter settlement – Villa El Salvador. This demonstrates the links between social, health and environmental action to improve the well-being of the community and underlines the value of integrative approaches. A large area of state-owned desert land has, over a period of 15 years, been transformed into a thriving, self-governing community of 300 000 people. At the heart of the development has been CUAVES (the Self-Management Urban Community of Villa El Salvador), Villa's own community organisation. The organisation's democratic structure gives representation to each block and a vast network of women's groups, through which citizens have planted 500 000 trees and built 26 schools, 150 day centres and 300 community kitchens. Training and education has reduced illiteracy to 3% and infant mortality to 40% below the national average. This is despite the fact that one-third of the residents live on lower-than subsistence incomes, compared with only 10% in Lima as a whole (Ekins, 1994). Though perhaps less dramatic in total impact, there are many examples of similarly successful community-based initiatives in the UK. Many of these, along with others from around the world, were detailed following the 1991 WHO Sundsvall Conference in Sweden (WHO, 1996). *Community Health Action*, the Journal of Community Health UK, dedicated its summer 1994 issue (32) to a wide range of 'settings-based approaches' to population health improvement including interventions in hospitals, places of worship, schools and workplaces. Evidence of population health outcome were not yet apparent, as the interventions were in relatively early stages, and poorly funded. However, recent policy commitments from the new Labour Government suggest that this situation may well change dramatically as the new health strategy, *Our Healthier Nation*, emerges.

CONCLUSION

There is considerable evidence to show that historical facts drawn from research evaluation make little difference to the practice of health care and, as Gray and Muir (1997, p 24) have observed:

> . . . there is no guarantee that any potential benefits identified within a research setting will be realized in practice, because outcome is also determined by the quality of management. To ensure that a population/group of patients receives the maximum health benefit at the lowest possible risk and cost from the resources available, both evidence-based healthcare and quality management are essential practices.

Perhaps the joint problems of what evidence there is in the world, and how it is used, are not amenable to separation. (This could be a variant of Heisenburg's (1927) uncertainty principle that 'objective' measurement itself changes the subject

(Heisenburg, 1927).) Popular paradigms of the notion of evidence insist that it can only be historical. The distinguished UK historian Edward Hallet-Carr (1989, p 654), commented that we owe our historical tradition to Voltaire (1694–1778). It is based on an empiricist/positivist theory of knowledge that presupposes a complete separation of subject from object. 'Facts, like sense impressions impinge upon the observer from outside, and are independent of his consciousness. The process of reception is passive: having received the data he then acts on them. . . . History consists of a corpus of ascertained facts available to the historian in documents like fish on a fishmonger's slab. . . .' Discredited as this view was to the discipline of history – even in the early 1960s, the evidence-based health care movement seems to have missed the implications, both here and from most of the post-modernist movement within a wide range of disciplines. The evaluation of past, and present, events is determined more by 'the gaze and cultural universe' of the viewer than from any supposed qualities intrinsic to the events themselves.

Perhaps a concept of *generative* evidence is more useful. This can be seen as evidence realised dynamically, *through* practice. It would draw on an active and integrated 'learning system' within the culture of the social system or organisation. Based on evidence of successful learning and innovation, its collective pursuit is likely to be more successful in capturing previous learning, transforming experience into knowledge and thus changing practice. Business approaches to what might be called 'evidence-based economic competitiveness' have already learned this lesson (Anderson & Johnson, 1997; Goodman et al., 1997; Kim, 1994). Implicit in the process is the transformation of social relationships within health care systems and the democratisation of meaning and knowledge without which the current irrelevant health investment strategies will not change.

The search for evidence-based health promotion is not primarily the pursuit of how effectively outcomes from discrete and specialist health promotion programmes can be achieved – this is a limiting conception inconsistent with the evidence on determinants of health. The search for evidence-based health promotion should be made wherever social processes can be identified that lead to health promoting change. Looking for evidence of effect in processes and outcomes of activities not culturally defined as health promotion will lead to useful insights. These can be gained particularly from within the domains of social system intervention.

A key goal of evidence-based health promotion activity must be to develop strategies for organisational change within the health care system. This must be a search for evidence-based health promotion intervention to increase the allocative efficiency of the whole health care system itself. Cost containment dilemmas experienced by health care systems throughout the world are simply not amenable to resolution within the current paradigm of neo-classical economics. Reinvesting in earlier more cost-effective interventions outside the health care system (associated with reduced cost and increased health outcomes) coupled with the development of social capital for health within institutions and communities, are the only sustainable solutions to this self-perpetuating problem. Health promotion must refocus its search for effectiveness within these domains.

As Weiss (1991) implies, integrity in the practice of evidence-based health promotion may involve the use of evidence itself within a similar framework to that of the judicial system. Here, evidence is openly sought to support competing views of truth whose nature is finally decided by consensus of a jury randomly drawn from the public. In the resultant marketplace of values and health investment choices, the role of health promotion will be to act as advocate of those evidential truths which support the promotion of social justice – from which equity in population health status is the principal outcome.

REFERENCES

Alkin M C et al. (1979) Using evaluations: does evaluation make a difference? Beverly Hills, CA: Sage.

Anderson V & Johnson L (1997) Systems thinking basics. From concepts to causal loops. Cambridge, MA: Pegasus Communications, Inc.

Antonovsky A (1996) The salutogenic model as a theory to guide health promotion. *Health Promotion International*, 11(1), 11–18.

Blane D, Brunner E & Wilkinson R (1996) Health and social organization: towards a health policy for the 21st century. London: Routledge.

Brunner E J (1996) The social and biological basis of cardiovascular disease. In: D Blane, E Brunner & R Wilkinson (Eds), Health and social organization: towards a health policy for the 21st century. London: Routledge.

Brunner E J, Marmot M G, White I R, O'Brien J R, Etherington M D, Slavin B M, Kearney E M & Davey Smith G (1993) Gender and employment grade differences in blood cholesterol, apolipoproteins and haemostatic factors in the Whitehall 11 study. *Atherosclerosis*, 102, 195–207.

Bulmer M (Ed) (1978) Social policy research. London. Macmillan.

Caplan N (1977) A minimal set of conditions necessary for the utilization of social science knowledge in policy formation at the national level. In: C H Weiss (Ed), Using social research in public policy making (pp 183–197). Lexington, MA: Lexington Heath.

Cooper C L & Payne R (1990) Causes, coping and consequences of stress at work. Chichester: John Wiley.

Deitchman S J (1976) Best-laid schemes: a tale of social research and bureaucracy. Cambridge, MA: MIT Press.

Dockrell W B (1982) The contribution of national surveys of achievement to policy formation. In: D B P Kallen et al. (Eds), Social science research and policy making (pp 55–74). Windsor: NFER-Nelson.

ECHHO (1997) European Clearing Houses on Health Outcomes Conference: Outcomes measures make sense – do they make a difference? International Meeting in Linkoping, Sweden 12–13 June.

Ekins P (1994) Wealth beyond measure: an atlas of new economics. London: Gaia Books Limited.

Evans R (1994) Why are some people healthy and others not? The determinants of health of populations. New York: De Gruyter.

Goodman D et al. (1997) Designing a systems thinking intervention: a strategy for leveraging change. Cambridge, MA: Pegasus Communications, Inc.

Gray J & Muir A (1997) Evidence based healthcare. How to make health policy and management decisions. London: Churchill Livingstone.

Grossmann R & Scala K (1994) Health promotion and organisational development. Developing settings for health. European Health promotion Series No. 2, Vienna: WHO.

Hallet-Carr E (1989) The historian and his facts: lectures from Trinity College Cambridge

1961. In: R Comley et al. (Eds), Fields of writing: readings across the disciplines. New York: St Martin's Press.

Handy C (1995) The empty raincoat: making sense of the future. London: Arrow Books.

Heisenburg W (1927) Quoted in: Mallet-Carr E The historian and his facts. Lectures from Trinity College, Cambridge, 1961. In: C Comley et al. (1989) Fields of writing: reading across the disciplines. New York: St Martin's Press.

Hertzman C (1996) What's been said and what's been hid: population health, global consumption and the role of national health data. In: D Blane, E Brunner & R Wilkinson (Eds), Health and social organization: towards a health policy for the 21st century. London: Routledge.

Kanter R M (1993) Men and women of the corporation. New York: Basic Books.

Kim D (1994) Systems thinking tools: a user's reference guide. Cambridge, MA: Pegasus Communications, Inc.

Knorr K D (1977) Policymaker's use of social science knowledge: symbolic or instrumental? In: C H Weiss (Ed), Using social research in policymaking (pp 165–182). Lexington, MA: Lexington Books.

Leff N (1985) The use of policy science tools in public sector decision-making: social benefit–cost analysis in the World Bank. *Kyklos*, 37, 60–76.

Limb M (1996) Health of the nation under scrutiny. *Health Service Journal*, 106(5529), 8.

Marmot M (1996) The social pattern of health and disease. In: D Blane, E Brunner & R Wilkinson (Eds), Health and social organization: towards a health policy for the 21st century. London: Routledge.

May A (1996) Forward thinking. *Health Service Journal*, 106(5510), 12–13.

Milgram S (1965) Some conditions of obedience and disobedience to authority. *Human Relations*, 18(1), 57–76.

Newell S (1995) The healthy organisation. London: Routledge.

NHS Executive (1996) NHSE aims and objectives. Taken from the NHSE web site accessed via www.jsj.macmillan.com

NHS Executive North West (1994) Strategic statement. Warrington: NHSE NW.

Peters T J & Waterman R H (1982) In search of excellence: lessons from America's best run companies. New York: Harper & Row.

Putnam R D (1993) The prosperous community: social capital and public life. *American Prospect*, 13, 35–42.

Putnam R D, Leonardi R & Nanetti R Y (1993) Making democracy work. Civic traditions in modern Italy. Princeton: Princeton University Press.

Ranade W (1995) From government to governance: implications for health for all. *Health For All News*, 32.

Real World Coalition (1996) The politics of the real world. A major statement of public concern from over 40 of the UK's leading voluntary and campaigning organisations. London: Earthscan.

Rich R F (1977) Use of social science information by federal bureaucrats: knowledge for action versus knowledge for understanding. In: C H Weiss (Ed), Using social research in policymaking (pp 165–182). Lexington, MA: Lexington Books.

Rose G (1993) The strategy of preventive medicine. London: Oxford University Press.

Schwartz F W & Bitzer E A (1997) Systems perspective of evaluation in health care. In: A Long & E A Bitzer (Eds), Health outcomes and evaluation: context, concepts and successful applications. Leeds: ECHHO.

Smee C (1995) Introduction. In: Riley et al. Releasing resources to achieve health gain. Oxford: Radcliffe Medical Press.

Smith P (1996) Measuring outcome in the public sector. London: Taylor & Francis.

Smith P & Cantley R (1985) Assessing health care: a study in organisational evaluation. Milton Keynes: Open University Press.

Syme S L (1996) To prevent disease: the need for a new approach. In: D Blane, E Brunner & R Wilkinson (Eds), Health and social organization: towards a health policy for the 21st century. London: Routledge.

Toth B (1996) Public participation: an historical perspective. In: C Coast et al. (Eds), Priority setting: the health care debate. London: Routledge.

Vang J (1997) Swedish policy on the evaluation of hospital performance. Workshop on evaluating hospital effectiveness and efficiency. Milan (Italy) 30 Sept–2 Oct. Geneva: WHO.

Weiss C H (1991) Policy research: data, ideas or arguments? In: P Wagner et al. (Eds), Social sciences and modern states. Cambridge: Cambridge University Press.

Weiss, C H & Bucuvalas M J (1980) Social science research and decision making. New York: Columbia University Press.

Wilkinson R (1996) Income distribution and life expectancy. *British Medical Journal*, 304, 165–168.

World Bank (1993) World Development Report. Investing in health. New York: Oxford University Press.

World Health Organisation (1984) Health promotion. A discussion document on concepts and principles. Geneva: WHO.

World Health Organisation (1996) European health care reforms. Analysis of current strategies. Summary. Copenhagen: WHO.

Section 6.2

Applying the Evidence to Workplace Catering

Jenny Poulter

ENVIRONMENTAL VERSUS EDUCATIONAL INTERVENTIONS

Catering represents one focus for the broad range of 'healthy eating' interventions which can be staged in a workplace setting (Glanz & Seewald-Klein, 1986). Efforts to encourage positive dietary behaviour fall roughly into two categories:

- *Environmental or structural strategies* increase opportunities to learn and make healthier food choices and reduce barriers to behaviour change. They may influence knowledge, awareness and behaviour. They focus on health improvement by changing the environment first, without requiring individual voluntary participation in educational activities. Examples include point of choice information, which can be placed in the workplace restaurant where nutrition information is presented on cards. Sometimes these schemes are teamed up with incentives to encourage usage by consumers (Mayer et al., 1986; Williams & Poulter, 1991). Changes can be made in the quality of foods available (e.g. reduced sugar custard) for selection in the workplace cafeteria, or in vending machines (e.g. adding in lower fat lines of crisps) (Farnon, 1981; Richmond, 1986). Foods can be positively promoted, including incentives, and policies can be implemented (Poulter, 1994; Poulter & Torrance, 1993).
- *Educational or direct influence strategies* to target staff – what they know and how they feel about food. This type of individualistic strategy involves the provision of nutrition information, persuasion, and behaviour change techniques either on a one-to-one basis or in groups. Examples include one-to-one dietary counselling, fact sheets on healthier snacks in the office, 'healthy eating' exhibitions and weight watcher groups.

The types of health promotion activity which can be achieved through catering are sometimes solely environmental (e.g. changing the menu to include a greater range and volume of healthier choices) or at times, direct influence and environmental strategies co-exist (e.g. menu labelling schemes where customers are provided

Evidence-based Health Promotion. Edited by Elizabeth R. Perkins, Ina Simnett and Linda Wright.
© 1999 John Wiley & Sons Ltd.

with nutrition information which directly relates to the menu items. The very process of nutrition labelling heightens awareness regarding the nutritional profile of the menu as a whole resulting in changes in recipe and menu mix). In short, healthier catering practice may encompass environmental and/or educational strategies.

There is a strong rationale for prioritising catering within a workplace setting. Firstly, there is the simple argument that the availability of healthier food within the workplace is the key enabling factor in helping employees to select healthier meals within this setting. Catering has been the Cinderella of workplace health promotion activity. A survey of UK workplace health promotion programmes in the mid-1980s suggests that interventions tended to centre on the traditional one-to-one model with little attention being paid to preventive measures which originate in the staff restaurant (McInerney & Cooper, 1989). Since then, there is a large amount of anecdotal evidence, which suggests that catering has become an acceptable focus for food/health promotion activity (Mock, 1989) and its growth may be due to the increasing body of effectiveness information (Contento, 1995). There is evidence that certain catering focused programmes are effective in influencing food choice (Roe et al., 1997). For example Liddell et al. (1992) demonstrated that simple changes in institutional catering practice can bring about positive changes. In their case study, the fat energy/energy percentage of meals purchased by students was reduced from 38% to 35% for the women, and from 42% to 33% for men. More detail on effectiveness is given in What Works (p 146).

Lastly, it could be argued that the potential for changing food intake through food accessibility is probably far greater than through food knowledge (Hunt & Macleod, 1987; Wright & Slattery, 1986). There is a wealth of qualitative information that suggests that people make decisions about food based on taste, family preferences and value for money; they are less worried about whether it is healthy or not (HEA, 1989; 1996) A recent effectiveness review conducted for the HEA (Roe et al., 1997) revealed fewer good quality quantitative studies showing behavioural change in workplace settings where programmes were solely concerned with educational approaches (either individual screening or counselling sessions) compared to environmental approaches.

For health promoters, the foregoing discussion has far-reaching implications and suggests that in a workplace setting it is potentially more effective to focus limited resources on changing the sorts of foods and how they are promoted to customers, than helping employees learn about nutrition and its relationship with health.

WHY PEOPLE EAT WHAT THEY DO?

It is important that those concerned with the promotion of healthy eating are familiar with the interplay of factors which affect food choice. Any single decision about choosing or eating food is the result of a whole jigsaw of conscious and subconscious influences (National Consumer Council, 1992). These influences are

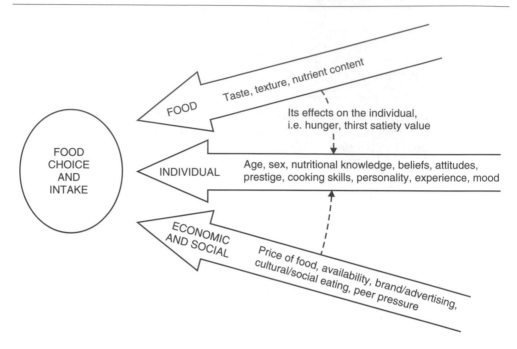

Figure 6.2.1 Some factors affecting food choice and intake

summarised in Figure 6.2.1. Models have been developed to further our understanding of food choice, including those which act directly on the individual and those which are the consequence of general public policy (Shepherd, 1990).

Although there is general agreement on the types of influences likely to be important, the integration of these factors remains an underdeveloped research area. Research has pursued two lines of inquiry (Leathwood, 1990):

- The experimental approach in which a particular factor like nutrient, drug or metabolite can influence some aspect of food intake or choice under experimental conditions.
- Understanding how different mechanisms are integrated under different circumstances, and demarcating the practical limits of their application, e.g. looking at how far price influences food choice, establishing links with income and availability of food.

Societal influences on food choice developed by Rozin and Fallon (1981) and extended by Fischler (1988) suggest that the behavioural mechanisms in food choice include innate preferences and aversions, innate behaviour patterns such as hesitant curiosity towards new foods and preferences for familiar foods. To some extent therefore we've all been programmed to eat the way we do. For healthy eating we need to break out and explore potential new foods, yet we are afraid of the unknown. These theories are built on a solid bedrock of experimental and circumstantial evidence and imply a vital role for catering to play in making new food more acceptable and familiar foods more exciting.

WHAT IS HEALTHY CATERING?

There is now a resounding consensus on the central direction for healthy eating (COMA (Committee on Medical Aspects of Food Policy), 1994; HEA, 1997):

- Eating lots of fruit, vegetables and starchy foods (much more than we currently eat)
- Adding in foods from the dairy and 'meat and alternatives' group of foods (including fish, eggs, nuts, peas and beans)
- Limiting fatty/sugary foods both in amounts and frequency (cutting back on current consumption).

Caterers can make a large number of changes in practice to help customers towards the style of eating advocated by COMA. These changes include:

- *Recipe development*:
  - Changing the proportion of ingredients or foods, e.g. increasing the amount of potato and decreasing the quantity of meat in a cottage pie or increasing the portion size of potato and vegetables and decreasing the portion size of meat components of roast meals
  - Cutting back on less healthy ingredients, e.g. decreasing the amount of sugar in puddings
  - Making swaps, e.g. using unsaturated margarine in crumble toppings instead of butter
  - Introducing new ingredients, e.g. adding in red lentils to bolognese sauce, which effectively dilutes the fat and increases the fibre content of the finished sauce.
- *Menu planning* (i.e. increasing the frequency and volume of healthier choices, e.g. adding pasta and rice-based dishes, limiting the number of fried and pastry items.
- *Promotion of healthier choices* through innovative marketing (e.g. pricing, presentation, merchandising) of healthier choices.

Integrating healthy eating into any catering operation involves many changes along the whole chain from purchasing of ingredients to service of products within the staff restaurant. A visual example of the broad range of changes which can occur in catering is shown in Figure 6.2.2. The example given is for providing a greater volume of healthier choices on a snack trolley, which is just one of the food outlets (serviced by caterers) within a workplace setting. Other food outlets may include a workplace restaurant, staff dining room or canteen, vending machines (snacks and drinks), snack bars, retail outlets (e.g. newsagent-type shops), bars, coffee shops, coffee points (e.g. electric kettle and biscuit tin).

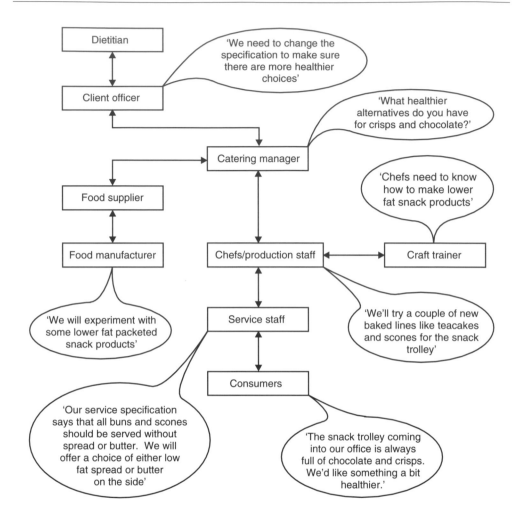

Figure 6.2.2   Integrating healthy eating into a workplace operation (from Poulter, 1994)

Workplace catering services are diverse. Increasingly they are run by contract caterers and controlled through a specification, which is managed by the parent workplace through a client or contracts officer. This specification is only as strong as the monitoring systems used to track and control the delivery of the service. If specifications do not address nutrition and set down how healthier choices are delivered and promoted to customers, then it simply won't happen. The catering specification and its monitoring is central to controlling healthier choices both in terms of volume and how they are marketed (or not) to customers.

Taken as a whole, the range of activities and quantity of effort involved in the delivery and marketing of healthier meals to customers looks pretty daunting and can develop into an amorphous feeling of powerlessness for all those involved in encouraging positive dietary behaviour in a workplace setting. So on a pragmatic level it's a question of where to start. As yet we have no reliable evidence on the relative effectiveness of different elements of the catering chain – i.e. we don't know whether there is potentially greater impact on customer fat and calorie intake by manipulating recipes or by, for example, merchandising healthier products which appear on a workplace menu. We do know that these tactics have impact but their relative strength remains unclear, mainly because researchers have used different indicators of outcome (Roe et al., 1997).

There has been some debate over the relative merits of different approaches to healthier catering practice including the:

- *Subversive approach* where subtle changes are made to recipes and the menu mix. These changes largely go unnoticed by consumers and even though the food they are choosing is healthier they are usually unaware that they are selecting lower fat products (e.g. swapping whole milk for semi-skimmed in sauces, using a reduced fat cheddar in lasagnas and cheese sauces).
- *Overt approach* which can include recipe and menu changes but also linked up to some sort of merchandising which promotes healthier choices to customers. Generally health is the underlying theme of the merchandising, e.g. healthy dish of the day, Heart Smart choice, Heartbeat choice, etc.

Given that most workplace catering operations are commercially driven, then deciding on the best approach is determined by the demand for healthier choices. A review of two major pieces of consumer research in the 'eating out' catering sectors indicates that the availability of healthier choices is not top priority. Taste and value for money are the most influential factors in consumer choice (HEA, 1996). Thirteen per cent of consumers are committed to eating healthily and will look for healthier options when eating out. In addition, a large number of customers (51%) have an open mind. Nearly all (97%) of the people questioned think that people should have a choice to eat healthily (BMRB (British Market Research Bureau), 1995; Scott, 1994) and this demand for healthier choices is probably much stronger in a workplace setting, where eating patterns are more 'every day' rather than something special. Nevertheless, this consumer research gives valuable pointers on how healthy eating should be handled by caterers:

- the main area of consumer interest is fat reduction
- presentation and menu descriptions are vital; taste concerns need to be addressed by using appetising descriptive terms such as 'freshly cooked' or 'tasty'
- discreet references to health are generally welcomed and tend to reflect well on providers. Uptake is likely to be higher if the healthier options are placed on the general menu rather than separated out, i.e. healthy choices are mainstream rather than something specialised for a specialised market

Table 6.2.1 Comparison of formative and summative evaluation

Formative evaluation	Summative evaluation
Mainly about process	Mainly about outcomes

Describes activity
   (e.g. reaction of catering staff to a menu
   labelling scheme which they are
   instrumental in developing and piloting)
	Seeks to quantify outcome
	   (e.g. number of people purchasing jacket
	   potatoes)

Understanding of effectiveness and insights
   on how success was achieved or missed
	Looks at achieved objectives, effects both
	   expected and unexpected

Qualitative methods (e.g. observation of
   activities, interviewing staff)
	Quantitative methods (e.g. before and after
	   study of consumer purchasing behaviour)

- communication about 'across the menu' catering changes needs to be handled vary carefully; there is evidently a danger that such changes may be perceived as detracting from meal enjoyment.

INDICATORS OF SUCCESS

Much has been written on the evaluation of healthy eating initiatives. Kemm and Booth (1992) have provided a clear evaluative framework by dividing evaluations into two main types:

- *Formative evaluation* involves collecting information while the programme is running and using it to develop and improve the programme.
- *Summative evaluation* involves collecting information about an established programme (or completed programme) in order to decide whether it should be continued (or repeated). This basic division is easily applied to healthy catering programmes and the characteristics of each are summarised in Table 6.2.1.

In practice there is considerable overlap between these two types of evaluation and most evaluations will have some of the characteristics of both types. Therefore indicators of 'success' for a healthy catering programme will vary according to a programme manager's interpretation of the word success. It could mean:

- What effect did the programme have (e.g. did a 'fantastic fish' promotion in a workplace restaurant result in employees eating more fish, and if so did this significantly affect their overall fat and energy intake?).

or

- How effective was the programme (e.g. do the promotional materials do what they set out to do, which is appeal to customers, communicate the messages clearly and appropriately?).

Theoretically, there are many different types of information which could be collected in order to assess the impact, or track the process, of a catering initiative (Kemm & Booth, 1992) and these are summarised below.

ITEMS OF INFORMATION (THE STUDY VARIABLES)

Awareness and agenda of catering teams

1. Perceived problems – what are caterers worried about with reference to healthy eating/catering?
2. Awareness of nutrition and health issues

Food knowledge and skills of production and service staff

3. Knowledge of links between food choices and health
4. Knowledge of food values (e.g. foods low in fat)
5. Craft skills/menu planning

Values

6. Cultural differences in cuisines
7. What caterers and customers say they value about healthy eating
8. Perceived credibility of sources of information – whom do people trust?
9. Role models – whom do people (chefs, service staff, customers) want to be like?

Behaviour of customers

10. Meal patterns
11. Frequency of consumption of different foods – how much? – how often?
12. Intake of nutrients (energy, fat, sugar, starch, fibre, etc.)
13. Purchasing patterns in staff restaurant
14. Weight and weight control

Availability

15. What foods are available in catering outlets – what price? – how visible are they? – what are the relative volumes of different lines?

Economic data of catering operation

16. Profit, turnover, food costs, labour costs

Different people have different expectations of what an evaluation should contain. The personnel manager may be keen to know whether the programme is easy or costly to organise, while the catering department may want information on how catering staff reacted to the initiative and how it affected business. Practical considerations (usually the budget!) will determine what can and cannot be done in terms of evaluation. Often there has to be a trade off between scientific rigor and grass roots feasibility. The skill comes in fitting the best quality methodology (either quantitative or qualitative) to the resources (e.g. budget, skills and man-power, equipment and technology) and making sure that something meaningful is done for the money. Applying the evidence in this sense means:

- Looking to see what the literature tells you in terms of effectiveness and impact.
- Gleaning information from others in the field. There is a wealth of formal and informal food and health networks in the UK including the British Dietetic Association, Hotel and Catering Institutional Management Association, Food For Health Network and the National Food Alliance. Within these groups there may be people who have tackled or are currently embroiled with the very evaluative questions which you face. There is much to be learnt from others and why reinvent the wheel?

WHAT WORKS?

Because nutrition is a science and nutrition practice is built on scientific consensus, where the controlled randomised trials are valued as 'the best', then this quality criteria is often applied to catering research. Quantitative outcome data, preferably from controlled experimental studies are perceived as the best indication of whether something 'is working', i.e. having effect.

At first glance, a scan of the available literature on catering interventions, which are designed to promote healthier eating practices, looks promising. There is a substantial review of nutrition at the work-site (Glanz & Seewald-Klein, 1986) which implies an exponential growth of food/health promoting activities in the workplace since 1980. Closer examination for clues on effectiveness and impact of catering-focused programmes are less promising. Many of the papers are descrip-tive and merely document elements of a particular programme (what we did) as opposed to examining outcomes (what effect we had). For example, Richmond (1986) describes a comprehensive cafeteria programme with training for cafeteria staff about heart healthy foods, recipe and menu development, changes in cafeteria layout and written information as handouts. Other companies have introduced modified cafeteria menu choices (King et al., 1983) and vending machines (Farnon, 1981). Point of choice, or point of purchase nutrition information has been used in vending machines (Larson-Brown, 1978) as well as employee restaurants (Williams & Poulter, 1991). The reviewers say that these approaches are gaining widespread acceptance, but in the absence of quality outcome data it is difficult to defend duplication of such programmes, other than on the basis of altruism.

A recent review of the effectiveness of healthy eating interventions in catering settings paints a gloomy picture regarding the quantity and quality of reliable evidence regarding healthy catering interventions (Roe et al., 1997):

- only 15 controlled experimental or quasi experimental 'healthy catering' studies were identified in the literature post 1985 – only two are from the workplace
- virtually all the data comes from US studies
- the overall quality of the studies was deemed mediocre – often no data on characteristics of the participants, or overall food consumption, sometimes studies used self-reported food intake which is notoriously unreliable and baseline data was sometimes incomplete.

The best workplace catering study was conducted by Jeffery et al. (1994) and involved increasing the number of fruit (by 50%) and salad choices (by 30%) and decreasing their price (by 50%) and resulted in a tripling of sales, which was not sustained beyond the intervention period. Fruit sales returned to baseline but salad remained 50% higher. The other workplace cafeteria study is less convincing and set out to assess the effect of providing nutritional signs for a number of items, both healthier and less healthy. This resulted in a decrease in fat intake from catered meals of 3g which did not reach statistical significance (Schmitz & Fielding, 1986).

A more global consideration of the catering interventions drawn from other settings is much more positive. Eleven out of the 15 showed a positive effect on food selection or nutrient composition, at least in the short term. One good quality study assessed changes in the selection of low-fat main courses after promotion on school menus (Whitaker et al., 1994) and showed an increase of 3% in proportion of total main courses. The intervention in university cafeterias (Davis-Chervin et al., 1985) provided nutritional information for all main courses; adding an explanatory poster showed no effect on the proportion of low-fat main courses chosen. Hidden changes to the recipes within a catering service in a boarding school (Ellison et al., 1990) showed a decrease in saturated fat intake in the entire diet of 2% of energy after eight months.

Four moderate quality studies evaluated the promotion of healthier choices in public restaurants (Albright et al., 1990; Colby et al., 1987; Mayer et al., 1986; Wagner & Winett, 1988). All these interventions resulted in increased sales in the short term, which varied between 2% and 12% of total market share for main courses, and a smaller increase for salad promotion of 13% above baseline sales. Two studies evaluated a change in the physical location of confectionery and crisps to make them less accessible, which reduced the selection of these items by individual participants to 13% and 15% of baseline levels, and in one study increased selection of healthier substitutes.

Two moderate quality studies from the schools sector, which were included in the effectiveness review, were concerned with changing recipes and menus (offering more low-fat choices) resulting in a reduction in the fat content of the school lunches by 6% to 12% of energy. However the authors fail to make any comment on whether this affected overall choice or diet of consumers (Snyder et al., 1992; Whitaker et al., 1993).

The review draws a question mark over the effectiveness of nutrition labelling. The best quality cohort study in two university cafeterias (Aaron et al., 1995) had a negative effect on individual food choice; that is, it led to an increase in fat intake from catered meals of about 2g versus controls. The Schmitz and Fielding (1986) workplace study is more positive regarding its effect on reduced fat intake for labelled catered meals; however the results did not reach statistical significance.

Examples of the most effective large-scale interventions showed that they need not be intensive but do require substantial workplace organisation and resources. The Treatwell nutrition programme (Sorenson et al., 1992) at 16 sites consisted of workplace events, cholesterol screening, classes and modification in cafeteria meals over 15 months. The intervention resulted in a net reduction in fat intake of 1% of energy but no change in dietary fibre intake.

So, what does this brief overview imply?

- There is very little good quality research to draw on, which gives pointers on what sort of healthy catering interventions have most impact.
- It is possible to change what people eat and choose to eat (at least in the short term) through catering mediated interventions.
- The increase in the total market share of promoted items ranged from 2–12% whilst the interventions were in place. Passive manipulations of food composition decreased the fat content of catered meals by 6–12% of energy intake.
- Interventions in catering settings which provided signs with nutrient data for all food items and assumed customers would compare them, were not effective, and in one study were counterproductive, i.e. nutrition labelling has to be selective and simple.

IN SUMMARY

- In a workplace setting it could be potentially more effective to focus limited resources on changing the sorts of foods and how they are promoted rather then helping employees learn about nutrition and health.
- Models of food choice provide a sound theoretical basis for catering/cuisine interventions as they tap into our 'innate preferences for familiar foods' and 'hesitant curiosity of new foods'.
- Catering interventions are broadly positive and there is good indication that they have the ability to influence both the food which people choose and what they eat.
- Promotion of healthy main courses led to increases in total sales proportions of between 2% and 12% but this increase seems to be short lived, i.e. promotions can shift purchasing patterns in a healthier direction but a variety of promotions need to be used and changed regularly.

- It is perfectly possible to produce recipe and menu items which are significantly lower in fat (changes in menus or recipes in school cafeterias reduced the fat content by 6% to 12% of energy intake), i.e. hidden approaches can get people to eat healthier foods.
- Taste and value for money are probably more effective handles for promoting healthier choices rather than selling food on the health ticket alone.
- For promotions in workplace catering:
  - there is most customer interest in fat reduction
  - presentation (i.e. appearance of menu products) and menu descriptions are vital
  - healthier choices need to be mainstream and not divided off into some specialist 'health bar or salad service'.
- Communication about 'across the menu changes' needs to be handled carefully – it is not simply a case of telling customers that unsaturated margarine and wholemeal flour is being used throughout, as this could be perceived negatively by many customers.
- If you are going to evaluate a healthy catering intervention, first learn from others, using both formal published sources and informal networks, which may yield 'hands on experience' from individuals who have conducted evaluative work in a similar arena.

REFERENCES

Aaron J I, Evans R E & Mela D J (1995) Paradoxical effect of a nutrition labelling scheme in a student cafeteria. *Nutrition Research*, 15 1251–1261.

Albright C L, Flora J A & Fortmann S P (1990) Restaurant menu labelling: impact of nutrition information on entree sales and patron attitudes. *Health Education Quarterly*. 17. 157–167.

BMRB (1995) Qualitative research conducted on behalf of the HEA. London: Health Education Authority.

Colby J J, Elder J P, Peterson G, Knisley P M & Carleton R A (1987) Promoting the selection of healthy food through menu item description in a family style restaurant. *American Journal of Preventive Medicine*, 3, 171–177.

Committee on Medical Aspects of Food Policy (1994) Nutritional aspects of cardiovascular disease. Report on health and social subjects No. 46. London: Department of Health.

Contento I (1995) The effectiveness of nutrition education and implications for nutrition education in policy, programs and research: a review of research. *Journal of Nutrition Education*, 27, 279–420.

Davis-Chervin D, Rogers T & Clark M (1985) Influencing food selection with point of choice nutrition information. *Journal of Nutrition Education*, 17, 18–22.

Ellison R C, Goldberg R J, Witschi J C, Capper A L, Puleo E M & Stare F J (1990) Use of fat modified food products to change dietary fat intake of young people. *American Journal of Public Health*, 80, 1374–1376.

Farnon C (1981) Let's offer employees a healthier diet. *Journal of Occupational Medicine*, 23, 273–276.

Fischler C (1988) Cuisines and food selection. In: Food acceptability (pp 193–206). London: Elsevier.

Glanz K & Seewald-Klein T (1986) Nutrition at the worksite: an overview. *Journal of Nutrition Education*, 18, S1–S16.

Health Education Authority (1989) Diet, nutrition and 'healthy eating' in low income groups. London: HEA.

Health Education Authority (1996) The national catering initiative. Offering the consumer a choice. London: HEA.

Health Education Authority (1997) Eight guidelines for a healthy diet. A guide for nutrition educators. London: HEA.

Hunt S M & Macleod M (1987) Health and behavioural change: some lay perspectives. *Community Medicine*, 9, 68–76.

Jeffery R W, French S A, Raether C & Baxter J E (1994) An environmental intervention to increase fruit and salad purchases in a cafeteria. *Preventive Medicine*, 23, 788–792.

Kemm J & Booth D (1992) Promotion of healthier eating (pp 11–15). London: HMSO.

King J C, Achinapura S & VanHorn L (1983) Nutrition in the workplace. *Journal of Nutrition Education*, 15, 59–64.

Larson-Brown L B (1978) Point of purchase information on vended foods. *Journal of Nutrition Education*, 10, 116–118.

Leathwood P (1990) Food intake and food choice. In: Why we eat what we eat (pp 50–59). London: British Nutrition Foundation.

Liddell J A, Lockie G M & Wise A (1992) Effects of a nutrition education programme on the dietary habits of a population of students and staff at a centre for higher education. *Journal of Human Nutrition and Dietetics*, 5, 23–33.

Mayer J A, Heins J M, Vogel J M, Morrison D C, Lankester L D et al. (1986) Promoting low-fat entree choices in a public cafeteria. *Journal of Applied Behavior Analysis*, 19, 397–402.

McInerney D & Cooper C (1989) Profiting from healthy staff. *Sunday Times*, 3 September.

Mock J (1989) Healthy eating – caterers' response. *Nutrition and Food Science*, July/August 1989, 6–9.

National Consumer Council (1992) Your food: whose choice? (pp 1–26). London: HMSO.

Poulter J (1994) Healthy eating at work. London: Health Education Authority.

Poulter J & Torrance I (1993) Food and health – the costs and benefits of a policy approach. *Journal of Human Nutrition and Dietetics*, 6, 89–100.

Richmond K (1986) Introducing heart-healthy foods in a company cafeteria. *Journal of Nutrition Education*, 18, S63–S65.

Roe L, Hunt P, Bradshaw H & Rayner M (1997) Health promotion interventions to promote healthy eating in the general population: a review. London: Health Education Authority.

Rozin P & Fallon A F (1981) The acquisition of likes and dislikes for foods. In: Criteria of food acceptance. Zurich, Forster Verlag 35–48.

Schmitz & Fielding (1986) Point of choice nutritional labelling – evaluation in a workplace cafeteria. *Journal of Nutritional Education*, 18, 565–568.

Scott K (1994) Qualitative research conducted on behalf of the HEA. London: Health Education Authority.

Shepherd R (1990) Overview of factors influencing food choice. In: Why we eat what we eat (pp 12–30). London: British Nutrition Foundation.

Snyder M P, Story M & Trenkner L L (1992) Reducing fat and sodium in school lunch programs: the LUNCHPOWER! intervention study. *Journal of the American Dietetic Association*, 92, 1087–1091.

Sorenson G, Morris D M, Hunt M K, Hebert J R, Harris D R et al. (1992) Work-site nutrition intervention and employees dietary habits: the Treatwell program. *American Journal of Public Health*, 82, 877–880.

Wagner J L & Winett R A (1988) Promoting one low fat high fiber selection in a fast food restaurant. *Journal of Applied Behavior Analysis*, 21, 179–185.

Whitaker R C, Wright J A, Finch A J & Psaty B M (1993) An environmental intervention to reduce dietary fat in school lunches. *Pediatrics*, 91, 1107–1111.

Whitaker R C, Wright J A, Koepsell T D, Finch A J & Psaty B M (1994) Randomised intervention to increase children's selection of low-fat foods in school lunches. *Journal of Pediatrics*, 125, 535–540.

Williams C & Poulter J (1991) Formative evaluation of a workplace menu labelling scheme. *Journal of Human Nutrition and Dietetics*, 4, 251–262.

Wright G & Slattery J (1986) Talking about healthy eating. Special report. Bradford: University of Bradford, Food Policy Research Unit.

A Workplace Stress Survey

Sue Hepworth

There had been longstanding trade union concern about stress levels amongst the 1400 staff at the head office of a large white-collar organisation. There was also a belief that there were particular pockets of stress and low morale. Some of the reasons given by the trade union officers for the perceived stress were the lower management style, low experience levels due to staff turnover, and the design of the office building. For her part, one of the senior managers suggested the causes were changes in the organisational culture, the relocation to the office of a significant number of staff, the style of management, and the feeling that staff were demotivated and felt trapped.

The trade union had prepared a questionnaire which they wanted to use for an investigation, but the resident psychologist staff counsellor saw the need for professional expertise in the design of a stress audit. Therefore, a joint committee of management and trade unions commissioned the survey from an independent occupational research psychologist.

The advantages of getting an outside consultant to do the stress audit were:

- that she would bring specialist knowledge and skills, and also a fresh eye to the situation
- staff should feel more confident that their responses would be confidential, and hopefully therefore give more honest responses
- the analysis and reporting of the final results should be more credible as independent of any interest group.

AIMS OF THE RESEARCH

A first step in any such exercise must be to agree the aims of the research. The researcher set these out and they were then agreed with all parties as follows:

Evidence-based Health Promotion. Edited by Elizabeth R. Perkins, Ina Simnett and Linda Wright.
© 1999 John Wiley & Sons Ltd.

1. To examine the scale of stress experienced by all staff, and to compare levels of stress and staff morale between individual departments.
2. To pinpoint the causes of any stress with the primary focus being on stress caused by factors in the work setting, though external stressors, such as financial or domestic worries, would also be touched on.
3. To compare, where possible, levels of stress, morale and other work attitudes with those of samples of similar workers based elsewhere.
4. To ask staff for suggestions on ways to remove the causes of any stress, or ways to prevent stress from occurring in the future.
5. To make recommendations for further action.

THE QUESTIONNAIRE

The researcher held informal individual conversations with a variety of employees at the site. These included the trade union officials, the staff welfare officer, and various managers and staff from most of the departments within the office. The researcher then designed the questionnaire with closed questions to yield quantitative data, but with two open-ended items included to give qualitative responses. The topics covered were:

- Issues arising in the informal conversations with staff, which included shift working arrangements, difficulties caused by staff in other departments, the accessibility and reliability of information technology, and tight deadlines which characterised a significant part of the work of some departments.
- Issues emerging from previous discussions of the joint management and trade union committee, mentioned above.
- Factors which the occupational stress literature had shown to be related to work-related stress, such as job satisfaction, lack of stimulation, role overload, uncertainty, supervisor support, communications and physical working conditions. These included items which had been used in surveys of similar samples of employees based elsewhere in the country. This was done to make comparisons more straightforward and valid.
- Worries about health problems, domestic/family problems, financial problems, the journey to/from work, and the economic climate.
- Demographic details.
- Two self-report measures of health, both of which are validated and published psychometric tests. The Somatisation scale from the SCL-90-R (Derogatis, 1983) measures distress arising from perceived physical symptoms which have been shown to be associated with some psychiatric disorders, though of course they may be reflections of true physical disease. It was included not as an absolute measure of health but so that various sub-groups within the organisation could be compared. The second measure was the 12-item version of the General Health Questionnaire, which was originally designed to be a self-administered screening test aimed at detecting psychiatric disorders in community settings

(Goldberg, 1978). The GHQ-12 has also been widely used as a general measure of psychological well-being – particularly in occupational settings (Warr, 1987) – and was included in this survey as a measure of stress.

THE SURVEY

The researcher having piloted the questionnaire elsewhere, the final version of it was distributed to all staff who were asked to return the completed questionnaire directly to the researcher. The accompanying letter, which was signed by the chief executive and the two trade union officers, pointed out that the questionnaire was anonymous, and that all responses would be treated in the strictest confidence. Staff were also told they could complete the questionnaire in work time. In addition, the trade unions sent a separate message to their members, encouraging them to respond to the survey. It was hoped by these means to encourage a good response from staff and to persuade them to be completely frank about their feelings and experiences. The survey was not called a 'stress survey', so as not to prompt over-reporting of the experience of stress. It was instead entitled a 'Survey of work, health and well-being'.

RESULTS

The response rate was 57%, which compared well with a response rate for the annual national organisation attitude survey of 53%. An analysis of demographic data showed the survey respondents to be representative of the staff in post. The questionnaire contained many items but space constraints here prevent the mention of more than a few results.

The Scale of Stress at the Site

The question which directly asked staff about their perceived job stress was phrased in the following way:

Which of the following statements more nearly expresses how you feel?

(a)   Generally speaking, the challenges and pressures in my job cause me too much stress.

(b)   Generally speaking, I enjoy the challenges and pressures in my job.

Seventeen per cent of staff agreed with statement (a), whilst the remaining 83% agreed with statement (b). Those staff who said the pressures and challenges of their job caused them too much stress had higher scores on both the symptom checklist and on the GHQ than those who ticked statement (b). The higher grades of staff were more likely to report stress than the lower grades and the former were also more likely to be suffering from stress as measured by the GHQ.

Did Morale and Stress Vary According to Department?

The stress audit found no evidence of pockets of stress, as suggested by the trade union, but there were some differences between departments in work attitudes. These were: job satisfaction; perceived supportiveness of line managers; optimism about chances of promotion; evaluations of staff–management communications; and lastly, staff in three departments were more likely to say that other departments did things (or didn't do things) that caused them difficulty.

These difficulties were related to work-related stress and the main causes were errors, inefficiencies and poor communications. Those complaining in two particular departments thought that other staff with whom they liaised neither understood their methods and procedures, nor realised the importance of accurate information and realistic timing for the efficient completion of the work of the two departments.

Comparative Stress Levels

If scores on the GHQ are taken as a measure of stress, then staff here were suffering less stress than other samples in comparable organisations for which figures were available. However, a national survey of the general population (Cox et al., 1987) showed *lower* 'stress' scores than those of some groups of staff in the present sample.

Morale

The level of morale at head office was comparable on most counts with that for staff in other parts of the organisation.

Physical Working Conditions

Physical working conditions were the source of a great deal of dissatisfaction amongst staff. The most serious problems for all respondents were – in terms of both frequency of mention, and also centrality to the well-being and efficiency of staff – unsatisfactory temperature and ventilation, and poor facilities for quiet work.

Causes of Stress

For those reporting job-related stress the most frequently given cause was dead-lines or not enough time to do the work, for example:

> Because of tight deadlines, and lack of staff, work is rushed and errors made creating more unnecessary work.

Staff thought the solutions lay in better planning, more resources, more time, and more realistic workloads and deadlines.

However, when those staff who said they *enjoyed* the challenges and pressures of their job were asked which single work pressure they saw as the most positive, the most popular pressure was working to deadlines:

> Working to deadlines keeps you motivated and gives you something to aim for.

It is quite striking that the work pressure most frequently seen as stressful by one group of staff should be seen in a positive light by the same proportion of another group. This serves as a salutary reminder both of individual differences, and also of the fact that some kinds of stress are not always negative. If 'unstressed' staff had not been questioned about positive work pressures, the conclusion might have been drawn that deadlines were always unwelcome.

Twenty-one per cent said that workload or shortage of staff was to blame for their work-related stress, and they saw the answers in an increase in staff numbers, better cover for key staff, training for all staff in all aspects of the work, and more staff available for special exercises.

All factors shown by this survey to be related to stress level were entered into a statistical analysis to discover their relative contributions. A multiple regression showed the best single predictor of GHQ score to be the frequency with which someone worried about domestic or family problems (accounting for 13% of the variance). The next best predictors were:

- whether the person said their job caused them too much stress (8% of the variance)
- their opinion about staff management communications (4%)
- how much they worried about their health (2%)
- whether they felt they had too much work to do (2%)
- their job satisfaction (2%).

All of these factors together only accounted for 32% of the variance in GHQ score, which reminds us of the fact that this survey only touched on *some* of the factors contributing to a person's psychological well-being.

AFTERTHOUGHTS

The use of a validated measure such as the GHQ made it possible to answer the central questions posed by those commissioning the stress audit. Comparisons between sample sub-groups could be made, and comparisons could also be made between the total group and other groups of employees for which data were available (for example, Jenkins, 1985; Jenkins et al., 1982; Orlans, 1991). This particular researcher was also fortunate to have access to confidential survey data from the rest of the same organisation, and also from a comparable one. Secondly, the fact that the survey was quantitative, with a relatively large number of respondents, made the differences found between departments open to testing for statistical significance.

However, quantitative surveys can only go so far. Closed questions tell you how many people feel a certain way but not *why* they feel it. For example, in this investigation, staff in one department reported lower job satisfaction and felt less positively about staff–management communications than did other departments. Why was this? To answer this question, other methods would be needed, such as semi-structured interviews, or focus groups. A stress survey is a tool not a solution; how it is used will depend on the political climate within which it is commissioned.

REFERENCES

Cox B D, Blaxter M, Buckle A L J, Fenner N P, Golding J F, Gore M, Huppert F A, Nickson J, Roth Sir M, Stark J, Wadsworth M E J & Whichelow M (1987) The health and lifestyle survey. London: Health Promotion Research Trust.

Derogatis L R (1983) SCL-90-R. Towson Clinical Psychometric Research.

Goldberg D (1978) Manual of the GHQ. Windsor: National Foundation for Educational Research.

Jenkins R (1985) Minor psychiatric morbidity in employed young men and women and its contribution to sickness absence. *British Journal of Industrial Medicine*, 42, 147–154.

Jenkins R, MacDonald A, Murray J & Strathdee G (1982) Minor psychiatric morbidity and the threat of redundancy in a professional group. *Psychological Medicine*, 12, 799–807.

Orlans V (1991) Stress and health in UK organisations: a trade union case study. *Work and Stress*, 5(4), 325–329.

Warr P B (1987) Work, unemployment and mental health. Oxford: Oxford University Press.

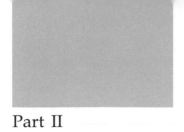

Part II

Evidence-based Work in Settings

Edited by Ina Simnett

Chapter 7

The Evidence Base of Work in Settings

Ina Simnett

You may wish to read Part II of the book because:

- you work in one defined setting and want to know about it
- you want to expand your activities into additional settings (for example, hospital outreach work; or community nursing reaching into schools or prisons)
- your job involves frequently moving on your work from setting to setting.

We aim to help those new to a setting to find out about it, rather than guess. It is equally important for those who work in only one setting to try and see it as 'foreign' in order to identify whether they are making assumptions which they should check out.

Health promoters are often required to work in settings which are not necessarily familiar to them – for example, a school nurse may be employed and trained within the NHS, but required to work within schools. Undertaking health promotion work in unfamiliar settings requires gathering evidence about each particular setting and is a necessary part of practice. Evidence-based practitioners will do more than just read about other settings and more than just reflect on how these are different from the one in which they usually work or were trained. In addition, they will gather evidence about the settings in which they are required to work, for example, about social, occupational or professional norms, customs, practices, beliefs, values, and behavioural styles, in order to understand the culture. Culture is 'the underlying bedding' which individuals make use of when they interact with each other (for further discussion about what we mean by culture, see Chapter 11 on working in hospital). Understanding the culture is essential for any change at all and will provide evidence about, for example, how difficult or easy particular changes may be, what might be the barriers and how they might be overcome.

Evidence-based Health Promotion. Edited by Elizabeth R. Perkins, Ina Simnett and Linda Wright.
© 1999 John Wiley & Sons Ltd.

EVIDENCE AND SETTINGS

Types of Evidence

Evidence-based health promotion practitioners can gather two main types of evidence about settings in which they wish to work:

1. Evidence about the setting itself – the culture (history, attitudes, norms, beliefs, customs and practices, etc.), the physical environment, lifestyles, and also evidence about the target group, such as what they need and want. It will also be necessary to collect evidence about what the purchasers and providers of health promotion (and other important groups of stakeholders) want.
2. Evidence about the effectiveness and efficiency of health promotion work in the setting (what works in practice, what is good quality, what provides good value for money).

We are here, therefore, mainly concerned with what could be described as 'social analysis': understanding how any proposed change or development can best fit in with the on-going activities and circumstances of its surroundings. By gathering evidence about the current situation (and the legacy of history) and then setting realistic objectives for the proposed change, it should be possible to gauge the effects that the change will have. It should also be possible to identify some of the risks and benefits of the change and this will assist in the management of the change process.

Given both the wide range of evidence, the differing objectives of different stakeholders and the underlying debates about what is health and what is health promotion – about which there is no general agreement (see Section 3.1 by Dale Webb in Chapter 3) – the evidence may be difficult to interpret. So, what can you, as a practitioner wishing to intervene in a setting, do? How can you best set about gathering the evidence you need? Whose evidence do you believe? Whose evidence should you act on? There are no easy answers to these questions, but the following guidance may help.

Issues and Topics on which You Might Collect Evidence

First, you will need to assess how you can gather the evidence you require about health promotion work in a defined setting. Some of the issues and topics on which evidence may be needed are set out below. This list should not be considered exhaustive and not all categories will apply in a given setting. Not all these topics will require rigorous research, but the list will help you to consider if and how much you know about them and what you intend to do about it if you don't!

- *The views of stakeholders*: these are people with a vested interest in an issue, who wish to influence what is done and how it is done. They are powerful forces in the setting and it is vital to identify which of the stakeholders could be allies and how to gain their trust. This means paying attention to their concerns, values, beliefs and behaviour patterns, and working through fitting in with these.
- *The views of local people*: the views of the target population or group, i.e. the 'end' customers – those who will 'use' or receive the health promotion you wish to provide in the setting, especially about their beliefs, attitudes, customs, norms, concerns, aspirations and history. You may find it useful to read Sections 14.1 and 14.2 by Linda Lawton and Heather Roberts in Chapter 14 on how best to assess local needs.
- *Quality of team working*: good teams allow responsibilities to be shared and provide a sense of purpose, belonging and ownership (Johnson & Johnson, 1991). Team working provides opportunities for knowledge and skills to be shared and enables organisations to respond swiftly to challenges and opportunities. It will be essential to establish whether teams working in a setting are effective. Key characteristics are discussed in Simnett (1995, Chapter 7).
- *Quality of health alliances* (agencies working together to achieve health gain, which the agencies working on their own could not achieve as effectively or efficiently). Successful health alliances do not 'just happen'. It will be necessary to gather evidence about how successful any alliance in a particular setting is. Key success criteria are set out in Ewles and Simnett (1998, Chapter 9).
- *The distribution of power*: language is the medium for operating the structuring and defining of power (Fairclough, 1989). Both those with power and those without it collude in this. In health promotion work we are often interested in gathering evidence about the degree of power sharing between the providers and receivers of interventions and in understanding how we could increase the power of receivers.
- *Levels of participation by the community*: some agencies are now attempting to move from various degrees of tokenism to genuine community participation (Nutbeam, 1996). Projects using this approach are not easy, quick or cheap. However, those involved are often convinced that the community-empowerment approach, with its key principles of starting with people's own concerns and working with them to build up skills and confidence, offers the best hope of improving health in areas of high health need (Ewles et al., 1996).
- *Timeliness, time-scales and resources*: it is important to consider when to introduce a change or when to delay. If people are already preoccupied with other major issues, it may not be the right time to introduce another change. Time-scales also need to be addressed – many health promotion initiatives will require considerable time before they show results. It is also important to gather evidence about resources – these are not just money, but competent staff with time to carry out activities, competent managers to monitor, control and audit progress, and facilities (for example, sound-proof rooms for counselling).
- *The physical and social environment*: for example, quality and quantity of facilities in a neighbourhood setting (such as health centres, leisure centres, play

areas, shops, roads, public transport, and housing) and issues such as road safety and drugs problems. (See Section 14.3 in Chapter 14 for an example of how evidence about the environment was collected and used.)

Sources of Evidence

One source of evidence is published documents. This paragraph highlights some key documents on 'what works' in a variety of settings. The Dutch guides (in English) to effectiveness in health education and health promotion cover a wide range of settings, through topics which include sexual health, patient education, mental health, drug abuse, school health, oral health, tobacco control, accidents, exercise and cancer (see Useful Addresses). Tones and Tilford (1994) contains chapters on the theoretical and practical aspects of work in schools, health care settings, workplace and community, with UK and international examples. Scriven and Orme (1996) has chapters on health promotion in different settings: health service, local authority, education and youth organisations, voluntary sector and workplace. The Health Education Authority have published guidance on developing a healthy workplace in the NHS (Health at Work in the NHS, 1995a) and on how to address organisational sources of stress in the NHS (Health at Work in the NHS, 1995b; 1996). Recent meta-analyses of health education and health promotion work also provide pointers to effective practice in a variety of settings (Kok et al., 1997).The contributions to this book, applicable to your setting, will also provide starting points.

You also need to be aware of what the published research in *related* settings tells you, and to reflect on how what was learned might apply in your circumstances (for example those practising in institutions of higher education could look at the research on health promotion in other educational settings).

Networks can also provide evidence. The Health for All (UK) network is the co-ordinating body for promoting health in urban settings ('Healthy Cities'). The European Network of Health Promoting Schools (ENHPS) is a collaborative research and development initiative funded by WHO, the European Commission (EC) and the Council of Europe (CE). The aim is to develop the effectiveness of schools as settings for the promotion of health. The HEA acts as the national support centre within the UK. 'Health Promoting Hospitals' is a WHO initiative designed to improve hospitals as settings for health promotion. An English Network of Health Promoting Hospitals is supported from Preston Acute Hospitals NHS Trust. These are national and international networks, but tracking down and joining local networks may be just as important. (Please see Useful Addresses at the end of this section for details of all the organisations above.)

Also, evidence is not confined to formal research by other people. Your own experience is important evidence, and if you plan carefully and evaluate or audit what you do, you will be building up your own body of knowledge. It is important that any work you do complements that of others working in the setting, so their views will be essential evidence. (See the discussion on practitioner knowledge in the section on the Tension between Different Types of Knowledge in Chapter 1.)

SCRUTINISING AND ACTING ON THE EVIDENCE

Having gathered some evidence about a setting, the next stage will be to scrutinise the evidence, in order to ensure that you draw sound conclusions from it on which to base actions (see Chapter 12 in Part III for a more extensive discussion of this). To do this you need to ask yourself a number of key questions (Simnett, 1995, p 26). These could include:

- What are the reasonable conclusions which can be drawn from this evidence?
- What would help those already working in this setting to improve their performance?
- What outcomes could realistically be attainable in this setting?
- Do these outcomes appeal to any of those with an interest (stakeholders or local people)?
- How high a priority does intervening in this setting have?
- What would work and what wouldn't work?
- What might be most appropriate, economical, good quality and practical?
- How long will it take to achieve the desired outcomes?
- What might be the potential 'value added' outcomes or 'spin-offs' from this intervention?

Can you think of any other important questions to ask?

In Summary

An important question to ask, when working in a setting, could be, *'How can health promotion help those already working in this setting to improve their performance, and achieve better health for their clients, in the most efficient way?'*

ACTIVITY

Gathering, Assessing and Acting on Evidence in Settings

Think about a specific setting in which you might wish to work or in which you are planning to work (and which is *not* your usual work setting), where you desire to make changes in a group or population of people. (For example, you might wish to introduce a fitness programme in a particular workplace, or a health promotion programme in a particular school, or a healthy eating programme in a hospital canteen, or an accident prevention programme in a particular neighbourhood. Or it could be that you are a

nurse about to start work on another ward, or a teacher about to take over a new class.)
Then answer the following questions:

1. What are the main topics on which I need evidence?
2. How should I set about gathering this evidence? What are the relevant sources for
    this evidence? How can I ensure that I gather the evidence systematically and
    comprehensively, so that I have all the relevant data? What might be the main
    pitfalls to avoid?
3. How could I best assess the subjective and objective evidence in order to form a
    judgement about whether it is reliable, whether it is biased (and if that matters) and
    whether it is valid?
4. How could I best use the evidence, in collaboration with all the people concerned,
    to help us to decide what to do?

VALUES, EFFECTIVENESS AND EVIDENCE

One of the things which may emerge from carrying out this activity, is that
decisions are a matter of judgement and that good judgements are not just based
on evidence, but are also based on a guiding set of principles and values. Health
promotion is driven by the interaction of both values and evidence (as discussed in
Chapter 1), so that there are two key questions: do we think we ought to do this
and will it work? (Seedhouse, 1997). The following paragraphs show how my own
values colour my approach to evidence-based practice in settings.

In my view, a central value for health promotion work is to help to give a voice to
those who are least heard. This means actively seeking out these people in those
places where they are to be found, whether it is on the streets, in prison, in deprived
communities or in institutions such as schools. The task is not only to listen to them,
but to enable them to shape the sort of health promotion they receive and to decide
for themselves whether and how much to participate in it. A critical and ultimately
political question is: 'Whose interests does the health promotion intervention
serve?'

In Chapter 10, for example, Section 10.1, written by Robin Burgess, demonstrates
that current health promotion interventions with offenders primarily serve the
interests of influential stakeholders, such as prison officers and politicians (themselves representing the interests of the general public) and may not serve the
interests of the offenders themselves. In a similar way, the Section 9.2 on detached
youth work in Chapter 9, by Beth Lindley, demonstrates that older members of
communities may pay scant attention to the needs and interests of their young
people and, for example, perceive young people on the streets as a problem to be
got rid of. In Chapter 8, Section 8.3, by Frances Hudson, vividly highlights how the
needs and interests of young people are not met by much of the sex and relationships education currently provided in schools.

I believe that the needs, interests, rights and responsibilities of those for whom health promotion is provided (the 'end customers') are paramount, and that the needs and interests of other groups of stakeholders are secondary. This is supported by business experience, and initiatives based on the theory of Business Process Re-engineering (BPR), which asserts that the ultimate test of the quality of a service is its effect on end customers (Coulson-Thomas, 1996, p 113). However, in order to get the opportunity to work with the 'customers' it is vital to understand the views of the providers, purchasers and other stakeholders. Often prior work with providers and other stakeholders will be necessary (so that they are sure that any intervention will 'add value') before it is possible to work directly with the 'customers'. These tensions between the views of customers/clients and those of other stakeholders will always be present, and effective work in settings means understanding them and if necessary compromising (so long as you do not betray essential values). This is discussed in depth by Sally Perkins in Chapter 10 (Section 10.2), related to working within prisons.

Meeting the needs and interests of a target group requires paying attention to how these people live their lives and to how their lives are shaped by the situations in which they live. Young people like to 'hang out' on the streets. Beth Lindley (Chapter 9, Section 9.2) demonstrates how it is possible for detached youth workers to understand them in this setting, and to work effectively with them. Unfortunately, projects like this are vulnerable to cuts (the project described has now suffered this fate) and the connection does not always seem to be made, by politicians and other stakeholders, that these are precisely the sorts of activity needed to prevent crime and drug abuse (perhaps because they do not come with a 'crime prevention' or 'drug project' label). However, the contributions in this part of the book show that projects which genuinely meet the needs of the group for whom they are provided, are also likely to meet the needs of the wider society (but perhaps not in the way envisaged by the general public). For example, a successful youth work project might make the streets safer for young people to hang out in, rather than go for the solution favoured by many older people: keeping young people off the streets. The important point is that successful work with young people allows the young people to identify their own needs and to find ways of meeting these needs by and for themselves. In this way it also meets the needs of society to nurture responsible citizens.

The standards of health promotion provided for young people are a cause for concern. Cale (1997), for example, argues that school health education is not in good health, and must fight for its survival in a rapidly changing educational climate. The UK signed up to the United Nations Convention on the Rights of the Child in 1991. Since then, the United Nations Committee on the Rights of the Child has been critical of progress in the UK (Lansdown, 1996), echoing many of the points made in this book. Lansdown emphasises that much remains to be done to ensure that the principles and standards of the Convention inform policy and thinking at a more profound level than is currently the case. Failure will be a betrayal of our children. Several of the contributions to this part of the book provide pointers about how we can improve health promotion work with children and young people.

Factors which Determine Effectiveness and Efficiency

Funders and purchasers naturally want to channel resources towards the most effective and economical interventions. However, health promotion work in many settings does not lend itself to *scientifically* rigorous evaluation (see Section 3.2 by Liz Rolls in Chapter 3). This may, unfortunately, have distracted attention from focusing on the factors which determine whether an intervention in a setting is likely to be successful and good value for money (about which more evidence may be gained from rigorous qualitative studies). This part of the book sets out to provide practical examples to purchasers and practitioners which demonstrate that we have a good deal of evidence about what these factors are. They include:

- Actively seeking out the groups with whom you are concerned, either through working in those localities where they are to be found, or through gaining entry into the settings which they use, or through creating environments which they find attractive, such as drop-in centres (see, for example, in Chapter 9, Section 9.1 on Informal Education and Health Promotion by Tony Jeffs and Mark Smith).
- Listening non-judgementally, and not making assumptions (see, for example, Section 8.3 in Chapter 8, by Frances Hudson, on Sex and Relationships Education in Secondary School).
- Focusing on the positive health needs, goals, interests and aspirations of the target group/s or population, rather than on the problems as you perceive them (which might be prevention of, for example, crime, HIV/AIDS, cancer or drug abuse) (see Section 9.2 on Detached Youth Work in Chapter 9).
- Focusing on the strengths and resources of the target group/s, and helping them to identify a first, small, safe step through which they can begin to act (see Section 9.2 on Detached Youth Work in Chapter 9).
- Ensuring that a detailed and qualitative needs assessment is undertaken which engages the interest of all those concerned (see, for example, in Chapter 11, Section 11.3 on Breast Health Awareness by Alison Mitchell).
- Understanding the culture and fitting in with it, rather than trying to change it, whenever possible (see, for example, Sections 10.1 and 10.2 in Chapter 10 by Robin Burgess and Sally Perkins, respectively, and in Chapter 11, Section 11.1 on Working in Hospital). Grand plans for transforming cultures will only be achieved with the active support of top management or community leaders within a setting.
- Considering the way the setting works as a whole and how to make every bit of the system influence the outcomes (see, for example, Section 8.1 in Chapter 8, Rationale of Work in School Settings and the practical examples of whole school approaches later in that chapter, both by Alysoun Moon).
- Making effective alliances with other agencies and people, both locally and further afield, so that you have access to a wide range of resources (see, for example, the case study in Chapter 8, Section 8.4 on Drug and Alcohol Education by Ruth Joyce, and in Chapter 11, Section 11.2 on Child Accident Prevention by Kathy Brummell).

• Planning, implementing, and evaluating or auditing collaboratively with those for whom the intervention is provided and with the other people in the alliance (see, for example, Section 11.3 on Breast Health Awareness in Chapter 11).

Factors in the Wider Environment Influencing Health Promotion Work in Settings

We have a long way to go yet in order to improve the links between health promotion and the criminal justice system, but nevertheless successful health promotion work is being delivered in very difficult circumstances (see Chapter 10). The report by the Public Health Alliance (1997) is a welcome contribution to this debate and it is to be hoped that closer working between the Department of Health, the Department for Education and Employment and the Home Office will begin to map out how we can make the criminal justice system genuinely more health promoting.

There is still a long way to go to achieve healthy public participation in the NHS. Chapter 11 shows us how it can be achieved in health promotion work, but this would be more effective if the NHS as a whole had more and better ways to involve the public in decision making. A report from the NHS Confederation (1997) calls for support for community development work and user groups so that people can develop their own ideas and agendas rather than simply being asked for their views in consultation processes.

In summary, if we really want to tackle inequalities in health, all of us working as health promoters must do our utmost to value those who are vulnerable, poor, discriminated against or on the margins of society. They must be able to make informed choices about their health, and be helped to do this through services which are confidential, accessible and flexible. Their voice must be an integral part of planning how best to meet their needs. The essence of what I mean by evidence-based practice in settings is gathering, assessing and using evidence in order to:

1. Understand the culture in which people are to be found and therefore how best to intervene.
2. Empower them to act.
3. Understand their environment and work with them to change it, to make it more supportive.

This approach is also illustrated by the contributions of Heather Roberts and Anne McClelland (see Chapter 14, Sections 14.2 and 14.3, respectively).

Collecting Evidence about what Works in Settings

Finally, we need to collect evidence about how far we are succeeding. It is hard to assess the impact of health promotion. The difficulties have already been highlighted in relation to *The Health of the Nation* strategy (Appleby, 1997). More evidence is needed about the underlying causes of changing trends in *Our Healthier Nation* and what mechanisms connect the underlying determinants of health with outcomes. It is equally difficult (but not impossible) for the front-line practitioner to know whether she or he is succeeding. This book is one contribution to attacking these difficulties. For example, the challenge and difficulties of assessment and evaluation in informal education is discussed in depth in Section 9.1 by Tony Jeffs and Mark Smith in Chapter 9. Beth Lindley, writing in the same chapter, demonstrates how informal education *can* be evaluated in practice. Another example is an overview of evaluation of community health development, with particular reference to a project in Corby, which has been provided by Luck and Jesson (1996). Chapter 16 in Part III of this book also addresses these issues.

What is clear is that while it may be easy to identify change, it is much harder to know what were the pivotal factors which brought about the change. In the face of these difficulties, it is vital that the benefits of health promotion work, carried out by competent practitioners, are not denied to those who most need it (for example, because funders believe that practitioners must prove 'scientifically' that they are hitting certain short-term targets). To ensure that health promotion plays an effective part in the new 'health improvement programmes' (HIPs) proposed in the Green Paper (Secretary of State for Health, 1998) we need evidence about what actually works in practice in particular settings. This means opening up our evidence-based practice for scrutiny.

REFERENCES

Appleby J (1997) Health promotion: feelgood factors. *Health Service Journal*, 107(5560), 24–27.
Cale L (1997) Health education in schools: in a state of good health? *International Journal of Health Education*, 35(2), 59–62.
Coulson-Thomas C (Ed) (1996) Business process re-engineering: myth and reality. London: Kogan Page.
Ewles L & Simnett I (1998) Promoting health: a practical guide. Fourth edition. London: Baillière Tindall.
Ewles L, Miles U & Velleman G (1996) Lessons learnt from a community heart disease prevention project. *Journal of the Institute of Health Education*, 34(1), 15–19.
Fairclough N (1989) Language and power. London: Longman.
Health at Work in the NHS (1995a) Working for health: a practical guide to developing a healthy workplace in the NHS. London: Health Education Authority.
Health at Work in the NHS (1995b) Organisational stress in the National Health Service: an intervention designed to enable staff to address organisational sources of work-related stress. London: Health Education Authority.
Health at Work in the NHS (1996) Organisational stress: planning and implementing a programme to address organisational stress in the NHS. London: OPUS/HEA.
Johnson D W & Johnson P F (1991) Joining together: group theory and group skills. London: Prentice Hall.
Kok G, van den Borne B & Mullen P (1997) Effectiveness of health education and health promotion: meta-analyses of effect studies and determinants of effectiveness. *Patient Education and Counselling*, 30(1), 19–27.
Lansdown G (1996) A model for action: the Children's Rights Development Unit. Promoting the Convention on the Rights of the Child in the United Kingdom. London: Unicef.

Luck M & Jesson J (1996) Evaluation of community health development. Bath: Community Health UK.

NHS Confederation (1997) The people's health service? NHS Confederation, Birmingham.

Nutbeam D (1996) Achieving 'best practice' in health promotion: improving the fit between research and practice. *Health Education Research*, 11(3), 317–326.

Public Health Alliance (1997) Framing the debate: crime and public health. Birmingham: PHA.

Scriven A & Orme J (Eds) (1996) Health promotion: professional perspectives. Basingstoke: Macmillan/Open University Press.

Secretary of State for Health (1998) Our Healthier Nation: a contract for health. A Consultation Paper. London: The Stationery Office.

Seedhouse D (1997) Health promotion: philosophy, prejudice and practice. Chichester: John Wiley.

Simnell I (1995) Managing health promotion. Chichester: John Wiley.

Tones K & Tilford S (1994) Health promotion: effectiveness, efficiency and equity. London: Chapman & Hall.

USEFUL ADDRESSES

For information about the Dutch guides to health education, contact:

Netherlands Institute for Health Promotion and Disease Prevention
De Bleek 13
Woerden
PO Box 500
3440 AM Woerden
The Netherlands
Tel: +31 348 43 76 00
Fax: +31 348 43 76 66

For information about the UK Health for All network, contact:

The Network Coordinator
Health for All (UK)
PO Box 101
Liverpool L69 5BE
Tel/Fax 0151 207 0919.

For information about work resulting from the ENHPS project, contact:

The Administrator
Young People and Schools Account
Health Education Authority
Trevelyan House
30 Great Peter Street
London SW1P 2HW
Tel: 0171 2225300

For information about the English network of Health Promoting Hospitals, contact:

WHO HPH Project Coordinator
North West Lancashire HP Unit
Sharoe Green Hospital
Fulwood
Preston PR2 8DU
Tel: 01772 711223

Chapter 8

Working in School Settings

Ina Simnett

INTRODUCTION

This chapter aims to help those from the NHS, and elsewhere, who wish to work effectively with schools. There is a tendency for people outside schools to feel that all (or many) of the problems encountered in adult work could be solved if only the schools did more. Whilst it is accepted that there is a continuing need for school-based health promotion, it is essential that outsiders understand the constraints and opportunities offered by the school setting. Education in schools is driven by the curriculum, but the curriculum alone cannot deliver effective health promotion to pupils – it needs to be supported by the whole ethos and functioning of the school as a 'health promoting community'.

The first section, *Rationale of Work in School Settings*, explains what is meant by a health promoting school and the principles behind it.

The second section, *Working in Primary School Settings*, explains why primary schools provide special opportunities for health promotion, and the pressures primary teachers are under as a result of the changes that have taken place in recent years. It provides guidance on how to plan and undertake effective work with primary schools including how to get started and how to deal with events and changes which could hinder your work.

The third section, *Sex and Relationships Education in Secondary School*, illustrates the shortcomings of much current sex education in schools, which results in continuing ignorance amongst young people about issues such as contraception and sexually transmitted diseases, and no help with preparation for the emotional side of relationships. However, evidence about what works in terms of effective sex education is already available and is vividly described in this section, along with examples of pockets of excellent work being done in secondary schools. Improving sex and relationships education needs to be at the top of the agenda if we are to provide the parents of the future with the abilities to be 'good enough parents'.

Evidence-based Health Promotion. Edited by Elizabeth R. Perkins, Ina Simnett and Linda Wright.
© 1999 John Wiley & Sons Ltd.

The final section, *Drug and Alcohol Education*, describes the progress made in drug and alcohol education, over a decade, through the work of a 'healthy alliance' in Cambridgeshire under the leadership of a drug education co-ordinator. The process of developing an alliance is described and key areas for development are highlighted including setting quality standards, agreeing contracts and monitoring (vital pieces of evidence if we are to demonstrate that we are 'doing the right things right'). If only we had more examples of getting a grip on sex and relationships education in a similar way!

Section 8.1

Rationale of Work in School Settings

Alysoun Moon

Health education has been present in some form in schools in the UK for the past 100 years or so, but until the 1970s had its main emphasis on physical health and the prevention of disease. More recently, the focus has moved to a more positive and holistic concept which also encompasses mental, social, spiritual and emotional aspects of health and well-being. Health education is concerned not only with attitudes and behaviour but has as its foundation the need for personal growth and the teaching of skills which will lead to the development of responsible, independent, confident and well-informed young people who are able to make rational and healthy decisions and choices.

Healthy attitudes and behaviours are usually established at a young age and this, together with the fact that schools provide settings in which the majority of children will spend a significant proportion of their time, provide the continued justification for school-based health education. Teachers increasingly recognise the role they have as health educators and health education, both formal and informal, is now an established part of the curriculum in most, if not all, schools in the UK, often as an integral part of personal and social education (PSE).

WORKING TOWARDS THE SCHOOL AS A HEALTH PROMOTING COMMUNITY

The 1988 Education Reform Act (Department for Education and Science, 1988) placed a statutory responsibility on schools to provide a broad and balanced curriculum which '. . . promotes the spiritual, moral, cultural, mental and physical development of pupils at the school and of society and prepares them for the opportunities, responsibilities and experiences of adult life.' It also recognised, however, that the curriculum alone cannot achieve this aim but will need to be supported by extra-curricular activities, the whole ethos and functioning of the school and by interaction and partnership with home and the community.

Evidence-based Health Promotion. Edited by Elizabeth R. Perkins, Ina Simnett and Linda Wright.
© 1999 John Wiley & Sons Ltd.

The influences which determine health, particularly for children, are wide ranging and include sex, age and hereditary factors, home influences, social and economic background and environment, parental and adult modelling and access to and use of health services. Few would accept that an individual's lifestyle is the only definer of health. In the same way, a school which sees itself as having an important contribution to make to the health and well-being of all who work in it through its environment, ethos, extra-curricular activities, policy making and management structures and practices is likely to have a much greater impact on the health and well-being of children. Curriculum content will be dictated by the needs of the children and their knowledge about health. Parents, working in partnership with the school, will have their concerns addressed and be fully informed of what is being taught in order to ensure a consistent approach. Links with the community and community involvement in school life will add a further vital dimension of support and co-operation.

The ethos of the school will be such that children and all staff – teaching and support – will feel a sense of belonging and of being valued. Policies, which have been agreed and formulated by all staff and, where appropriate, pupils, will reflect the positive and caring ethos in the school. Everyone's self-esteem will be fostered and built up through day-to-day practices and the skills needed to make healthy choices – self-awareness, self-discipline, critical thinking, decision making, discernment, taking responsibility, assertiveness, negotiation, assessing outcomes – will be integrated both in the curriculum and through extra-curricular activities. The school's physical environment will be one that promotes health – suitably clean, safe, hygienic, stimulating, well-kept with plenty of fresh air and places for rest and contemplation as well as activity.

A health promoting school is likely to be an effective school as it seeks to develop individuals to their full potential. While there has been no specific research within this context, there is evidence to show a correlation between personal and social development and academic achievement (Barber et al., 1995). External interventions have an important contribution to make but will need to ensure that they support the development of a health promoting school through a whole school approach and the principles which underlie it. This will provide a firm foundation for future health promotion in schools.

REFERENCES

Barber M, Stoll I & Mortimore P (1995) Governing bodies and effective schools. OFSTED. London: HMSO.
Department for Education and Science (1988) The Education Reform Act. London: HMSO.

Section 8.2

Working in Primary School Settings

Alysoun Moon

Primary schools may be labelled county, grant maintained, grant aided or church schools – titles which largely reflect the way in which the school is funded. The majority, county schools, are funded by the Local Education Authority (LEA). In some parts of the country there will be first (ages 4–8 years) and middle schools (ages 8–13 years) or infant (ages 4–7 years) and junior schools (ages 7–11 years).

Whatever their status, primary schools are special places.

- Primary teachers often have a special relationship with the children in their care and possess unique knowledge and understanding of their backgrounds and health needs.
- There is usually a close relationship between school and home, parents and families. Primary schools are non-threatening places and there are many opportunities for co-operation, mutual support and working in partnership.
- The size of primary schools means that teachers and other staff, particularly the school nurse, are well placed to observe changes relating to health and well-being in children.
- Staff get to know each other well and support staff can be more actively involved in planning, policy making and in the classroom.
- The age and stage of development of primary children provides unique opportunities for health education.
- The care of young children is seen as a partnership and there are many formal and informal opportunities for co-operation between school and community, e.g. the police, health service and social services.
- The child-centred ethos and some flexibility with time enables a more informal approach in which visitors are welcomed and involved.
- The nature of the curriculum facilitates the development of cross-curricular health education programmes and a whole school approach.

Primary teachers, as with all teachers, are under considerable pressure as a result of the changes that have taken place in education over recent years. These include

Evidence-based Health Promotion. Edited by Elizabeth R. Perkins, Ina Simnett and Linda Wright.
© 1999 John Wiley & Sons Ltd.

major curriculum reform, new legislation relating to school management, the introduction of league tables, the change to OFSTED (Office for Standards in Education) inspections and greater accountability to LEAs and parents demanded by successive governments. Those contemplating working in schools need to be aware of these pressures and understand something of their potential influence and effect on practice. Time is at a premium in all schools and this will influence their willingness to participate in health-related projects or external interventions.

LOCAL MANAGEMENT OF SCHOOLS

Based on the concept of pupil-led funding, local management of schools took effect in primary schools in April 1994. LEAs are required to allocate a minimum of 80% of a school's delegated budget to the school governors to manage. The number of pupils registered is a major factor in the amount of funding granted to a school, along with size and provision for children with special educational needs, and headteachers will wish to develop a good reputation and present a positive image to potential parents and the community at large. Bad publicity must be avoided at all costs. The way the school is managed will affect the resources available to support health education initiatives. There may not be any!

THE NATIONAL CURRICULUM

This consists of ten core and foundation subjects, together with religious education and five cross-curricular themes – Economic and Industrial Understanding, Careers Education and Guidance, Health Education, Citizenship and Environmental Education. The cross-curricular themes, including health education, are not compulsory and primary schools are not required to cover modern languages. However, the Framework for the Inspection of Schools as set out in the OFSTED Handbooks (1995) includes reference to personal and social education, sex education and drugs misuse education, all of which are expected. Schools are required by law to have a sex education policy, although primary school governors can choose not to cover the topic in their school.

Each core and foundation subject has attainment targets which are divided between four key stages. Key Stages 1 and 2 cover the primary school age group and Key Stages 3 and 4 those in secondary schools. Pupils are tested in each subject, usually at the beginning of the summer term, using Standard Attainment Tests (SATs). It is wise to avoid interventions during this period, especially as teachers will also be in the process of completing reports and profiles for their pupils!

OFSTED INSPECTIONS

These are undertaken every six years by teams of qualified inspectors – more often if a school is deemed to be failing – and can last for a week or more, depending on the size of the school. Much rests on the outcome of the OFSTED report and, with the increasing profile given to falling standards, the inspection represents one of the most stressful procedures for staff. Preparation for the inspection can be all consuming and requests to work in schools during this time are likely to be given short shrift!

LEAGUE TABLES

League tables put considerable pressure on teachers to produce good academic results and this can mean that outside interventions which are not closely linked to academic subjects are less likely to be accepted. Press reports and complaints from industry and academia about falling standards increase the pressures.

THE ROLE OF GOVERNORS

This role has become much more significant in recent years and, whilst most will work closely with school staff, the governing body can over-rule on the content of health education, e.g. sex and drugs education, and make final decisions on matters relating to initiatives within school.

CHANGES IN PERCEPTIONS AND EXPECTATIONS OF TEACHERS BY PARENTS AND THE GENERAL PUBLIC

Considerable changes have been taking place over recent years. There is an increasing lack of respect for teachers in society and the high profile given to perceived failures has led to extra sensitivity and caution by teachers in becoming involved in external projects and interventions, particularly where there are potential sensitivities, e.g. sex education. Parents are encouraged to become more actively involved in their children's education and many will complain more readily if time is spent on non-academic subjects.

OTHER DEMANDS

Many teachers feel that their role has increasingly become one of honorary social worker as they struggle with children who are suffering from the effects of changes in family life and society. The number of children who are depressed or suffering from eating disorders has grown, even in primary schools. While most teachers care deeply about those they teach and seek to do their best for them, there will be some for whom involvement in a health education project or intervention is just an extra 'burden' which they would rather do without.

EFFECTIVE WORKING IN PRIMARY SCHOOLS

There are a number of ways in which outsiders wishing to work in a school setting can facilitate effective working and prevent problems arising. The following tips have arisen out of experience and been proved in practice.

If you plan to use more than one school in a LEA, approach the Chief Education Officer for permission to work in schools. She or he is likely to refer you to individual headteachers but this is a matter of courtesy. It sometimes helps to be able to reassure a headteacher that the LEA knows of your plans and has given you permission.

Plan thoroughly – remember the degree of success is proportional to the amount and depth of preparation:

- Consult early with educational advisers, the head teacher and staff at the school(s) you intend to involve – make it a partnership from the beginning and give the school ownership of the project; try to identify teachers who are keen to be involved, while at the same time giving everyone opportunity to participate.
- Find out what has already been done in school which relates to the project and where pupils are likely to be in their knowledge and experience. Plan to use pupils' own starting points and build on their experience wherever possible. Try to link what you do with topics being covered already in school.
- Be realistic, rigorous and detailed in your planning of the intervention.
- Have a clear purpose and expected outcomes – don't build in failure by expecting too much but equally, provide a challenge.
- Identify workable and achievable aims and objectives which everyone understands and key players have agreed.
- Select appropriate methods – for example, don't incorporate role play in the first session if teachers do not like it but try something else.
- Identify realistic time-scales – try not to underestimate, allow more time than you think is necessary, particularly for the consultation and setting up periods.
- Decide the degree of pupil involvement and criteria for selection.
- Plan staff involvement – don't take anything for granted but talk to the headteacher and key staff members first.
- Identify members of the community who may wish to be involved in the project, either as consultants, resources or contributors. Check out any school sensitivities first.
- Identify resources you will supply and how they will be funded.
- Identify resources you wish the school to supply – you will need to discuss this with the link person, headteacher, etc. – don't expect much but *always* ask!
- Build in methods for monitoring and evaluating the success of the project – relate these to purpose and expected outcomes, aims and objectives – keep it simple!
- Think about the presentation of outcomes and results and the distribution of the final report – who, what, why, when?

- Plan a whole school approach in which curriculum development goes hand in hand with policy development, training and parental and community involvement. (See Figure 8.2.1.)

Getting Started

Arrange a Meeting with the Head by Writing in the First Instance

Introduce yourself and state clearly why you want to come. Follow-up by telephone, fax or E-mail. Be prepared to persevere! When you meet, explain your plans in detail, including intended outcomes and potential benefits. Indicate the degree to which the project will involve staff and pupils and discuss concerns you or the headteacher may have. State where there are 'unknowns' and be prepared to make cuts. Acknowledge possible pressures on teachers and be flexible. Send a revised plan for agreement.

Offer a Range of Dates for the Project

Very few dates are immediately acceptable – parents' evenings, in-service training, exams, school plays, open days, school trips, celebrations, policy writing – and more – can all present problems for planning.

Offer a Small Incentive in Recognition of the School's Involvement

This might be a teaching resource, free in-service training or a small gift, e.g. £100 worth of book tokens.

Check out any Particular Sensitivities for the School

These might include cultural or religious issues or may relate to the recent death of a pupil or member of staff.

Be Flexible

Try to identify what could be omitted from the intervention without damaging it. Be prepared to modify aims and objectives. Build relationships, work for success – and pave the way to a welcome back into the school to carry out a much larger intervention.

Another example of a whole school approach is set out in Figure 8.2.2.

Be Prepared to Address Pupils, Staff, Parents or Governors' Meetings

This will give you the opportunity to explain the plans in detail and involve everyone at an early stage.

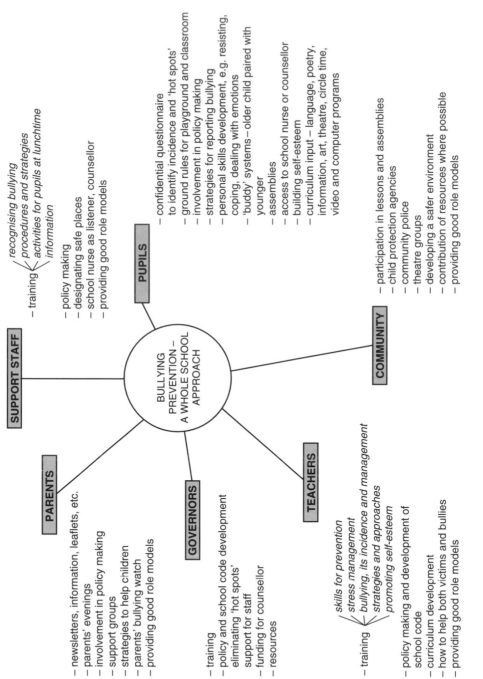

Figure 8.2.1 Bullying prevention – a whole school approach

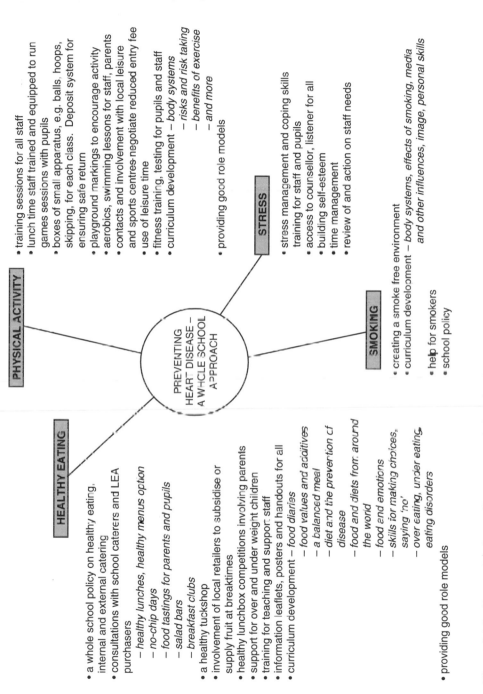

PHYSICAL ACTIVITY

- training sessions for all staff
- lunch time staff trained and equipped to run games sessions with pupils
- boxes of small apparatus, e.g. balls, hoops, skipping, for each class. Deposit system for ensuring safe return
- playground markings to encourage activity
- aerobics, swimming lessons for staff, parents
- contacts and involvement with local leisure and sports centres-negotiate reduced entry fee
- use of leisure time
- fitness training, testing for pupils and staff
- curriculum development – *body systems*
  – *risks and risk taking*
  – *benefits of exercise*
  – *and more*
- providing good role models

STRESS

- stress management and coping skills training for staff and pupils
- access to counsellor, listener for all
- building self-esteem
- time management
- review of and action on staff needs

SMOKING

- creating a smoke free environment
- curriculum development – *body systems, effects of smoking, media and other influences, image, personal skills*
- help for smokers
- school policy

HEALTHY EATING

- a whole school policy on healthy eating, internal and external catering
- consultations with school caterers and LEA purchasers
  – *healthy lunches, healthy menus option*
  – *no-chip days*
  – *food tastings for parents and pupils*
  – *salad bars*
  – *breakfast clubs*
- a healthy tuckshop
- involvement of local retailers to subsidise or supply fruit at breaktimes
- healthy lunchbox competitions involving parents
- support for over and under weight children
- training for teaching and support staff
- information leaflets, posters and handouts for all
- curriculum development – *food diaries*
  – *food values and additives*
  – *a balanced meal*
  – *diet and the prevention of disease*
  – *food and diets from around the world*
  – *food and emotions*
  – *skills for making choices, saying 'no'*
  – *over eating, under eating, eating disorders*
- providing good role models

PREVENTING HEART DISEASE – A WHOLE SCHOOL APPROACH

Figure 8.2.2 Preventing heart disease – a whole school approach

Be Well-informed, Confident and Enthusiastic

Convince the school of the benefits of participating and demonstrate your own commitment.

Check your Insurance Cover for Working with Children

If schools are included in your job description, you may be covered by your employer's insurance. The school may be covered if you are working there with their permission.

WHEN THINGS GO WRONG

However detailed and thorough the planning, all may not go according to plan. Schools are dynamic institutions and it is important to be prepared to adapt or change aspects of the programme at short notice. Examples of the sorts of things that could go wrong are set out below.

EXAMPLES OF EVENTS AND CHANGES THAT COULD HINDER YOUR PROJECT

Sudden and unplanned changes in priorities within the school, e.g. your link person goes on long-term sick leave and others are reluctant to deputise.

A flu epidemic resulting in half the staff and many pupils being away at a key time.

Changes in key staff, e.g. a new headteacher whose main focus is academic achievement or a member of staff carefully selected by you passing the job onto someone else because of other priorities.

Messages not being passed on.

Parental protest. This might take the form of concern about time taken away from academic subjects or sensitivity about the project content, e.g. an HIV/AIDS prevention initiative.

Staff who for various reasons do not follow instructions, e.g. in the administration of a questionnaire, resulting in biased outcomes to the project.

And more

There is no set formula for dealing with these kinds of things which, however justified, can be extremely frustrating. Talk them through with your manager, the headteacher and your link person. The key to success is willingness to change and adapt as necessary without compromising your project. Never show irritation but try to achieve an acceptable compromise through diplomacy and discussion.

Remember, you are a guest in school. The results will usually be very rewarding. Detail all changes to your original plan and the reasons why these have occurred in your report.

REFERENCES

OFSTED Handbooks (1995) Nursery and primary schools, special schools and secondary schools. London: HMSO.

Sex and Relationships Education in the Secondary School

Frances Hudson

INTRODUCTION AND DEFINITION

Personal and Social Education (PSE) encompasses a wide range of aims, subjects and learning methods. In recognition of this it is sometimes referred to as Personal and Social (Health/Moral) Education (PSH/ME), but is commonly known as Sex Education for short. Unfortunately, this shortening belies the purpose of both the subject matter and the aims.

The 1996 Education Act, quoted in the Sex Education Forum's briefing paper on sex education (1997a), requires all maintained secondary schools to make provision for sex education for all pupils, and defines sex education as having to include:

1. education about HIV and AIDS, and
2. any other sexually transmitted disease.

It is the duty of the governing body to form the policy and monitor its delivery and to do this in consultation with the head, the police and others in the community including parents.

In addition, all maintained schools are required to offer a curriculum which:

1. promotes the spiritual, moral, mental and physical development of pupils at the school and of society; and
2. prepares such pupils for the opportunities, responsibilities and experiences of adult life.

Such a programme should be given 'in such a manner as to encourage those pupils to have due regard to moral considerations and the value of family life' (Sex Education Forum, 1997a).

Evidence-based Health Promotion. Edited by Elizabeth R. Perkins, Ina Simnett and Linda Wright.
© 1999 John Wiley & Sons Ltd.

In this section I first illustrate how the health (in its widest sense) of children in the secondary school is not always well promoted. There follows a discussion of aspects of sexual health promotion which appear to be effective in the classroom.

DIFFICULTIES FOR SCHOOLS

Time

Most aspects of Personal and Social Education ('sex education') are not part of the national curriculum; only the biological facts related to reproduction remain, in science. The demands of the main subjects invariably have the effect of marginalising PSE.

Teaching

Where sex education consists of delivering biological and hormonal facts, there is little problem; facilitating discussion of children's and young people's opinions, hopes, expectations, fears, etc. regarding relationships is another matter. Not all teachers are willing, prepared or competent to do this. Health education is not a main subject in the undergraduate curriculum for teacher training. Where outside speakers are engaged the same time constraints apply. Family planning and school nurses are often invited to run sessions, and may or may not have had special training in teaching, or indeed in dealing with groups of young people in helping them to learn about these sensitive issues. Many schools operate their PSE programme with the nurse coming in for medical input. Both teachers and nurses may thus have had inadequate training, and have unmet needs for continuing supervision and support.

Parents may withdraw their child from all or part of sex education which does not form part of the national curriculum. Many teachers still do not understand what they may legally teach and, fearing parents' complaints and dissatisfaction, they worry about answering pupils' contraception queries, confidentiality, under 16s, and homosexuality. These concerns date from the Gillick controversy in the mid-1980s (Gillick versus West Norfolk and Wisbech Health Authority 1986, referred to in Bibbins, 1995), Section 28 of the 1988 Local Government Act (clause prohibiting the promotion of homosexuality) and the diversely interpretable wording of the Circular 5/94 (Department for Education, 1994).

Parents

The family is still expected to be the seat of information and moral training for children's sexual development and understanding. However, research shows that 94% of parents prefer sex education to be the responsibility of schools (Allen,

1987). Indeed, many children feel unable to discuss sexual relationships with their parents. And yet schools fear a moral backlash from parents and naturally feel cautious. Sex education policy and practice must take parents with them if a programme is to be effective.

DIFFICULTIES FOR CHILDREN

The constraints on schools and staff mentioned above have the effect of limiting the promotion of children's health and social education: their sense of worth, their confidence, relationship skills, even their knowledge – the very aspects which the 1996 Education Act (Department for Education, 1996) was designed to foster – are thus undermined.

Recent research undertaken in the Avon area (Hudson & West, 1996) which asked young people aged 13–21 about their sexual health provision found that, in spite of a well-thought out school policy and the goodwill of teachers, most respondents found education about sex and relationships inadequate. The following points from this research are not new; they have been made many times elsewhere:

- Too little, too late.
- Negative focus on prevention (pregnancy and HIV/AIDS).
- Real ignorance of other sexually transmitted diseases.
- Too many videos; little or no discussion.
- Little or no opportunity to talk or explore ideas or opinions.
- Groups are too large, inhibiting discussion.
- No help with preparation for the emotional side of relationships.
- Sessions insufficiently comprehensive, and inconsistent throughout the school career.
- No opportunity to acknowledge, let alone discuss, sexual orientations.
- Due to emphasis on reproduction and thus on heterosexual relationships, alternatives to vaginal sexual penetration are taboo.
- In spite of emphasis on prevention, programmes rarely include information as to the whereabouts of local clinics providing means of prevention of unplanned pregnancies and sexually transmitted diseases.
- Widespread ignorance among young people about emergency contraception and the anatomy of the opposite sex.
- No opportunity to reconcile the different attitudes to sex and relationships of young men on the one hand and young women on the other.
- Young people generally experience and expect adult disapproval for their behaviour.
- Boys particularly recognise the paucity of their sex education.

The young people felt short-changed. On the whole they felt they had some factual knowledge about contraception, including the condom, but none which helped them in a practical way to negotiate their relationships, none which helped them to ask for help, advice, support, little which informed them where to go, let alone help them negotiate the threshold. One young woman, aged 14, said: 'I knew there's a clinic in our area, but I wouldn't know what to do when I got there, and anyway I'm not 16 so I'm too young.'

This and many other examples demonstrate the huge potential gap between what information is made available ('There's a clinic in . . . Street, it's open between 5 and 7pm for family planning on Tuesdays and Thursdays') and what is accessible to those targeted. Are the words 'clinic' and 'family planning' appropriate to young people, for example? What happens there? Who will they have to see and how long will it take? The young people may not have their concerns addressed, such as: 'What will I be asked?' 'Does my mum have to find out?'

Gate-keeping is always a problem in targeting a particular group, especially when the group is children. What happens is that, while aiming to protect, we are in grave danger of ending up by ignoring, disempowering and actually handicapping the very children we purport to help. An example of this is a hard-pressed teacher with a list of PSE topics to deliver with a year 10 class, say. The class of 30 is mixed. The teacher is able to tick off her checklist as each topic is dealt with over the course of the programme. Occasionally, if the teacher is ill, a cover teacher will show, as instructed, a video; the chances are that this same video has already been seen by the group who, as before, have little or no opportunity to discuss the contents or style of it or relate any of it to their own lives. Apart from which, the relevance of any of the lesson is dependent on what is going on for each of the class members that week, that day, that hour, at home, at school; also what point on the scale in terms of sexual development and experience each child has reached.

It is all too easy to make assumptions. We talk, explain, repeat; it can still be misunderstood. The boy who went home and asked his mother why he hadn't started his periods yet; the boy whose mother revealed at a parents' evening that her son understood he could not use the sexual advice help-line because if he did they would think he had been abused. Children take what they can at any given time. A 14-year-old had heard that emergency contraception was equivalent to abortion and dared to say so in a PSE lesson. The teacher simply said it was not, backed this up with an explanation and moved on, hoping the matter had been dealt with. However, when the question came up again in a small group sex education lesson at the secure unit, where he was placed, he was still agitated. Using his experience, we were able to discuss choices, timing, responsibility, mistakes, and the needs of children, parents and families (Hudson & Manderfield, 1996). This tiny example shows how complex an issue is the whole business of 'sex education'.

As a result of the research previously mentioned, a telephone help-line was set up for young people with any question or issue about sexual health or related matters which they felt they could not discuss with anyone. As with other similar help-lines, it closed prematurely due to lack of calls. One of the reasons for this may well be a mismatch between what was attempted to get across to the target groups –

and what was actually received and understood. Although information about the line and the scope of its services reached schools, the heads, deputies, PSE teachers and school nurses made their own decisions about how to disseminate it. Some schools chose to put the flyers and cards advertising the help-line in the sixth form block only; others set the package aside until they had time to think what best to do with the information; others again were embarrassed about the information being seen by parents, governors or councillors coming into the school, and did nothing. One school nurse kept the cards in her drawer 'to hand out when she felt a child needed this sort of help' (Personal communication, school in North Somerset), and in the same school a teacher walked into his maths lesson to find a giggling group of 13–14-year-old boys round one boy who was handing out the help-line cards; when they saw 'Sir' they tried to hide them. He managed finally to explain that this was not a *sex* line but a *help* line. For all the explanation, they had misunderstood the nature of the help on offer. Possibly the adults concerned had equally misunderstood.

Young people need information which is easily accessible and posted anonymously round the school about how to access services for them outside school, to supplement the sex education within the school: which advice centres or clinics are open for them, who and what is available there, when they are open, what they offer, etc. In addition, access to the help must be straightforward. There are many stages for youngsters wanting to take responsibility for their sexual relationships: decide on protection, know where to go and when, pluck up courage to go (make an appointment? keep it?), ask their questions, obtain what they need, negotiate with the partner, use it effectively. Adults often fail to realise that saying 'where the clinic is' is not sufficiently encouraging.

We can see, therefore, how easily young people may be kept in ignorance. What they want most of all is someone to listen to them – unfazed, non-judgemental and with time to listen (Hudson & West, 1996).

SOCIETY'S AMBIVALENCE

Anomalies are widespread in the policy making, delivery, availability and accessibility of sex, relationships and general health education in secondary schools. While the government's intentions have been to reduce the incidence of teenage pregnancy, sexually transmitted diseases and other evils, there appears to be no coherent strategy for attaining such improvements. And teenagers' own concerns seem still to be at variance with goals dictated by government and health officials (Jacobson & Wilkinson, 1994) and what schools offer. Health professionals must realise that their efforts at promoting health and good relationships in the classroom pale into insignificance alongside the influence of peer group pressure, advertising, parental models, the need to experiment, and an impression of a 'mature' self-image (Macfarlane, 1993). The fact that sexual and health and relationships education as a whole subject is not part of the national curriculum (as it has been in Sweden, for example, for over 30 years (Genius & Genius, 1995)) is indicative of our society's covert lack of commitment to our children's physical and emotional well-being.

There are a number of different approaches to health education which need to be addressed together here. The *medical* approach aims for healthy lives free of disease and premature encumbrances (pregnancy); the *moral* approach is full of 'shouldn'ts' and 'oughts', doubts about the legitimacy of adolescent sex, protection of women and children and expectations that boys will be boys (i.e. unreliable); the *educational* approach tries to marry the two, and to provide factual information appropriately targeted – an impossible task, bearing in mind our traditional double standards. The hypocritical way in which we expect our young people to behave responsibly while withholding from them the resources for doing so beggars belief. It is not surprising to learn, therefore, that evaluations of school sex education programmes – few in number though they are – tend to show that they are frequently inadequate (Bagnall & Lockerbie, 1995).

WHAT WORKS

First and foremost, 'active learning' is an essential ingredient for what I call the 'Three Rs' (Respect, Responsibility and Relationships). Learning is:

> . . . that reflective activity which enables the learner to draw upon previous experience to understand and evaluate the present, so as to shape future action and formulate new knowledge (Kirby, 1995).

Active learning processes include group building, repetition, reinforcement and a 'ritual' lesson structure; working step by step at the students' pace; using simple creative activities where students can work together and learn relationship skills; not rushing students or answering for them; making it fun so students don't realise they're learning; or, most importantly, if they are aware of their learning, that they enjoy it.

Programmes must aim to counteract myths; encourage discussions; develop a shared understanding between males and females; facilitate later negotiations between couples; involve pupils in identifying their own health education needs and wishes, boys as much as girls, and encourage them to work in small 'friendship' groups which meet regularly; and include parents as partners in the learning process. (See Examples of Good Practice later in this section for illustrations of some of this.)

Making time to listen, making no assumptions about young people's preferences or behaviour, checking that educational messages have been both received and understood are vital to the process. Linking school programmes openly with local community health services is part of this overall care for children's welfare, and something which is mentioned time and again as evidence of good practice (Hudson & West, 1996; Sex Education Forum, 1997b).

All the above provide models of 'good enough parenting' which is what, after all, is needed if our children are to grow up into responsible and caring adults. If we were to learn to treat our bodies and emotions with as much respect, and give them as much attention, as we give to the traditional three Rs (reading, writing and sums), we would be much better equipped for relationships in general and the responsibilities of adulthood. It is curious that, as sexual beings from birth, we are left to grope in the dark and learn 'on the hoof'.

EXAMPLES OF GOOD PRACTICE

However, in spite of the double standards to contend with and an appalling lack of funds and time, there are throughout the UK pockets of excellent work being done in secondary schools.

The 'A PAUSE' project began in 1992 in Exeter with the aim of teaching a whole school sex education programme which would lead to a decrease in sexual activity. It is in my view one of the best programmes in terms of style and approach; the built-in evaluation is a vital aspect. The effectiveness of a programme can only be measured if it is regularly evaluated or audited.

Teachers in this programme are specifically trained for delivering the main bulk of the programme, with a doctor providing the medical component; this medical input results in greater credence in the programme as a whole. Peer education is also an important part of this project, and training for this is built in. The results are distinctly positive, with feedback from students, older peer leaders, teachers, school management, governors and education providers (Tripp & Mellanby, 1995). It is extremely encouraging that a programme of this calibre is available to an increasing number of school pupils. It is disappointing, however, that it has to be bought in. It is a model of such excellent practice that all schools should be doing something similar, with the will and the finances to fund it.

A sex and relationships education programme run at a secure unit by outside specialists (Hudson & Manderfield, 1996) has had some of the advantages mentioned above, in that we have small groups (up to eight, average five) of boys aged 13 to 17. The programme is run by a trainer/counsellor and a family planning nurse, both with long-term experience with young people and sexual health from different perspectives. They run the programme together (as team facilitators) for seven sessions over a term. Each group moves at its own pace, according to the individual's needs.

The experience of the trainer corroborates the findings of much of the research regarding yawning gaps in knowledge and relationship skills, reliance on myths and lack of emotional/cognitive connections with relationships generally. Feedback from staff and students tells us that this kind of approach works, in that it enables students to explore some of their own thinking and feeling. The young men have particular needs and the atmosphere, pace, style and content of the sessions have encouraged them to engage in the subject matter as it relates to them, to talk freely, to think aloud without being sniggered at, and to respect their mates' points of view.

Such a programme comes for many too late and it is too little. However, it is better than a one-off visit, which is sadly the policy of far too many schools even today. Anyone who has read Carol Lee's *The ostrich position* (1983) and *Talking tough* (1993) will appreciate the expertise and effectiveness of the experienced sex educator who sees groups of young people regularly over a period of time. The majority of young people are not so fortunate.

Other Examples of Current Practice

One outside educator tells how she was invited into one particular school as a speaker to a large year group of 80 plus. Her job was not to give information, rather to operate as a catalyst for discussion, providing stimulus and provoking thought. The large group then divided into small groups for an hour's discussion, each with a member of staff who had heard the speaker. During the rest of the half term further discussion was generated in tutor groups. She would hold forth to fourth, fifth, lower and upper sixth year pupils (now years 10, 11 12 and 13). She saw her role 'not as teaching but as opening up the knottier aspects, dealing with the bit they found difficult – talking about relationships'. Each year the pupils met her again for more, and the discussions continued in small groups, and in a different gear. As a programme she felt this was as effective as any, given the usual financial and timetable constraints. There was never any evaluative assessment of her input.

In another example, a family planning nurse doubles as outreach worker, going into schools and youth groups for one-off sessions with groups of about 20. In one school the teacher continues the sex education with her own follow-up – thus two sessions. This meagre input is not evaluated. With young men in a youth justice centre, working in small groups, she has a much better feel of the efficacy of her input. Feedback via probation officers is positive, but again the programme is not formally assessed.

In a comprehensive school on the city margins, catering for children on a large housing estate with typically few resources and high unemployment, the teacher in charge of PSE throughout feels strongly that school is not the right setting for 'sex education'. Such basic, holistic, all-encompassing, life determining matters should be the responsibility of all professionals, all adults, all parents. Sex education should not be made the burden of the few, reliant on scant resources meted out by an authority itself constrained by budgets and politics. However, given the limitations of the timetable, this teacher has achieved over the years what often seemed like the impossible. A play about HIV/AIDS, 'Positive Vibes' was a social and cultural innovation in an area which saw little creativity. The players performed in several schools in the county, and parents were enthusiastic about this way of disseminating information. The young thespians learnt a great deal, gaining insight and responsibility as well as information; doing drama is cathartic, and of course it was enormous fun to do. They also developed a sense of pride in themselves and respect for the wider issue of sexual diseases and a more tolerant view of the sufferers. It is generally thought that parents profited at least as much as the pupils by this exercise, enabled as they were to gain more understanding of the issue without having to admit to their ignorance. Out of this came the video, which has been widely circulated, and T-shirts.

Another creative activity which pulled many pupils together in a school was making a quilt in memory of those who had died of AIDS-related diseases. This inevitably became a cross-curricular, multi-subject exercise, bringing freely to discussion such otherwise uncomfortable issues as illness, infectious diseases, death, taboo, prejudice, homosexuality, sex, contraception and parenthood.

CONCLUSIONS

Such cross-curricular activities, invading and dissolving in every subject, surely replicate the place of sex and sexuality in human life. It is bizarre that the most basic and powerful force in our lives has no place at the top of the official education and health agenda for children and young people. One school nurse at a comprehensive school is resignedly pessimistic about her role. She is listener, comforter and adviser to those youngsters who stray in her direction; and she has her practical input on the PSE programme throughout the school – which she sees as positive and useful, albeit limited. However, she has to divide her time between schools, and is currently part of a restructuring process which will spread her time even more thinly in future. She is aware that children's sexual information and emotional needs are not met at home, that school (along with the local health clinic) really should be much more clued up in order to make up for the gaps at home.

Her observations echo those of so many who strive to encourage and enable children to come to terms with their sexuality in a confusing society of media pressure, sexual double standards, moral dicta – and uncanny silence. We know that what young people get is not sufficient for their needs, but this evidence is for the most part anecdotal – with due respect to those evaluative studies which do show evidence of good practice. What is needed is more evaluative work on current PSE programmes so that future funding will be seen to be clearly worthwhile. Many serious studies have highlighted the need for a flexible, open, holistic approach to sex education (Ingham, 1993; 1997 and others; Peckham, 1992; RCOG (Royal College of Obstetrics and Gynaecology), 1991). The target for *Health of the Nation* (Department of Health, 1992) to reduce the number of pregnancies to the under 16s (to take but one) is far from being reached. It would be exciting to see the government taking these and other studies seriously and corporately, with the Departments of Education and Health together taking the lead in schools and putting PS(H/M)E at the top of the national curriculum agenda. Meanwhile there is much that still needs to be done in order to gather evidence of what works, how and why.

REFERENCES

Allen I (1987) Sex education and personal relationships. London: Policy Studies Institute.

Bagnall G & Lockerbie L (1995) HIV/AIDS education: are senior pupils losing out? *Education and Health*, 13(3), 37–42.

Bibbins L (1995) Gender, sexuality and sex education. In N Harris (Ed), Children, sex education and the law: examining the issues. London: National Children's Bureau.

Department for Education (1994) Circular 5/94. Education Act 1993: Sex Education in Schools. London: DfE.

Department for Education (1996) 1996 Education Act. London: DfE.

Department of Health (1992) The Health of the Nation: a strategy for health in England. London: HMSO.

Genius S J & Genius S K (1995) Adolescent sexual involvement: time for primary prevention. *The Lancet*, 345, 240–241.

Hudson F & Manderfield M (1996) Vinney Green PSE Programme. Unpublished report. Bristol: Vinney Green Secure Unit.

Hudson F & West J (1996) Needing to be heard: the young person's agenda. *Education and Health*, 14(3), 43–47.

Ingham R (1993) Can we have a policy on sex? Setting targets for teenage pregnancies. Occasional paper. Institute of Health Policy Studies, University of Southampton.

Ingham R (1997) When you're young and in love. Southampton: University of Southampton.

Jacobson L D & Wilkinson C E (1994) Review of teenage health: time for a new direction. *British Journal of General Practice*, 44, 420–424.

Kirby D (1995) Editorial. *British Medical Journal*, 311, 7002.

Lee C (1983) The ostrich position: sex, schooling and mystification. London: Unwin.

Lee C (1993) Talking tough: the fight for masculinity. London: Arrow Books.

Macfarlane A (1993) Health promotion and children and teenagers. *British Medical Journal*, 306, 81.

Peckham S (1992) Unplanned pregnancy and teenage pregnancy: a review. Occasional Paper, Institute of Health Policy Studies, University of Southampton.

Royal College of Obstetrics and Gynaecology (1991) Report of the RCOG Working Party on unplanned pregnancy. London: RCOG.

Sex Education Forum (1997a) Factsheet 12, Education Act 1996 – briefing paper on sex education. London: Sex Education Forum.

Sex Education Forum (1997b) Factsheet 13, Sex Education Matters. London: National Children's Bureau.

Tripp J and Mellanby A (1995) Sex education – whose baby? *Current Paediatrics*, 5, 272–276.

Drug and Alcohol Education

Ruth Joyce

HISTORICAL CONTEXT

In 1986, the Department for Education and Science (as it then was) supported the development of drug education by part funding drug education co-ordinator posts in all Local Education Authorities. This was the first of a range of department initiatives heralding a core drug education entitlement for young people in schools. This access to core drug education took ten years to achieve and happened in September 1996, as part of the Department for Education and Employment's work within the Government strategy 'Tackling Drugs Together'.

Until 1986, drug and alcohol education had been developing in schools and the youth services, but often in a haphazard and unco-ordinated way. If a school had a query, problem, or wanted support they had turned to the few services who were able to offer anything. Sometimes the police were asked, the local drug agency (if one existed), or local doctor or pharmacist could be called on for their expert and sometimes differing advice.

For the education authorities who were able to employ a drug education co-ordinator, it was, for many, the first time that a lead person was able to offer expert educational support. Schools were needing to address a rise in the number of young people who were using substances at an increasingly young age while at the same time feeling the need to deliver a preventive educational programme to all pupils.

The author of this section spent her early days of working as a drug co-ordinator for Cambridgeshire Education Authority focused on setting up the inevitable systems necessary to function. But it also required something much more critical – the building of relationships within the education service and, more particularly, outside the service.

A range of other bodies had already developed links with schools around drug and health issues. Much work was already going on in the county, but provision

Evidence-based Health Promotion. Edited by Elizabeth R. Perkins, Ina Simnett and Linda Wright.
© 1999 John Wiley & Sons Ltd.

was far from being equable throughout all schools. This was not surprising with three health authorities sometimes serving one county, but neither was it helpful in the move towards developing consistent practice in all the county's schools.

Schools in the south of the area were offered a very different service from those in the north, with very little being offered to schools in the central area. There was little consistency in either the message or the approach and, as the increasing number of schools requiring help rose, the variations and inequalities were becoming more apparent.

From my drug education co-ordinator's view it was this often patchy and some-times contradictory drug advice that had, historically, been offered to schools that was of greatest concern.

Health authorities were also becoming more interested in ensuring that the drug services they purchased were effective and this also had an effect on the quality and level of provision for drug education.

THE PROCESS OF DEVELOPING AN ALLIANCE

This pressure on education and health services, coupled with the need to develop consistent provision for all schools led to the first stages of the partnership working which became known as 'The Alliance in Drug and Alcohol Education'.

As the newly appointed drug education co-ordinator it was my task to develop a coherent and consistent message to all schools. It was also apparent that there needed to be a clear understanding and definition of what was meant by 'quality'. For too long, support for drug education had suffered from a range of approaches, with little account taken of their effectiveness, often with no clear views of the aims of the model adopted and certainly little attention paid to monitoring and evaluation strategies. It was this particular development, to identify and develop good practice, that was the main focus of the work of the alliance.

It became increasingly apparent that schools wanted assurance that anyone they asked for support should be able to offer work of defined quality and that health purchasers needed assurance that the time taken up supporting schools was being spent in the best possible way. The stages in the development of the alliance are set out below.

STAGES OF DEVELOPMENT OF ALLIANCE IN DRUG AND ALCOHOL EDUCATION

- Need identified
- Steering group identified
- Key groups contacted as potential partners in the alliance
- A literature search to explore effectiveness of various models of drug education

- Meetings fixed
- Papers circulated describing the model, potential contents and the process of development
- First meeting – quality issues debated, a list of criteria for effective interventions in schools identified, and quality assurance standards drawn up
- School/service contract designed and piloted
- Partners asked to circulate service descriptions within their own teams for approval and signatory commitment
- Visits and training offered to all potential partner organisations
- Group reconvened to discuss the draft alliance document
- Draft rewritten
- Final draft circulated for approval in all partnership organisations
- Document redrafted, printed, launched and distributed to schools
- Monitoring process
- Rewrite and update

KEY AREAS OF DEVELOPMENT

There are six key areas in this process of development:

1. Partners
2. The literature search
3. Quality issues – quality standards and quality assurance
4. Contract
5. Training programme
6. Monitoring process

Each of these is discussed in turn.

Partners

The key potential key members of the alliance were identified by the steering group – from the education service, police service and health services. This included drug services, health promotion units, voluntary agencies and the local prison service. Senior staff from primary and secondary schools were also invited.

The Literature Search

This was managed through the services of the Institute for the Study of Drug Dependency (ISDD) (see Useful Address at the end of this section) where key pieces of research were studied.

Key points which identified the elements of quality provision were identified from these documents (ACMD (Advisory Council on the Misuse of Drugs), 1993;

Coggans at al., 1991; De Haes & Schurman 1975; Dorn & Murji, 1992). They were used as the basis for a briefing paper which was distributed to all the potential partners. This formed the source of good practice which each member of the alliance was being asked to support in their work in schools.

Quality Issues – Quality Standards and Quality Assurance

The alliance agreed a set of standards which are set out below.

- The role of the alliance partners was *not* to undertake direct teaching in schools, but to offer appropriate support that reflected the skills of their service
- The alliance partners would not support 'one off' input
- Shock/horror approaches would not be used
- Pupils needed accurate information about the law, physiological and psychological effects of drugs and a realistic account of the positive and negative implications of drug misuse for the individual, the family and society
- The main aims of drug education should be to provide accurate information, emphasise the benefits of a healthy lifestyle and to provide the knowledge skills and attitudes challenges which lead young people to make informed decisions
- Teachers must always be present at pupil sessions to support the learning experience during and after any visiting support
- All approaches to drug education should be regularly monitored and rigorously evaluated

The alliance also developed and agreed commitments about quality assurance. The agreements are set out below.

QUALITY ASSURANCE AGREEMENTS OF THE ALLIANCE PARTNERS

- Regular appraisal
- Receive and read relevant government documentation
- Use the contract form
- Evaluate the sessions
- Keep the alliance directory up to date
- Meet on an annual basis with all the alliance partners

Contract

The contract form (the 'request form') was developed to ensure that anyone offering a service to a school would have a basic set of information before they

SECTION 5

Request Form

Request form for service involvement in Drug Education in Cambridgeshire schools, colleges and youth services

- Please photocopy this form and retain a blank for future use

- When you have completed the form, please keep a copy yourself

- Please answer the following questions and return the form to the service you have chosen from the Directory section of this booklet

The Healthy Alliance in
Drug & Alcohol Education

EDUCATION FOR
YOUNG PEOPLE IN
CAMBRIDGESHIRE
SCHOOLS

Organisation

| Address | *Willowbank School Lower Road Ely, Cambridge* |

| Post Code | *CB4 8SJ* | Telephone number | *01353-678935* |

| Name of member of staff making request | Ms | Miss | Mrs | (Mr) | *Tony Davies* |

Target Group

Please check/enter relevant information in boxes below

Student Age/Year Group	*14/15 yrs.* *Year 10.*
Youth Group	*N/A*
Parents	*N/A*
Governors	*N/A*
Staff	*N/A*
Others (Please state)	

Practical Details

Time of session	*9.30 a.m. → 10.20 a.m.*
Number in group	*26*
Space available	*Classroom — semi circle chairs (no tables)*

—— **Education for Young People in Cambridgeshire Schools** ——

Aims – What are the aims of the session?

- to introduce pupils to local support services for drug and alcohol provision

Organisation – If the support is for students, which area(s) of the curriculum (e.g. Science PSHE) is the session part of?

P.S.H.E. — although the factual side is complemented by the science curriculum

Prior Education – What Drug Education have the group received so far?

8 lessons in yr. 10
3 in yr. 9
3 in yr. 8

Follow Up – How will the session be followed up immediately?

from 10.20 → 10.45 — general discussion self study exercise — to discover national support services

Future Plans – What are the future plans for Drug Education with this group?

To develop a peer information leaflet on 'here's who to help if you have a problem'

Other comments

The students will introduce you and manage the session with my support — I will be there all the time — please remember the evaluation we discussed over the phone

Signature of applicant ___Tony Davies___

Signature of appropriate manager ___Mr J. Gawthrop-Hay___

Date 6.3.96

Thank you for filling in this form. We hope it will provide a better service for you. Please keep a photocopy of this form and send the original to the support agency

— Education for Young People in Cambridgeshire Schools —

went in to work with the school. It also gave schools the opportunity to be clear about what they really wanted. It proved invaluable in bringing clarity to members of the alliance and has subsequently been adopted by other areas of health education as a key way of maximising opportunities to support schools.

Training Programme

A training programme offered to the partner agencies ensured that all individuals understood the principles of the alliance. The police offered a four-day programme to 20 officers which they were required to complete before they were able to work in the school classroom. The voluntary alcohol agency used the opportunity to extend the session to all their staff to ensure they all offered a consistent message. The three drug agencies shared training sessions.

Monitoring Process

The success of the alliance depends very much upon the commitment and support of individual members. Although a formal evaluation has not been undertaken, regular monitoring is done by logging the contract forms by each partner and by an annual review meeting of the partners which considers progress over the year and new research and developments in drug education. These, and other necessary updates, are integrated into the alliance document which is reprinted and redistributed to all schools in the county.

Of course the work of the alliance has its critics and of course it isn't perfect – but as an exercise designed to develop a consistent and quality approach to school support on drugs issues across a large, mainly rural area there has been a measurable improvement in the level and quality of the provision.

Relationships between partners in the alliance have been enhanced and we are much more aware of our own boundaries of expertise and more aware of what other services can, and should, be offering to schools. Undoubtedly we are all aware that joint working takes a great deal of time – but we acknowledge the benefits to those to whom we are accountable, to those who receive our support and to ourselves. The alliance has increased all our understanding about the range of services which are available to schools to support them in playing their individual significant part in helping young people deal with their world, where the presence of a range of drugs is a fact of life.

REFERENCES

Advisory Council on the Misuse of Drugs (1993) Drug education in schools: the need for new impetus. London: HMSO.

Coggans N et al. (1991) National evaluation of drug education in Scotland. Research Monograph No. 4. Scotland: ISDO.

De Haes W & Schurman J H (1975) Results of an evaluation study of three drug education methods. *International Journal of Health Education*, 18, 1–16.

Dorn N & Murji K (1992) Drug prevention: a review of the English language literature. Research Monograph No. 5. London: ISDD.

USEFUL ADDRESS

Institute for the Study of Drug Dependency
32–36 Loman Street
London SE1 OEE
Tel: 0171 928 1211

Chapter 9

Working in Informal Settings

Ina Simnett

INTRODUCTION

This chapter aims to help those who wish to work effectively in informal settings. While formal education is a major force, most people are not engaged in it and the pattern of inequality in learning echoes, in many respects, that in inequalities in health. So, in order to engage with those people most in need, health promoters must work with them in a variety of informal settings, often alongside informal educators such as youth workers. Informal educators work at two levels: directly influencing the behaviour of people and developing knowledge and understanding; or through strengthening the capacity of communities to respond to learning. The latter involves helping to repair the social fabric of society by building 'social capital': communities characterised by high levels of trust and many overlapping and diverse networks for communication and exchange of information and ideas.

The first section of this chapter describes what we mean by informal education, and suggests that informal education forms part of the bedrock of democratic societies. It describes the problems of assessment and evaluation in these settings, and how the solutions of managers can undermine the benefits of informal education. It highlights potential areas of tension between health promoters and informal educators.

The second section focuses on detached youth work and highlights how this differs from outreach work in projects with a specific remit (such as alcohol and drugs). It continues by describing one initiative, 'Positive Options', based in a disadvantaged part of Middlesbrough. It describes the role of health promotion in detached youth work and the outcomes of group work with young people. It concludes with practical guidance on how to go about it.

Evidence-based Health Promotion. Edited by Elizabeth R. Perkins, Ina Simnett and Linda Wright.

Informal Education and Health Promotion

Tony Jeffs and Mark K. Smith

The size and scale of the formal educational system is awesome. Over eight million youngsters attend UK schools where they are fed, taught and administered by around 500 000 adults. Post school a million or so students attend universities and colleges; and around four million adults enrol for part-time courses each year. All this activity, all these people following curricula, being tested and collecting certificates, help convey an impression that education is something that takes place in schools and colleges. When education is discussed it is usually what is, or is not, happening in schools and colleges that is the focus. The significance and value of formal education should not be underestimated. Success in the system correlates with benefits such as higher life-time earnings, more secure employment, greater longevity and improved health status.

However, education is not the sole prerogative of formal institutions. Children, young people and adults alike continuously engage in learning experiences outside the classroom. Learning from each other in conversation, from their experiences and from books, posters and television. At any one time 10% of adults in the UK are trying to teach themselves something informally – at home, at work or elsewhere (Sargant et al., 1997). Since the onset of mass schooling, during the early part of the nineteenth century, many educators have perceived the importance of work beyond the 'school gates'. Their reasons for doing so, not least in relation to health issues, have remained remarkably consistent.

WHY LOOK BEYOND FORMAL EDUCATION?

First, while formal education is a major force, the majority of people are not involved in it. If we turn to some of the classic indicators a familiar pattern emerges. For example, Sargant et al.'s (1997) study found that significantly more women (41%) than men (31%) report undertaking no (organized) learning since leaving full-time education. They also found that over half of upper- and middle-class (AB)

Evidence-based Health Promotion. Edited by Elizabeth R. Perkins, Ina Simnett and Linda Wright.

respondents were current or recent learners compared with one-quarter of unskilled working-class people and people on limited income (DE); and that there were marked regional differences in participation in organised learning. The pattern of inequality in adult learning echoes, in many respects, that in health. For example, those areas with the lowest participation rates in adult education appear to have the highest rates of infant mortality (Dorling, 1997; Sargant et al., 1997).

For those concerned with young people, there can be a desire to reach those alienated from school – those who may attend in body but are absent in spirit, as well as their peers who truant. The fear, often exaggerated, is that this cluster includes those most likely to succumb to health-threatening behaviours, or in the case of young women, become pregnant. Truants are, in most respects, boringly similar to their peers who regularly attend (O'Keefe, 1993). However, those not attending are missing out on learning opportunities. Also, disproportionately present in their ranks are those who are victims of bullying (which is linked to a higher frequency of illness and disease, Balding et al., 1996); and under-achievers (who are more likely to attempt suicide, smoke cigarettes, use alcohol excessively and be sexually careless, Blum, 1987).

Health educators can often only engage with these adults and young people by seeking them out. This entails working in those localities where they are to be found – the street, shopping mall, youth and community projects or at home, or through creating environments which they find attractive. This might mean drop-in centres, youth clubs and cafes, where the worker can build relationships which have an educational element. As with the school setting either trained health professionals can operate in such places alongside informal educators or the latter can be equipped to better incorporate a health promotion component within their practice.

Second, what is taught in schools and other institutions is circumscribed by law and the perpetual threat of external interference regarding both content and mode of delivery. For decades Victorian prudery made it impossible to discuss matters relating to sexual health in schools just as today the law prevents open and honest deliberation on sexuality. The constraints on honest and open presentation do not, it seems, evaporate over time but merely change their focus. Candid dialogue regarding drug use is also inconceivable. Students know that for teachers to keep their jobs many, perhaps even the majority, are obliged to lie about their own tastes, preferences and usages. Fear produces the 'I smoked but never inhaled' type response to direct questions which invariably insult the intelligence of the audience and demean the teacher (Allen, 1987). It also kindles a reliance on pre-packaged teaching materials and presentational styles which focus on information giving, both of which predictably thwart dialogue.

Perhaps not surprisingly, one study found that less than half of one per cent of young people felt confident about sharing a 'health problem' with a teacher, whereas approaching a third, by the time they left, would take a 'career problem' to them (Balding, 1995; 1996). Those seeking 'honest' answers, particularly in relation to drugs and sexual health therefore rightly seek out alternative sources of advice, information and support. For the majority friends, siblings and the media (TV, films, books and magazines) 'teach' them what they need to know (Balding, 1996). Many health educators are aware of the limitations of both school-based strategies and the laissez-faire substitute (Dennehy et al., 1996; Mellanby et al., 1995; Nutbeam et al., 1993). This awareness creates a willingness to exploit alternative modes of intervention and educational practice – such as peer education, the visual arts and informal education – as a means of influencing behaviour and developing understanding.

Third, the concepts and information encountered in formal approaches frequently lack relevance. A class or year group contains students in possession of a wide range of experiences and understandings. Commonalities of age or locality can never be assumed to guarantee a heterogeneity of understanding. Material relating to sexual health, child care or drugs, for example, may have little meaning to some at the time of delivery. Relevance may not be apparent until certain experiences or encounters have taken place. Hendry et al. (1995) found many young people, and one suspects adults would have responded similarly if asked, professed to have no recollection of encountering health education in school even though this was unlikely to have been the case. Others seemed to have all the 'information' but needed assistance regarding interpretation, appraisal and application.

This takes us into the classic domain of experiential learning – learning arising out of a direct encounter with a phenomenon. Here the central concern is how experience can be enlarged and emancipated (Dewey, 1933). It is all too easy to 'repeat our mistakes'. If there is to be development, then feelings have to be entertained and experiences revisited. Connections have to be made and theories developed about why we acted in this way or that. If this is done effectively then the evidence suggests that in comparison with the information assimilation process prevalent in formal education, experiential learning is likely to last longer and to provide an intrinsic motivation for learning. People are immediately working on what they see as problematic (see Boud et al., 1993). However, such learning is ultimately dependent upon intervention from others and here informal educators work at two levels. They may engage directly with people – helping to clarify, re-enforce and make sense of previous learning. Or they may seek generally to strengthen the capacity of people in communities and networks to respond to each other in ways that foster learning.

Fourth, and linked to the last point, formal education remains firmly locked into individualised learning. Even where groups are used there is a tendency to look to changes in individuals rather than the ability of the group to function for the benefit of its members. A key strand in informal education has a been a concern for interaction and for communities of learners. Informal educators operate with people who share interests, life experiences or friendships. For example a worker might specifically target young people with a common sexual orientation in order to address health or social needs that might be disregarded or marginalised by mainstream agencies (Batsleer, 1996). They work in settings in which young and old alike are more likely to be both more relaxed and receptive to learning. While they may be concerned with what individuals are learning, they will also have an eye on the capacity of the group or network. Informal educators will look to both strengthen the way in which people relate to each other and to deepen the knowledge and skills held within those relationships. They focus on people as members of groups and communities, they look to 'the whole person acting in the world' (Lave & Wenger, 1991). This is of particular interest in relation to health, given the extensive use of, and reliance upon, informal networks by people for information, support and practical help. An approach that focuses on such networks not only provides for the possibility of earlier guidance and care, it also actively fosters health with its concern for relationship and emotional under-standing.

WHAT IS INFORMAL EDUCATION?

So far we have been using the term 'informal education' without saying in any detail what we mean by it. Part of the problem is that the dominant language in this area is administrative. A common categorization involves formal, non-formal and informal education. In this approach informal education is the lifelong process in which people learn from everyday experience, and non-formal education is organised educational activity outside formal systems (Coombs & Ahmed, 1974). Formal education is linked with schools and training institutions; non-formal education with community groups and non-governmental organisations; and informal education covers what is left. This is an unhelpful way of looking at educational activity. A lot of 'organised educational activity' takes place in families and everyday settings and is not sponsored by any formal institution (Henze, 1992).

Informal education is perhaps better approached through process – and seen as part of a continuum. We have looked to formal education as essentially curricula-driven. In other words, it entails a plan of action and defined content. It also involves creating a particular social and physical setting – the most familiar example being the classroom. In contrast, informal education is driven by conversation. It is not tied to particular environments so it can happen anywhere (Jeffs & Smith, 1990; 1996). Whether we are identified as a formal or informal educator we will use a mix of the formal and informal. What sets the two apart is the relative emphasis placed on curricula and conversation, and the range of settings in which they may work.

Informal education tends to be unpredictable – workers do not know where it might lead. In conversation they have to catch the moment where they can say or do something to deepen people's thinking or to put others in touch with their feelings. This 'going with the flow' opens up all sorts of possibilities. On one hand, educators may not be prepared for what comes, on the other, they can get into rewarding areas. There is the chance, for example, to connect with the questions, issues and feelings that are important to people, rather than what they think might be significant. This is also likely to take educators into the world of people's feelings, experiences and relationships. While all educators should attend to experience and encourage people to reflect, informal educators are thrown into this. For the most part, they do not have lesson plans to follow; they respond to situations, to experiences (Smith, 1997).

So what is informal education? From what we have looked at so far we can say the following. Informal education:

- works through, and is driven by, conversation.
- involves exploring and enlarging experience.
- can take place in any setting.

However, there is more – purpose.

At one level, the purpose of informal education is no different to any other form of education. In one situation we may focus on, say, healthy eating, in another family relationships. However, running through all this, we argue, is a concern to build the sorts of communities and relationships in which people can be happy and fulfilled. John Dewey (1916) once described this as educating so that people may share in a common life. Those working as informal educators have a special contribution to make here. First, a focus on conversation is central to building communities. The sorts of values and behaviours needed for conversation to take place are exactly what are required if neighbourliness and democracy are to flourish. What is more, the sorts of groups informal educators (such as youth and social action workers) work with – voluntary, community-based, and often concerned with mutual aid – are the bedrock of democratic societies (Jeffs & Smith, 1996; Smith, 1997).

THE CHALLENGE OF ASSESSMENT AND EVALUATION

Even in the context of a school, where feedback can be built into a session and the participants are legally forced to attend and thus 're-visited' to assess knowledge acquisition, attempts to measure the effectiveness of health education programmes have proved 'notoriously difficult' (Hendry et al., 1995). How and when knowledge or an educational experience changes behaviour cannot, if at all, be readily assessed. As an unusually progressive secondary headteacher explained to one of the authors in a recent interview, his school had for over 30 years repudiated physical punishments, developed a strategy for controlling bullying by staff and students alike and consistently sought to encourage behavioural norms which eschewed aggression and violence. Reflecting on whether this had been a success he answered that it was impossible to judge because the school could not for example ever know if their ex-students 'were better, more considerate, less violent parents, husbands and neighbours than they would have been if they had gone to another school' (interview). The absorption of information and facts can obviously be tested but social and health education will always be based on an act of faith.

In the formal sector governments have become obsessed with the measurement of educational outcomes as a means of conveying an impression that they wish to secure both heightened efficiency (value for money) and greater control over teachers. An inevitable by-product of the imposition of testing, a national curriculum and school league tables has been a mounting pressure upon educators to focus their efforts on what will be tested rather than what they might perceive it to be their duty to teach. Frills like health and social education, the liberal arts and sports have inevitably been marginalised; sacrificed at the altar of spurious vocationalism. In part informal educators have been beneficiaries of this myopic attention on the 'core' curriculum. It has forced health managers to look beyond the school if they are to meet key targets in relation to young people. Those seeking to promote health have, much as those seeking to develop in the young an interest in the sporting, artistic and spiritual aspects of life, found that they cannot rely on the schools to give adequate attention to these matters. However, they, like their compatriots in education, have not been immune from those imperatives and pressures which are increasingly obliging schools and colleges to limit their vision and educational ambitions. For health promoters have more and more been encouraged to set and enforce definite outcomes and measures of the value-added element of an educational programme. This inevitably encourages face-to-face workers to focus their attention on what can and will be measured in the short-term and seek out the more receptive in order to achieve their pre-ordained outputs. Consequently as those promoting health education have looked towards the informal sector as a potential ally, so they have often threatened to undermine its effectiveness by imposing inappropriate funding and managerial constraints upon practitioners.

Unfortunately within the informal education sector attempts to measure outcomes have generally ranged from the pathetic to the ludicrous. Great play is made in recent literature of the need to provide 'output indicators', 'qualitative criteria' (Huskins, 1996), 'objective success measures' (France & Wiles, 1996), 'adequate assessment criteria' (OFSTED, 1997a) and evidence of how 'young people have developed personally and socially through participation' (OFSTED, 1997b). However, advocates of such measures tend to be strong on exhortation but uniformly deficient when it comes to moving beyond bland generalisations to the specifics of how these measures of effectiveness might operate. The problem is, of course, of attempting to assess the unassessable.

First, the variables which influence a given behaviour cannot be simplistically disaggregated. You can certainly test to see if teen crime is higher on an estate where the youth club is open every weekday evening compared to a locality which lacks such provision, but what will the difference, if it even exists, prove? For given the oft-cited links between youth crime and school ethos (Graham &

Bowling, 1995), early years intervention (Graham & Bennett, 1995), family support (Lally et al., 1988: Schweinhart & Weikart, 1993) and policing practice it rapidly becomes impossible to assess the impact of a single informal education project.

Second, the members of the community 'worked with' frequently cannot be easily isolated because contact with a worker takes many varied forms such as individual and group conversations, festivals, activity weekends, counselling, supporting self-help and peer education programmes and providing the infrastructure which will allow formal inputs to take place in the form of adult classes and discussion groups. Also 'clients' may be highly mobile, the intensity of relationships are highly variable and in many settings the identity of contacts may remain unknown. It is, therefore, impossible to construct even a meaningful assessment procedure based on 'client satisfaction'.

Third, change can rarely be monitored even on an individual basis. For example, an informal educator who decides to focus on alcohol abuse within a particular group or community faces an insurmountable problem if subsequently challenged to provide evidence of success. For they will be unable to ascertain use levels prior to intervention, during contact or subsequent to the completion of their work. In the end all the worker will be able to offer is vague evidence relating to contact or anecdotal material. Attempts by the government in Northern Ireland to impose, for political reasons, a youth work curriculum serve to illustrate the inherent difficulties which flow from any attempt to measure what is achieved in this sector. For as one report explained, 'clubs and organisations are becoming more adept at report writing showing programmes met funding criteria rather than the needs of individual young people and their communities' (Milburn et al., 1995). It also led to work being focused on 'clubs' and 'centres' where contacts could be monitored and numbers counted to prove work had taken place. Inevitably this led to a decline in the volume of work undertaken with those groups or individuals who were unattached or more difficult to reach.

Last, but not least, there is an issue with time-scale. Change of the sort with which informal educators are concerned does not happen overnight. With shifts into short-term project funding around defined issues, the length and variety of relationship that has been involved in locally-based community education and youth work is less likely to occur. Through reflection on changing relationships and upon how people respond differently to situations some assessment of progress was possible over time by both educators and participants. Indeed, this process of reflection was central to the work. However, what this process tends to do is to identify the change – it is much harder to identify in any detailed way what the pivotal factors were in the change for the reasons outlined above.

Both in relation to health promotion and crime reduction funders have sought to find a solution to the innate problem of an inability to measure outcomes. In doing so they have tended to create 'extremely tight contracts' (Nettleton & Burrows, 1997) which focus on process rather than outcomes. If you cannot quantify product, then ensuring they give value for money by controlling their time and movements seems to increasingly be the approach of those funding health promotion initiatives. Workers have, as a consequence, been burdened with excessive amounts of paper work to first secure funding and then post-hoc to justify it. Also their practice has been subjected to increasingly intrusive monitoring by managers endeavouring to monitor that they are 'doing health promotion when they are supposed to be doing it'. All this activity tends to discourage work with those who are the most difficult to reach and challenging. Equally it creates a danger that the benefits of informal education will be sacrificed to meet the needs of funders who believe they must prove they are doing something specific. It is important therefore that health promoters reflect on why they turn to informal education in the first place. In particular they need to acknowledge the unique strengths of good informal education which enable effective workers to create learning relationships with many who have previously been most resistant to any engagement with educators operating in formal settings.

CONCLUSION

The influx of health promotion funding into informal education appears to have been universally welcomed. Many practitioners seem to have encountered no ethical or moral difficulties in taking and employing it (Jeffs & Smith, 1999). On the surface complete co-terminosity of aims seem to be shared by health promoters looking to disseminate their message and informal educators searching for ways to fund their work. Real dangers do, however, lurk within this cosy arrangement, especially for the latter.

Earlier campaigns by health educators and social hygienists manipulated the youth work and community movements in order to suppress masturbation, alcohol and tobacco consumption. There is always the possibility of informal educators allowing themselves to be manipulated by the agenda of outsiders (Wagner, 1997). The historical tendency of health educators to focus on personal responsibility, advocate restrictive controls on individual behaviour particularly in relation to the access of people to drugs, alcohol and tobacco products and to adopt a condemnatory stance towards young single mothers, all hint at a source of potential tension between health promoters and informal educators.

The danger for health promoters is that if they engage with what runs through informal education – dialogue, a focus on people in community, and a concern for democracy – then they will be faced with some fundamental questions. As Weare (1992) put it:

> The language of autonomy and empowerment falls easily from the lips, but the practice is never easy or comfortable . . . the logical consequence of accepting autonomy as a goal is to agree that if . . . people choose to act in an unhealthy way then, provided it does not impinge on the freedom of others, this must be seen as an acceptable end result of an educational process.

Informal education is not a 'method' that can be simply used to promote health, it is a set of relationships and commitments that can radically alter the initial concerns of those who participate in it.

REFERENCES

Allen I (1987) Education in sex and personal relationships. London: Policy Studies Institute.

Balding J (1995) Young people in 1994. Exeter: Schools Health Education Unit.

Balding J (1996) Young people in 1995. Exeter: Schools Health Education Unit.

Balding J, Regis D, Wise A, Bish D & Muirden J (1996) Bully off: young people that fear going to school. Exeter: Schools Health Education Unit.

Batsleer J (1996) It's all right for you to talk: lesbian identification in feminist theory and youth work practice. *Youth and Policy*, 52, 12–21.

Blum R (1987) Contemporary threats to adolescent health in the United States. *Journal of the American Medical Association*, 257, 3390–3395.

Boud D, Cohen R & Walker D (Eds) (1993) Using experience for learning. Buckingham: Open University Press.

Coombs P H & Ahmed M (1974) Attacking rural poverty. How non-formal education can help. Baltimore: Johns Hopkins University Press.

Dennehy A, Smith L & Harker P (1996) Not to be ignored: young people, poverty and health. London: Child Poverty Action Group.

Dewey J (1916) Democracy and education. An introduction to the philosophy of education. New York: Free Press.

Dewey J (1933) How we think. A restatement of the relation of reflective thinking to the educative process. Boston: D.C. Heath.

Dorling D (1997) Death in Britain: how local mortality rates have changed – 1950s to 1990s. York: York Publishing Services.

France A & Wiles P (1996) The Youth Action Scheme. London: Department for Education and Employment.

Graham J & Bennett T (1995) Crime prevention strategies in Europe and North America. European Institute of Crime Prevention and Control Publications Series (28). New York: Criminal Justice Press.

Graham J & Bowling B (1995) Young people and crime. Home Office Research Study (145). London: Home Office Research and Statistics Directorate.

Hendry L, Shucksmith J & Philip K (1995) Educating for health: school and community approaches with adolescents. London: Cassell.

Henze R C (1992) Informal teaching and learning. A study of everyday cognition in a Greek community. Hillsdale, NJ: Lawrence Erlbaum.

Huskins J (1996) Quality work with young people. London: Youth Clubs UK.

Jeffs T & Smith M K (Eds) (1990) Using informal education. An alternative to casework, teaching and control? Milton Keynes: Open University Press.

Jeffs T & Smith M K (1996) Informal education – conversation, democracy and learning. Ticknall: Education Now Books.

Jeffs T & Smith M K (1999) 'Tainted money': ethical dilemmas in the funding of youth and community work. In: S Banks (Ed), The ethics of youth work. London: Routledge.

Lally J R, Mangione P L, Honig A S & Wittner D S (1988) More pride, less delinquency: findings from the the the ten-year follow-up study of the Syracuse University Development Research Program. *Zero-to-three*, 8(4), 13–18.

Lave J & Wenger E (1991) Situated learning: legitimate, peripheral participation. Cambridge: Cambridge University Press.

Mellanby A R, Phelps F A, Crichton N J & Tripp J H (1995) School sex education: an experimental programme with educational and medical benefit. *British Medical Journal*, 311, 414–420.

Milburn T, Clark J, Forde L, Fulton K, Locke A & MacQuarrie E (1995) Curriculum development in youth work. Edinburgh: Scottish Office Education Department.

Nettleton S & Burrows R (1997) Knit your own without a pattern: health promotion specialists in an internal market. *Social Policy and Administration*, 31(2), 191–201.

Nutbeam D, Macaskill P, Smith C, Simpson J M and Catford J (1993) Evaluation of two school smoking education programmes under normal classroom conditions. *British Medical Journal*, 306, 102–107.

OFSTED (1997a) The contribution of youth services to drug education. London: The Stationery Office.

OFSTED (1997b) Inspecting youth work: a revised inspection schedule. London: The Stationery Office.

O'Keefe D (1993) Truancy in English secondary schools. London: Department for Education.

Sargant N, Field J, Francis H, Schuller T & Tuckett A (1997) The learning divide. A study of participation in adult learning in the United Kingdom. Leicester: National Institute for Adult Continuing Education.

Schweinhart L J & Weikart D P (1993) A summary of significant benefits: the High/Scope Perry Pre-School Study through age 27. Ypsilanti, Michigan: High/Scope Press.

Smith M K (1997) Introducing informal education. *The informal education homepage*, http// :www.infed.org/i-intro.htm

Wagner D (1997) The new temperance: the American obsession with sin and vice. Boulder, Colorado: Westview Press.

Weare K (1992) The contribution of education to health promotion. In: R Bunton & G Macdonald (Eds), Health promotion: disciplines and diversity. London: Routledge.

Detached Youth Work

Beth Lindley

What is youth work? Contrary to many people's assumption the core of youth work is personal development and informal social education, not ultimately the provision of sport or leisure activities. In the main youth work is funded directly or managed by the local authority and as such it has a statutory obligation to provide an appropriate service. Resources vary from authority to authority and this leaves providing an appropriate service open to interpretation, of course, by adults. Some youth service staff are fully occupied with running youth centres, others offer flexible access to a service which encompasses a variety of approaches to young people, including detached work (i.e. 'detached' from a centre) and short-term project work. This style of work is, in the opinion of the author, geared to respond to the changing needs of young people.

Under Section 55 of the Further and Higher Education Act (1992), youth work that is funded or managed by a local authority, or an independent voluntary organisation which receives some financial or other assistance, i.e. training or managerial support, from a local authority, may be inspected by Her Majesties Inspector of Schools, known as OFSTED (Office of Standards in Education). The purpose of the inspection would be to report on the quality of the service and the standards achieved.

Detached workers meet young people who are often alienated and vulnerable on their own terms, on their own territory – street corner, school field, parks, bus stops and in fact anywhere where young people congregate. The aim of the workers is to provide a two-way relationship built on trust, thus enabling development of skills and abilities which will assist during transition to adulthood – the emphasis being to empower young people to make informed decisions.

Detached work is often unseen by adults in the community and therefore misunderstood. Often when an adult community encounters detached workers it is assumed they are agents of social control and should rid the streets of young people. This is inappropriate and impossible. Only one in five young people attend a youth club, whereas 'hanging around' with friends is the most common way

Evidence-based Health Promotion. Edited by Elizabeth R. Perkins, Ina Simnett and Linda Wright.
© 1999 John Wiley & Sons Ltd.

young people utilise their leisure time. Concerns for young people's safety are often excluded from community safety initiatives. However, there is the assumption that adults need to be protected from young people and not the other way around.

Measuring standards of success or achievement when working with young people is quite difficult but not impossible. If a young person attends a youth centre three or four times a week it would be easy to say they were showing commitment and loyalty to that particular centre. If, however, they were also growing in confidence, influencing decision making and taking some responsibility by supporting staff and other young people, a significant achievement would have been made and should therefore be recognised. Detached workers offer a universal service to the young people they encounter, therefore it is even more difficult to qualify achievements. Contacts are logged on recording sheets at the end of each session and achievements recognised when evaluating the work.

Young people are a target group for many health agencies, especially those with sex, drugs and rock 'n' roll in their remit. Youth outreach workers for these projects vary tremendously from those of detached workers because they have a direct responsibility for passing on pieces of information to young people. I believe there is great value in workers from youth services and health agencies coming together to share their expertise and work collectively to offer a holistic approach to young people's needs, using the four yardsticks of the national curriculum: education, empowerment, participation and equality of opportunity.

POSITIVE OPTIONS – A CASE STUDY

Positive Options was a City Challenge funded project based in Middlesbrough – an area of disadvantage with high unemployment (10.5%), high truancy figures, 80% attendance at a local secondary school, and poor health. The project was managed by the local authority's youth service from November 1993 to March 1997, when funding ceased.

The team offered information, advice and a listening ear to young people in the geographical area known as East Middlesbrough. It also offered a flexible programme of activities which encouraged participation in planning and organising. In the main the work concentrated on face-to-face work with young people wherever they were, the street, schools and also within a drop-in facility. Often work was done in conjunction with agencies that had a specific remit to reach young people. Positive Options offered an approach to youth work which aimed to address a diversity of needs, both practical and physiological, amongst a group of young people marginalised for a variety of reasons from mainstream provision. The work was aimed at 14–21 year olds. As in many areas young people were seen as a threat and nuisance, and listening to numerous elderly persons who used the community centre, many wished for the return of the days when young people were seen and not heard, or even better not seen and not heard.

Many of the young people we came into contact with had no dreams and no aspirations, just a sense of inevitability that they would learn about life behind bars. They escaped the tedium by experimenting with drugs, alcohol and crime. For example, seeing how many codeine they could take before they became itchy and nauseous and daring each other to see how far they could take it before inducing vomiting; sometimes thinking, perhaps this time they wouldn't bother and just sit and hope quietly, in the back of their minds, that they would become immune to it.

Crime featured heavily in many of their lives. They did, however, have codes of conduct. Many would not burgle a house, but sadly cars were seen as fair game. The buzz of driving a car on the grass, doing a handbrake turn and showing off to their mates made it worth the risk. They also ran the risk of court, prison and, of course, the risk of taking a life, maybe even their own.

The pain, turmoil, confusion and anxiety of growing up in today's society was and still is an extremely heavy burden for many young people. The work was challenging and exhausting, but building a close relationship with young people reminds you of their energy which is all so often suppressed.

In a study of Positive Options in 1995 it was found that, 'In fact, all respondent service users admitted to consuming alcohol and smoking cannabis.' In another study, in 1996, 'Alcohol was clearly viewed as a necessary social activity by those wandering the streets of East Middlesbrough.' The sample maintained that the detached workers gave them advice on alcohol and drugs without using melo-dramatic shock tactics. All users felt that any information offered by Positive Options was well received and welcomed. Probably the most important facet of Positive Options was counselling and advice. Although this was a central part of the project it was conducted subtly in the various activities offered.

Informal Education in Detached Work

Using staff recordings it was found on average that nine out of ten sessions would have included in them some element of health education. The workers' overall aim was to give young people accurate accessible information so they in turn could make informed choices about their lives. It is generally accepted by detached workers that they are unlikely to stop drug and alcohol use, tobacco smoking or underage sexual activity, so they work within a harm reduction framework. Young people from the age of ten upwards openly drank alcohol on the street. Cannabis was also smoked in small groups and the young people we encountered used a vocabulary that intimated an in-depth knowledge of illegal drugs and how to use them.

Building relationships with young people based on trust gives the worker the chance to pass on information about the consequences, both physically and morally, of drug and alcohol use. The project had a large bank of leaflets from Manchester Lifeline and also a Tees Health Production comic book, *Sorted*, with drugs education as a focus. Both publications gave accessible information in the form of comic strips, they used language that young people could relate to and humour, but most importantly they got over correct information.

Detached Work with Small Groups

Detached work is often spent with small groups; those groups will have similar interests and this will give the workers a focal point when chatting to them. In the Priestfields area of Middlesbrough a group of young men aged 14–19 were met on a regular basis. HIV/AIDS and drug use were talked about regularly. In the autumn of 1995, a local AIDS support agency offered young people a chance to take part in a peer education project to celebrate World AIDS Day. With the assistance of the workers the group secured £500 funding to organise a poster campaign aimed at schools, colleges and youth centres. The group of ten then met at a Youth Centre that had computer facilities. The first session was to ensure they had correct and relevant information and they invited a worker from the AIDS agency along. At the end of four sessions, two posters had been picked for printing into A3 posters and postcards. The young people then organised a week of events that included hand delivering the posters and postcards and red ribbons to all youth centres in Middlesbrough. The content of the poster caused a lot of discussion, as the one with a picture of Jesus holding a sign saying, 'For Christ's sake use a condom' had the Benetton effect. However the young people were confident in making a stand to get a positive message across. At the evaluation session, before we went out for a pizza, a treat for the young people's hard work, two of the young men commented: 'It [Positive Options] gives you things to do and learn, we have a chance to do what we want to, instead of doing the same things all the time' and 'It's nice here [Priestfields], but we're here all the time, so we get bored of it; it's nice to go to different places.' In March 1996, this group successfully negotiated a room in the residents' association building for one night a week over a six-week period so they could produce their own version of a drugs education comic. They also began training with a disabled basketball team, who needed groups to practise with, and learnt a lot about disability and blisters on the palms of their hands when tackling in a wheelchair. This group of young men continued to work with the project until it closed.

Group Work

Detached work may often lead to groups of young people asking for something more. Positive Options ran several girls' and young women's groups and interest groups particularly connected with arts and sports. Thorntree girls' group, 'The Gang', met on a weekly basis at the community centre. It has to be acknowledged that within this situation the role of the worker changes. Rules of the centre have to be adhered too, so no smoking, drinking alcohol or taking drugs in the sessions can be allowed. Importantly, the group themselves need to make ground rules for their session and often, 'no bullying', 'wash your own pots' and 'respect each other and the workers' crop up. A programme of activities was drawn up in consultation with the young people and visits to the Drugs Advisory Service, Alcohol Counselling Service for information and advice were two of the most popular. A family planning nurse was invited in and the group took a practical first aid course with the help of the St. John Ambulance Brigade. The group responded well to being treated as adults; most of them were aged 13–16. What seemed to make users want to listen and participate wasn't so much the content of the talks but the way they were delivered. Contrary to popular belief that young people aren't interested, they are if treated with respect and maturity.

Drop-in Service

A drop-in service was also undertaken by the project staff. This ran for three afternoons a week in the community centre. It was aimed at school leavers. However, it also attracted non-attenders. After discussions with the young people and local schools, negotiations allowed the non-attenders to attend the drop-in if they attended school in the mornings. The sessions held were informal, a safe place to have a coffee and a chat, listen to some music or have a group discussion. It soon became clear that users wanted more information about a variety of issues but did not have the confidence to use agencies in the town centre or with those whom they saw as 'formal agencies'. Staff then invited agencies to attend the drop-in, Drugs Advisory Service, Family Planning Service and a Probation Service funded employment agency became involved on a regular basis and with pleasing results. The drop-in facility was always well attended and seen as a great loss when the project closed.

School Work

This was carried out in a local secondary school. Initially the team would enter the school at break times to be available for information and advice or occasionally to act as advocate on behalf of a young person experiencing a problem at school. As the project grew so did the work in schools. Staff would deliver personal and social education classes on issues identified by young people. Abuse, racism, sex and bullying were the most requested issues and are worrying to young people. They needed space to air their feelings. Positive Options afforded them a forum to discuss such subjects.

Teachers were glad of the support and expertise it lent to the schools and, furthermore, teachers felt that young people who rarely joined in activities had been encouraged by the youth workers to open up and join in. Once again, the way the users were treated was revealed in evaluation. One pupil said, 'She [the youth worker] came into school and talked about bullying, pressure and that, she treat us dead mature, not like teachers.'

HOW TO GO ABOUT DETACHED YOUTH WORK

What are the guidelines? Many factors, obviously, determine where geographically you would work. Once that has been decided, it is important to spend some time surveying the area.

Reconnaissance

Observe where young people are seen and where they hang around unseen. Explore and investigate parochial boundaries. It may be that a secondary school is in the area and spending time in the lunch breaks introducing yourself, and the nature of the project, is a useful tool in the route to gaining young people's trust and being seen as a safe adult. It is not, I believe, beneficial to go into an assembly as this puts you in a position of authority. A non-authoritarian approach may encourage young people to make a move towards you when first on the street.

Cold Contacts

Don't come on too strong at first; keep your introduction simple. Don't ask too many questions as this arouses suspicion. However, be aware that your first contact may include the young people asking you lots of personal questions.

Personal Safety

With that in mind, do not share personal information such as home phone numbers. Have calling cards with office contact numbers on. Sharing common experiences may be appropriate later in the relationship, but be aware that 'befriending' is very different to 'being a friend'. Always work in pairs, never alone. You will appear less vulnerable and will have each other for mutual support. It is also useful to get two points of view at the end of a session. Practically, don't carry a bag with valuables in it. Wear comfy shoes and sensible clothing. Also find safe places to go in case of an emergency. Introduce yourself and the nature of your work to local shopkeepers. Don't deliberately put yourself at risk.

Identification

Always carry an identification card with a photograph on it. However, I wouldn't advise you to wear it around your neck. Identification cards are advantageous if adults or parents are suspicious of your movements. It may be of value to contact the local community liaison police officer and community or neighbourhood councils to avoid suspicion. Arrange a meeting to discuss the work and its aims. It may be possible to come to an arrangement for local police officers to keep a discreet eye open for you, particularly when working in potentially explosive situations.

Recording

At the end of each session it is important to record the session's events, including number of contacts, balance of age groups, male/female balance, etc. Youth workers will also need to record which areas of the national curriculum have been covered and which topics discussed. A section on action to take place is also essential, as is confidentiality, which would need to be discussed at length with any inter-agency work.

Finishing a Session

Spend ten minutes or so with your co-worker evaluating and reflecting on the session. Ensure your written recordings are accurate. Put in individual feelings and thoughts. Often a worker is taken on one side by an individual for a private discussion, so both workers will have different perspectives on the session. Make sure the young people know you are finishing by telling them when and where you will be available. This could mean giving them a time in your office to come and see you, or just to inform them of the next street session. Ensure the information you give them is as accurate as possible and never set up expectations you are unlikely to fulfil.

Support and Supervision

These are essential for the development and maintenance of effective work. It is up to you to ensure that you have access to a supervisor whom you trust and respect. It is vital to the success of any work that supervision is planned to be comfortable and constructive. During the session explore your anxieties and feelings, as well as your achievements. Using your recording sheets, notch up issues to discuss and ensure they are covered. At the end of a session, explore how the session went and discuss it with your line manager.

Inter-agency Work

Positive Options undertook inter-agency work from its conception. What emerged from qualitative data was that Positive Options was innovative, in that it accepted a policy of inter-agency working and had a firm commitment to consultation with users. Derived from interviews with the users of the service was a distinct feeling that the Positive Options team were not merely paying lip service to service consultation. The key aspects of interagency working are set out below.

CHECKLIST FOR INTERAGENCY WORKING

- In the initial stages, set clear aims and objectives.
- Identify what may be conflicting policies and how to deal with them.
- Reaffirm joint policies and procedures, e.g. around child protection issues.
- Use expertise available to offer the best service to young people.

PRACTICE POINTS

- Treat young people as equals, autonomous to make decisions and confident to choose activities and to make suggestions.
- Treat your user group as if they are adults and accepted members of the community.

This point of view contrasts with current perceptions, as Brown et al. (1995) say in their article about youth provision in East Middlesbrough, *Nobody Listens*:

> The cultural and political preoccupation with youth as a problem for communities, rather than young people as citizens of communities, is the most enduring.

REFERENCE

Brown S, Heald M & Sallans C (1995) Nobody listens: problems and promise for youth provision. Middlesbrough: Middlesbrough City Challenge/Middlesbrough Safer Cities.

Chapter 10

Working within the Criminal Justice System

Ina Simnett

INTRODUCTION

This chapter aims to help those who wish to work effectively within the criminal justice system. Offenders are at higher risk of poor health, but until recently there have been few attempts to improve their health. Concern about the risks of the spread of HIV from the prison population has brought about a belated interest in the health of offenders, although this is largely focused on protecting the general public rather than on promoting the health and well-being of the offenders themselves. Health promotion work with offenders presents unique challenges, related both to access to them and how best to work with them.

The first section of this chapter, *Health Promotion with Offenders*, describes the distinguishing factors which shape the delivery of health promotion activities to offenders. It moves on to discuss current practice in health promotion with offenders, including opportunities for work with groups in the community and in prisons. The research evidence about the features of effective health promotion with offenders is outlined and the implications for practice are discussed, including resources available to measure behavioural, attitudinal and knowledge change. Finally, the particular barriers to working with women offenders and young offenders are highlighted and the huge opportunity for effective work with the latter group in residential homes and secure or custodial settings is outlined.

The second section of the chapter focuses on HIV prevention work within prisons. It starts by setting the context of HIV work in prisons, including the development of policies and practice against the background of a rapidly rising population, security problems, management changes and a troubling increase in suicide. It moves on to discuss the role of outside agencies in prison HIV prevention work and the practical effects of recent changes in legislation. It continues by describing how primary HIV prevention work differs, in the prison setting, from that in the community. The setting up of multidisciplinary AIDS management teams with a remit including the organisation of sexual health and risk reduction training programmes for prisoners is described and the section ends with a guide to co-operative work between prison staff and outside agencies.

Evidence-based Health Promotion. Edited by Elizabeth R. Perkins, Ina Simnett and Linda Wright.
© 1999 John Wiley & Sons Ltd.

Health Promotion with Offenders

Robin Burgess

Offenders have rarely been considered as a specific group in health promotion literature, neither as offenders in the community nor in prison. Neither has literature related to the needs of offenders shown very much interest in their health needs. Recently however there has been an increasing interest in relation to specific areas of health, such as drugs, mental health and HIV, which in turn has led to consideration of offenders' broader health needs.

Specific client groups such as offenders are undoubtedly at higher risk of poor health: on almost every indicator they demonstrate high levels of problematic health behaviour or conditions. Mental health, suicide, stress, poor diet, drug or alcohol misuse, sexually transmitted diseases, and indeed other health issues associated with poverty and such subsidiary causes as homelessness, are far more likely amongst offender populations. This has been known for a very long time (Guibord, 1917). Despite this, there have been few attempts to improve poor health amongst offenders. Even today there is a shocking lack of concern with their health. Even such bodies as the Penal Affairs Consortium (1997) have failed to call for health promotion activity for offenders as a right. There are signs of change in those bodies responsible for the welfare of prisoners however, as illustrated by Ramsbottom (1996). However, whilst there are the first stirrings of concern for the health of prisoners, although less concern with offenders in the community, there is less evidence of health promotion or of its effectiveness.

The answers for the current surge of interest in offender health and the lack of literature in the past lie not with the interests of those concerned with penal reform but with the needs of government and broader society. Guibord, in arguing that ill-health directly caused offending, illustrated that what matters most is the effect the 'bad health' behaviour of offenders has on society, not their own health *per se*. Two health areas illustrate this point.

Initially, HIV prevention messages took a broad, whole community approach, but more recently it has become clear that some groups are particularly at risk, pose

Evidence-based Health Promotion. Edited by Elizabeth R. Perkins, Ina Simnett and Linda Wright.

risks for the broader population and should be priorities for specific attention. Prisoners, because they do not have access to condoms and are more likely to engage in homosexual activity, are one such group who are considered to pose serious risk of 'contamination' to the broader community. Accordingly, their status as an at-risk group *who are incidentally offenders*, makes them a target community for specific health promotion.

The second major health issue relates to the inexorable rise of drug and alcohol problems. Offenders are overwhelmingly likely to have problems with drug or alcohol misuse. This has been known for at least 30 years, but the sheer scale of drug-related crime and its effect upon the broader community has been one major factor in promoting responses designed to reduce the scale of drug taking amongst offenders. Even before this, the belief that drug users posed major risks in relation to trans-mission of HIV was a further stimulus to activity designed to improve their health behaviour.

Both of the above factors are different from client-centred motivatory factors that prompt health promotion activity. The drug taking activity of offenders can be understood as a health-related behaviour that will have negative effects upon longer term health and well-being. However, the prompt for intervention against it is the consequent harm from that unhealthy behaviour to the broader society.

This point is crucial for it illustrates that the health of offenders had historically not been high on the agenda, until their unhealthy behaviour posed a risk beyond themselves. The consequences of this are that the *shape* of both health care and health promotion strategies for offenders are distorted by other concerns related to the well-being of society. If this is the primary and distinguishing factor concern-ing health promotion with offenders, there are a number of other points that can be made.

THE APPROACH TO HEALTH PROMOTION

If we relate the concern to address health behaviours of offenders to ideologies of health promotion found in the literature, it is clear that offender practice is less concerned with the client than with the functioning of the system of penal affairs. In the typology advanced by Ewles and Simnett (1995) of different purposes in health promotion, the purpose of the activity is not primarily to enable the recipients to live more healthy lives out of choice, but is motivated by a com-mitment to ensure that their behaviour does not hurt others. It is not health for health's sake. The identity of offenders as *offenders* whose behaviour *ought* to be changed rather than ordinary, high risk individuals and groups dominates the discourse. Accordingly health promotion in such settings is not essentially client centred and neither does it seek to change the environment in which offenders operate; it seeks, within that system, to change their behaviour.

COMPULSORY PARTICIPATION

The second issue is one of definition and access. Offenders become a unified group by virtue of their collective status as offenders. At home, going about their ordinary lives, they are part of the general public. Collectively, they attain a different status. However, they come together collectively only through compulsion – through forced attendance predicated by a particular order of the court, or by custody. They can only be reached *as offenders*, in settings that they attend compulsorily. This has potentially profound repercussions for their ability or potential to learn, or to change behaviour.

GENDER

A third distinguishing feature is the issue of gender. Overwhelmingly, offenders are male, and men traditionally have shown little interest in health issues. Masculinity and offending are profoundly linked in a destructive, unhealthy way (Newburn & Stanko, 1994). As men, their health issues are also specific, commonly related to issues of consumption and smoking. The dynamics of health promotion inter-ventions to those with men are very different with women.

OFFENDER HEALTH ISSUES

The issue with which offender health is concerned are issues which involve much more than simple reliance upon fact and factual education. Education with offenders who misuse drugs is as much concerned with attitude change as it is with acquisition of knowledge. Factual programmes have a particularly poor record with offender groups (Baldwin, 1990). Models of successful practice par-ticularly in relation to drugs and alcohol have developed approaches located in a broader arena that emphasises attitude and value to a greater degree. Such health promotion is required to lay greater stress on beliefs and values, and frequently to occur within highly directive and therapeutic frameworks. This involves the use of health promotion techniques within a discourse dominated by a moral framework. This may seem incongruous to some models of health promotion but the need to tackle underlying beliefs and values is congruent however with the model of health promotion proposed by Downie et al. (1997). Indeed, all health promotion is driven by values, whether or not this is openly acknowledged.

LITTLE FREEDOM OF CHOICE

Offenders are uniquely badly placed to act on messages of health promotion. This may be because of addiction, but it is more likely to be because of the more generally chaotic and disordered life that is the feature of so many offender lifestyles in the community. Likewise prisoners are almost uniquely unable to enact change in their lives. An environment is which they cannot change diet, have limited access to exercise, are at real risk of violence, exploitation, brutality and fear, is hardly one conducive to behavioural change, nor is it a realistic environment to practise changes that will be much harder on the outside.

POLITICAL INTERFERENCE

Interventions within the criminal justice system have been subject to sustained political manipulation over many years. The Conservative administration of 1979–1997 emphasised punishment and incarceration. There are tokenistic signs of change in the current Labour administration, but there remains a legacy from that period in profound sea changes in the style of intervention with offenders in probation practice (Harris, 1992; Jones et al., 1995). Such services as work with offenders are no longer concerned with the whole person, but are increasingly only concerned with offending behaviour and its management and, as such, the opportunity to address broader welfare concerns of offenders, including health, is eroded. Particularly, as indicated above, there is no method of access to offenders other than through probation or prison attendance, thus allowing less opportunity for health promotion to occur.

HEALTH PROMOTION IS OUTCOME LED

Health promotion with offenders, because of all the above points, is inevitably outcome led. It becomes concerned with measurable behavioural change in relation to specific areas of concern such as drugs or alcohol. The educator is primarily concerned with encouraging the individual to change their behaviour, not with pursuing an 'informed choice'. In this context, given the proven harm (an offence that is related to drugs) that may have resulted from the unhealthy behaviour, there is an explicit desired outcome of change.

HEALTH PROMOTION IS SECONDARY TO TREATMENT

Health promotion with offenders is often placed in a secondary capacity to their treatment or therapeutic needs given the greater propensity to more serious problems found in offender populations. Offenders who are drug users for example are often felt to be 'beyond' the educational stage.

These eight factors shape the delivery of health promotion activity with offenders and, in some ways, create a bleak picture. It is arguable that the adoption of a more client-centred approach would be more likely to be effective, allowing as it would, greater autonomy and self-confidence to offenders and thus freedom to control health aspects of their lives. This would require fundamental changes to the justice system to allow greater offender power and self-determination in environments in which they are currently deliberately denied them. Nonetheless where the constraints detailed above are accepted and understood it is possible to identify successful, evidence-based examples of effective practice which can change the health of offenders considerably.

CURRENT PRACTICE IN HEALTH PROMOTION WITH OFFENDERS

As noted above, offenders require more than simple factual information, and indeed not just a caring, loving social work environment in order to change. A simple understanding of health psychology reveals the complex web of belief and attitude that acts to prevent behavioural change. In practical terms this affects the way we conduct health promotion and how healthy behaviour can be stimulated. It is necessary to accept that behaviour is most likely to be changed by a model of intervention which reflects that it is caused by a complex interaction of cognitive, behavioural, motivational and value-based processes and transactions. In relation to drug-taking, accepting a social learning model of alcohol and drug behaviour requires recognition of a cognitive and attitudinal framework that underpins change behaviours.

One such structure is provided by the work of Prochaska and DiClemente (1986). Their simple model, originally derived from studies of smokers, has been massively influential upon practice with drinkers and drug takers. It posits the important concept of pre-contemplation, the state of not having an attitudinal commitment to change nor set of beliefs or knowledge that will facilitate change. The majority of individuals who engage in continuing use of substances can be categorised as being pre-contemplative or contemplative. They lack either the life experience, exposure to negative viewpoints or circumstance, broader perspective or simple sense of value to motivate change. Offenders are even more likely to be pre-contemplators. Their offending has led to arrest, conviction and punishment. This is likely to have interrupted a career of drug taking. Consequently they are in custody or on probation frequently without having naturally reached a point of willingness or motivation to change.

Health promotion activity with offenders has to work within this framework. Whatever messages it delivers will be received by people who need to be convinced to change. It therefore requires a content that reflects this requirement. A further consequence of the point about compulsion is that there is likely to be additional resistance on the part of consumers within the criminal justice system to imposed messages. Coupled with pre-contemplator status this requires a further complexity and sophistication of message.

An important point about health promotion with offenders is that there is a fine balance between health promotion and treatment. It is often erroneously believed that the sole needs of offenders in relation to such matters as drugs or mental health is treatment, i.e that they are already so advanced in their conditions as to require complex therapeutic interventions rather than education designed to prevent such consequences. So dominant and entrenched is this belief that much health work with offenders is structured around presumed therapeutic needs. This rightly reflects the priority upon achieving behaviour change and the presence of very serious problems for many offenders. It is important however to recognise that pre-contemplator status, and indeed lesser levels of problematic drug or alcohol use are also present in many offenders and as such they may require a less therapeutic approach. This is particularly the case with young offenders. However, it is sometimes impossible to reach offenders without 'riding on the back' of treatment priorities.

REACHING OFFENDERS IN THE COMMUNITY

In this section I shall concentrate on the possibilities for health promotion with 'adult' offenders aged 17 and over, as the circumstances for 'juveniles' are rather different and are addressed in a later section. The literature of health promotion with offenders in prison is small enough but that of work with offenders in the community is even smaller. This is probably because it is difficult to find mechanisms that reach offenders whose contact with the system is frequently on a one-to-one basis with police and Probation officers. Their attendance at the police station or the Probation office may be fleeting. In this context posters and literature may not only be the sole method possible but may also have little impact given that they are not directed at individuals with a leisured reflective opportunity to consider behavioural change. Probation officers may incorporate health promotion within their casework with offenders, as police officers may do in custody suites, but such work is by circumstance, individualised and occurring in a setting that does not encourage reception of health promotion messages. Custody suites may be a useful location to encourage attendance and contact with treatment services, but they provide limited opportunity for absorption of structured health promotion. As a result of this we have to look for specific interventions that allow greater potential for more sustained intervention.

The traditional opportunity for health promotion activity in the community with offenders is the group. Probation groups have been run for very many years, some on a voluntary attendance basis, but increasingly within a compulsive framework, revised by the Criminal Justice Act of 1991, under a 1a2 or 1a3 (day centre) version of a standard Probation order. These two orders give considerable opportunity for health promotion activity with offenders in the community, particularly concerning drugs (Hart & Webster, 1991). Under a 1a2 order, offenders are required to attend for six or eight sessions of about two hours each. The content of such programmes needs to reflect the therapeutic priorities given above but research has demonstrated that health promotion can be a useful component of such groups. Such groups are designed to tackle entrenched behavioural problems that cause offending, commonly including anger, sexual attitudes and behaviours, alcohol and drugs. They are most particularly suited to addressing the frequently shared patterns of drug-related behaviour and attitude that lead to drug-related offending. As such there are almost no restrictions on the content of such groups other than that they must have demonstrable effects upon such behaviour or attitudes. In this context research (Baldwin, 1990) suggests that any programme needs to have the following.

FEATURES OF EFFECTIVE HEALTH PROMOTION WITH OFFENDERS

- An environment that is open and supportive and non-threatening to individual group members. It has to be a led or structured group
- It must contain factual information that will enable strengthening of motivation and resolving of ambivalence
- It must address the belief systems of the group
- It must give analytical skills to the consumer to evaluate their own behaviour
- It must help give practical coping skills that can be used by participants
- Because it is related to the offending of participants, such groupwork must address the linkage between problematic behaviour and offending
- It must reflect to participants the effects of problematic behaviour on others

---

Such groupwork is clearly concerned with a mixture of skills, attitudes, values and knowledge; attempting via a cognitive/behavioural methodology to challenge value systems, attitudes, ignorance and lack of skills that lead to problem behaviours. Within this framework, health is a positive value that can be used to motivate against ambivalence, encourage motivation, and support efforts to change. The achievement of good health, or its maintenance, is one factor in motivating non-drug behaviours. It is an easy 'way in'.

The above points may include items which are untraditional to health promotion, and which may seem akin to moral or judgemental education. However, it should be remembered that such education occurs inevitably because the only reason the group is called together is because of morality expressed in law; and the inclusion of material that addresses such concerns is a requirement of practice within the criminal justice framework. The intended behavioural outcome of reduction in alcohol or drug use requires a broad range of interventionist methodologies far beyond the non-moralistic arena of provision of facts. Nonetheless, factual material should have a significant part in such groups, as it can have value in raising understanding of the effect of intoxication, for example, on offending.

Effective programmes have been written and evaluated by Baldwin (1990), Baldwin et al. (1988) and Purser et al. in relation to alcohol (1989); and by Burgess et al. (1993) in relation to other drugs. The resource by the present author includes a comprehensive evaluative structure to measure behavioural, attitudinal and knowledge change.

Day centre programmes (1a3 orders) present different opportunities. At one time Probation day centres promised a great opportunity to address the broader welfare needs of clients through group and individual work (Priestly et al., 1984). Such centres seemed to offer considerable hope of effective intervention in welfare, anger management, offending behaviour, and health generally as well as specific issues such as drugs and alcohol (Mair, 1988; Vass, 1990). By offering a far greater amount of time to reach offenders, and by the development of a supportive, friendly, non-abusive environment, such centres can provide opportunity for more generic, less goal-oriented health promotion, good examples of which are to be found in the literature (for a collection of useful examples, see Brown & McCaughan, 1991). However, many factors have conspired to make their promise unfulfilled. Firstly, such centres, operating with offenders who would otherwise be in prison, have received less referrals in an era where it is believed that prison 'works'. Secondly, they are as expensive as prisons at a time when resources within Probation are tight. Thirdly, their broader, more social-work oriented, welfarist approach is increasingly out of line with the ethos of offender management of modern Probation practice. Lastly, Probation officers themselves consistently fail to refer clients to groupwork resources, a factor that also affects 1a2 groups. All this means that the day centre movement is in decline, with many centres closing, which removes an important environment in which constructive health promotion work can take place.

Drugs and alcohol most clearly lend themselves to outcome led groupwork of this sort. Handling of offenders with mental health problems is very different. Individual work clearly incorporates promotion of good mental health through counselling on self-esteem, etc., but opportunities to promote good mental health as opposed to early intervention with those who are already sufferers are very limited. 1a2 groups are not suitable for this type of offender, who are primarily dealt with in the criminal justice system through individual work, often through diversion from prosecution. Whilst mental health promotion can occur in such settings, the 'treatment first' rule applies here even more, and offenders are extremely unlikely to be identified as being at risk of mental health problems before such systems identify them as *already* suffering from serious problems.

Community work with offenders comprises work in police contexts, individual work with Probation or social work staff, Probation groups and day centres. Having looked at all these, prison also provides an environment in which health promotion with offenders can occur.

PRISON-BASED HEALTH PROMOTION

Prisons are not healthy environments. The very physical dereliction of many prison buildings, coupled with overcrowding, lack of proper diet, exercise and clothes, means that even before the culture of prison life is considered, there are profound reasons why prisons are not good places to practise health promotion. Prison life is brutalising, an environment designed, through punishment and inmate culture, to increase stress, to dehumanise, and to destroy self-esteem. Nonetheless, for the first time there are real opportunities. In the past, medical provision was distinctly unsuitable as a mechanism for promoting health (Sim, 1990). Medical care was linked to punishment systems, and implicated in control and abuse of all kinds, such as prescribing unsuitable drugs and so on. The burgeoning size of the prison population and the concern over HIV and drugs has however led to some imaginative changes. The prison is a captive community in which many offenders can become fanatical about maintaining and improving health, and become single minded in achieving personal change. This gives scope for distinctive practice.

Firstly, there is continued opportunity through Probation practice, particularly in groupwork. Secondly, there is motivation through prison staff and management to address health needs on induction and rehabilitative education and in throughcare.

Lastly, there is determination to address drug issues through education and treatment. Whilst all work in prison is done within a culture that is brutalising and coercive, there is no compulsory linkage between discipline and education and health care in many prisons. Accordingly programmes developing at the present time frequently have no linkage between discipline and attendance. There is increasing motivation for employment or engagement of health professionals, either from within the prison medical service (Wilmott, 1992) or externally within health authorities, to undertake such work (Heyes & King, 1996) and for such workers to be skilled in health promotion. There is evidence that such work can yield productive results (Peterson & Johnstone, 1995) and tackle broad health needs.

Again such work can take the form less of health promotion than of provision of health care with those already engaging in unhealthy behaviour or suffering ill-health (Yates, 1994); given the pressure of work in treating individuals with identified health needs there may be little time for health promotion. Nonetheless there may be opportunities via a number of routes. Theatre, writing groups, education and drug treatment programmes all provide opportunities for communication of healthy messages to other prisoners and engagement of prisoners in promoting good health to others. Prison drug programmes, often structured around drug-free environments where there are benefits for living without drugs, provide good opportunities for a graduated range of drug-related interventions including intense therapeutic work at one end (Burgess et al., 1998) through to education at the other with less seriously involved individuals.

WOMEN OFFENDERS

As noted above, health promotion with men is very different to that with women, but the structure for carrying out practice with either gender is shaped by the same systems although they are potentially worse for women.

Firstly, there are less women offenders; this means that it is often extremely difficult if not impossible to structure single sex groupwork in the community for reasons of timing, volume and distance. Whilst the presence of women in mixed groups undoubtedly changes the attitudes and behaviour of male offenders, it is frequently a difficult and solitary experience for women whose specific needs are likely to be unmet given the volume of male issues to be considered.

Secondly, female offenders are still likely to be treated differently by the criminal justice system to men, through prejudice, bigotry and demography. Women are more likely not to be put on Probation, but more likely to be sent to prison, particularly for less serious offences. The decline of community day care and the shift either towards custody or community service (which has almost no opportunity for educational imput on health), has meant that potential examples of good empowering practice that addressed women's needs, including health (Mistry, 1989) have been lost.

This again, leaves prison. Female prisons are just as barbaric and brutal as men's. However, women's prisons do provide opportunities for gender specific groupwork, education and theatre, using the same opportunities as were given above, that are not available in the community, and which may benefit women more because women are more prepared to engage in prevention and health promoting programmes (Peterson & Johnstone, 1995).

YOUNG OFFENDERS

Offenders under age 17 in the community and age 17–21 in custody are treated in different ways to older offenders and therefore this provides different opportunities to promote good health.

First time or very young offenders are likely not to be prosecuted; rather, they are likely to be diverted out of custody, dealt with by virtue of a caution, and in some cases and in some areas, by reparation schemes. These seek to create greater dialogue between victim and offender and allow the offender to make amends for what they have done in a way related more clearly to their offence. Comparatively fewer younger offenders are prosecuted and sentenced. If they are, the structure of that response is more oriented towards a social work ethos than with adults; although, as with adult offenders, increasingly occurring within a context that emphasises punishment to a greater degree. In the community there are the same individual opportunities as for adults to help young people change and grow through individual counselling or education. There is however less opportunity to practise groupwork. Because it is believed that less engagement with the criminal justice system is better in terms of not leading to exposure to other offenders or attitudes and opportunities, groupwork with young offenders in the community is almost unpractised (in contrast to the highly participative, group environment of intermediate treatment of the 1970s). Other than where diversion schemes are prepared to offer limited groups to offenders who are already known to one another, in the community such opportunities found with adults are almost non-existent.

In custody or within residential care, opportunities are much greater, as education in such settings rarely is required to follow the same approaches as such offenders would receive in mainstream state schools. Within residential homes and secure or custodial settings there is huge opportunity to conduct imaginative education that promotes good health and does so through a framework that reflects the social milieu of offenders and the causes of crime (Eaton, 1994). Whilst programmes of this sort were rare in the Ramsbottom Report of 1996, given the freedom to experiment with material, the opportunity to look at such causes as self-esteem and masculinity that are so causative of ill-health and other behaviours, and the support of the prison service to encourage such practice, there is no reason to doubt that they can be effectively expanded and developed.

CONCLUSION

Interest in the health of offenders is a recent discovery which gives all sorts of challenges for the provision of health promotion. Clearly this is a client group with a very great need for work to tackle destructive personal health behaviours, yet also hard to access, to reach and communicate effectively with. In seeking to base practice on evidence of effectiveness there is limited written material which helps shape effective work. In relation to drugs and to alcohol there is however a tradition and model of practice which has been demonstrated to achieve behavioural change, knowledge and attitudes that affect drug or alcohol consumption. There is a small but growing literature which reflects new opportunities to undertake health promotion practice with incarcerated offenders.

REFERENCES

Baldwin S (1990) Alcohol education and offenders. London: Batsford.
Baldwin S, Wilson M, Lancaster A & Allsop D (1988) Ending offending. Glasgow: Scottish Council on alcohol.
Brown A & McCaughan N (Eds) (1991) Various articles. *Groupwork*, 4(3).
Burgess R, Davies L & Dilley C (1993) Drugs and offending. Northampton: CAN.
Burgess R, Houlihan A & Grant L (1998) Drugs and offending: therapeutic resources for work with prisoners. Northampton: CAN.
Downie R S, Fyfe C & Tannahill A (1997) Health promotion, models and values. Second edition. Oxford: Oxford University Press.
Eaton L (1994) Health and young offenders. *Nursing Times*, 90(24), 32–33.
Ewles L & Simnett I (1995) Promoting health: a practical guide. Third edition. London: Ballière Tindall.
Guibord A (1917) Physical states of criminal women. *Journal of the American Institute of Criminal Law and Criminology*, 8, 82–95.
Harris R (1992) Crime, criminal justice and the Probation service. London: Routledge & Kegan Paul.
Hart D & Webster R (1991) The revolving door stops: the Criminal Justice Act – new opportunities for drug users. London: SCODA.
Heyes J & King G (1996) Care and control: implementing a prison drug strategy. *Druglink*, pp 8–10. London: ISDD.
Jones A et al. (1995) Probation practice. London: Pitman.
Mair G (1988) Probation day centres. London: HMSO.

Mistry T (1989) Establishing a feminist model of groupwork in the Probation service. *Groupwork*, 2(2), 145–158.

Newburn T & Stanko E (Eds) (1994) Just boys doing business. London: Routledge.

Penal Affairs Consortium (1997) Crime, drugs and criminal justice. London: Penal Affairs Consortium.

Peterson M & Johnstone B M (1995) The Atwood Hall Health Promotion Program, Federal Medical Center, Lexington, Kentucky. *Journal of Substance Misuse Treatment*, 12(1), 43–48.

Priestly P, McGuire J, Flegg D, Hensley V, Wellham D & Barnitt R (1984) Social skills in prisons and the community. London: RKP.

Prochaska J O & DiClemente C C (1986) Transtheoretical therapy: towards a more integrative model of change. *Psychotherapy, Theory, Research and Practice*, 19, 276–288.

Purser R et al. (1989) Drink-related offending. Coventry: Council on Alcohol.

Ramsbottom D (1996) Patient or prisoner? A new strategy for health care in prisons. London: Home Office.

Sim J (1990) Medical power in prisons. Milton Keynes: Open University Press.

Vass A (1990) Alternatives to prison. London: Sage.

Wilmott Y (1992) Career opportunities in the nursing service for prisoners. *Nursing Times*, 88(37).

Yates S (1994) Promoting mental health behind bars. *Nursing Standard*, 8(52), 18–21.

Section 10.2

HIV Prevention Work within Prisons

Sally Perkins

A ROUGH GUIDE TO THE PRISON SERVICE

There are two prison services in mainland UK; the Scottish prison service, which is operated by the Scottish Office, and the English and Welsh prison service, which comes under the jurisdiction of the Home Office, and is the area discussed in this section. At the end of 1997, there were 135 prisons holding between 62 000 and 64 700 people in custody, and that number continues to rise. The majority of these were men, although the small number of women who did appear before the courts were dealt with fairly severely. Black people were over-represented in this population. The 136 prison establishments included remand centres for unconvicted prisoners and institutions of varying degrees of security, from open prisons to top-security establishments.

Women are held separately from men, but sometimes in units contained within male prisons, and at three prisons mothers are allowed to keep their babies with them, up to the ages of nine or 18 months. There is an increasing number of young people held in prison in this country, and they are normally held in Young Offender Institutions (YOIs) or housed separately within adult prisons. (Young offenders are also held in secure units and residential homes, which are under the jurisdiction of the social services rather than the prison service, and to which juveniles can be sent by a court.) Foreign detainees held under the Immigration Act are generally housed in designated detention centres.

Overcrowding is a problem, and has automatically worsened with the increased prison population, and integral sanitation or 24-hour access to sanitation is not yet available at every prison.

WHY PROMOTE HEALTH IN PRISONS?

In the UK, the promotion of health within particular settings has been established over the last decade, with the acknowledgement that the environments in which

Evidence-based Health Promotion. Edited by Elizabeth R. Perkins, Ina Simnett and Linda Wright.
© 1999 John Wiley & Sons Ltd.

people exist play an important part in their overall health. The government paper, *The Health of the Nation* (DOH, 1992), identified several target settings for the promotion of health, one of which is custodial environments. The problems associated with HIV, AIDS, and sexually transmitted diseases (STDs) were highlighted within that document as one of the five key areas to be earmarked for special attention. In 1998, the health minister announced her intention to further illuminate that key area by publishing separate guidelines on STDs, HIV and AIDS.

HIV transmission via sexual activity is one of the main ways in which the virus spreads. In prisons, where the majority of prisoners are young, male and sexually active, HIV may be spread through unprotected penetrative sexual intercourse; this occurs among gay prisoners and also among prisoners who identify as heterosexual outside prison, and who will continue heterosexual activity on release. Transmission of HIV through sharing needles and injecting paraphernalia (spoon, water, filter, etc.) must also be seen in sharper relief in the context of prison; as this setting certainly offers some increased opportunities for risky incidents whilst severely limiting access to the harm minimisation interventions which are offered in the community outside. So risks inside prison may include unprotected penetrative sex, sharing injecting equipment, sex attacks, tattooing, and bloody fights. Other problems can also arise within a closed community from fear of HIV and AIDS through lack of correct information, or the circulation of false information. It is important to remember that the prison population is constantly changing as individuals enter or leave custody, underlining the risk of transmission in prisons as an issue of general public health.

Prisons are also recognised as an important context for HIV and AIDS prevention at an international level, and in 1993 the World Health Organisation published the *Guidelines on HIV Infection in Prisons* (to be updated in 1998). The first general principle states that:

> All prisoners have the right to receive health care, including preventive measures, equivalent to that available in the community, in particular with respect to their legal status or nationality.

It is worth noting that some people who enter custody may not have previously had the opportunity or the desire to access information about health promotion or healthier lifestyles. Prison is essentially a boring environment with little to occupy the time for many inmates; educational resources are often limited and the available work can be repetitive. Perhaps the prison setting offers a good opportunity for health promoters to work with clients they may not otherwise encounter.

The prison setting is also a workplace, for prison officers, managers, educators, social workers, maintenance people, nurses, doctors, administrators and others. Prison staff, for the same reasons as everybody else, are vulnerable to infection or the fear of infection, in their private lives, and have the added dimension of a work environment already often perceived as dangerous. Clear knowledge of the real risks of transmission of communicable diseases can be as important for staff as it is for prisoners. Occupational health and safety is an everyday live issue in prisons, where staff as well as prisoners have been under attack, from flying fists, the contents of a 'slop out' bucket, or a blood-filled syringe used as a threat.

PRISON SERVICE INITIATIVES

Since 1987, the Directorate of Health Care for Prisoners (DHC) has launched several initiatives aimed at HIV prevention and the support of those who are infected:

- The issue of Circular Instruction 30/91 (CI 30/91, Directorate of Prison Medical Services, 1991), a series of recommendations to prison governors and staff regarding the management of HIV.
- Training programmes in multi-disciplinary AIDS management team formation (updated from 1997 to include some other communicable diseases), officer training in pre- and post-test counselling skills, incident management, and specialist medical training for some prison doctors.
- The creation of two training packages comprising films and training manuals: *AIDS inside and out*, and *Talking about AIDS* (Perkins & Robinson, 1995a; 1995b).
- An unlinked anonymised HIV prevalence study being carried out by the Public Health Laboratory Service.
- A knowledge, attitudes and behaviour study conducted by the Institute of Psychiatry.

Prior to CI 30/91, prisoners with HIV, or those suspected of seropositivity, were often kept apart from the rest of the prison population in a misguided attempt to control the spread of the virus. This was permissible under the prison ruling 'Viral Infectivity Restriction' (VIR), which was also applied to prisoners with other diseases such as hepatitis. It is clear that the prison service has come a long way on the issue of HIV and AIDS policies since then, and this must be acknowledged. However, it must also be understood that policy is not always translated into practice at a local level. As with most large national organisations, there is a great deal of discrepancy in the way that policy is interpreted from one location to another. Prisons and their managers must deal with HIV and AIDS among many other competing priorities, whilst considering the constant priority: security.

In recent years, prisons have had to deal with a rapidly rising population which has led to severe overcrowding in places, a troubling increase in suicide (and with it the development of a suicide prevention strategy) privatisation of part of the service, changes in the planning of budgets, and a drugs strategy which includes mandatory drugs testing for prisoners. These are some of the problems facing those who work or live in prisons, and are realities which must be faced by outside agencies or individuals wishing to work in this setting.

THE DEVELOPMENT OF THE ROLE OF OUTSIDE AGENCIES IN HIV PREVENTION WORK IN PRISONS

Across the prison system, there are a number of examples of prisons and outside agencies working together on HIV prevention, although an overall picture is difficult to document for the following reasons:

- There is no co-ordination or available register of such work.
- Many agencies are suffering severe funding problems and are prioritising other work areas.
- Ambiguity in funding arrangements has made it unclear whether DHAs have an obligation to facilitate prison work.

There are a number of useful roles which outside agencies could and occasionally do play in prevention of HIV and health promotion in a prison setting. District health authorities (DHAs) or prison governors could commission projects for prison establishments from community agencies, individuals, or health promotion units. DHAs and agencies could liaise with individual prison establishments and Prison Service headquarters to promote a co-ordinated approach to prevention work. Staff from the community could share their skills as members of multidisciplinary AIDS management teams. Healthy alliances could be formed between internal and external organisations interested in different aspects of health promotion in prison. There are a number of almost traditional cultural differences between the prison service and external agencies which may arise. These must be carefully considered, and will be discussed more comprehensively below.

In terms of one-to-one work it can be very important for an individual in prison to gain the support of an outside agency worker, who can help with advice, counselling and in practical ways. Some prisoners, although by no means all, feel more secure about confidentiality when discussing their health status with someone who is not employed by the prison service – although it must be said that prison officers are the people who spend the most time with prisoners, and have the best opportunity of getting to know individuals. Sometimes, the best way of gaining access to prisoners is to offer advice sessions for individuals via an appointment system.

LEGISLATIVE CHANGES AND THEIR PRACTICAL EFFECT

In promoting health in the prison setting, it is vital to be fully aware of legislation or prison rules which affect health and prevention initiatives, either adversely or otherwise. The prison service Directorate of Health Care for Prisoners has stated that prisoners should receive an equivalence of care to that received in the community. For various reasons, mostly connected with security, some of the prevention strategies permitted in custody are very different from those accepted outside:

Condoms are not freely available in prisons, despite recommendation by the AIDS Advisory Committee (1995), as the then Home Secretary did not approve this measure. As a matter of urgency, the DHC issued an instruction to prisons in the accepted format of a 'Dear Doctor letter'. Prison doctors were advised that they are '. . . free, in the exercise of their clinical judgement, to prescribe condoms for individual patients' (Director of Health Care, 1995). This advice is interpreted in different ways throughout the prison system, as research has shown (Perkins, 1998). In one prison, condoms were not permitted at all, as they are perceived as a threat to security by the management – drugs may be concealed in a condom and swallowed by a prisoner. In another, the prison doctor had delegated respon-sibility for the distribution of condoms to prisoners to a nurse. In this case, inmates could approach this member of staff in confidence.

There is no prison in the English/Welsh system which operates a *needle exchange* scheme. Again, in the *Review of HIV and AIDS in Prisons*, the AIDS Advisory Committee (1995) recommended that, for the purposes of harm minimisation, 'cleansing agents (washing up liquid and Milton sterilising tablets) should be made easily available to prisoners together with clear instructions and education about the importance of clean injecting equipment and of the methods for doing this . . .'

Although the Home Secretary authorised this recommendation, and cleansing agents were distributed around the prison system in the form of sterilising tablets, these were withdrawn fairly quickly after questions regarding health and safety from staff. In January 1998 there was still no indication of when they will be redistributed, although the National AIDS and Prisons Forum (NAPF) has received assurance from the DHC that this will happen.

Mandatory drug testing, which is now a routine part of the prison service Drug Misuse Strategy, also has potentially serious implications for the prevention of HIV in prisons (Perkins, 1996). In brief, at each prison, a percentage of prisoners is chosen, mainly at random, to be urine-tested for illegal drugs. Penalties including extra days of imprisonment are meted out to offenders. A further exploration of this can be found in the *AIDS Reference Manual* (Perkins, 1997). The problem is that the 'soft' drug cannabis, which is normally smoked by users, may be detectable in a urine sample for up 30 days, whilst heroin and cocaine – both injectable – leave the body's system relatively quickly (Shapiro, 1994). Some observers feel that this may lead to individuals giving up cannabis for more harmful drugs, which if injected also carry a risk of blood-borne infection.

The Circular Instruction 30/91 described the main aims of the prison service policy in relation to HIV and AIDS, which are to:

- Prevent the spread of infection
- Protect the health of inmates and staff
- Provide care and support for those infected.

CI 30/91 went on to describe measures in progress – staff training, education for prisoners, prevention of transmission, condom policy, illicit injecting equipment policy, blood testing policy, management of infected inmates and the recommended discontinuation of VIR in advance of the *Review of HIV and AIDS in Prisons*, and discussed the benefits of linking with external agencies. The CI also recommended the setting up at each prison establishment of a multi-disciplinary AIDS management team (AMT), described below as an example of good practice.

EXAMPLES OF GOOD PRACTICE

Primary HIV prevention, which focuses on attempting to halt the spread of infection to uninfected people, usually means education about the routes of transmission of HIV, sex education, promotion of the use of condoms, the provision of needle exchanges, and education about risk taking. As the distribution of condoms is not permitted in prisons, apart from an individual prescription item, and as there is no plan at the time of writing (January 1998) to allow needle exchanges in any prison, primary HIV prevention in a prison setting is not equivalent to prevention in the community. Nevertheless, there are pockets of good practice to be observed throughout the prison system, which may be studied and improved upon.

One of the most important and innovative internal strategies for the prevention of HIV in prison was the setting up and training of the AIDS management teams (AMTs). This project was a DHC initiative, and was introduced in 1990, when *HIV and AIDS: a multidisciplinary approach in the Prison Service – a working manual* was published by HM Prison Service. This manual was a collection of papers which aimed to 'identify the important interface between HIV infection and imprisonment', and contained a section on care in the prison community, which stressed the importance of the involvement of different disciplines in managing HIV in a custodial setting. A suggested format or blueprint for the operation of AMTs was attached, which was open to adaptation locally. From 1997, the remit of AMTs had been broadened to include the management of other communicable diseases such as tuberculosis, hepatitis B and hepatitis C.

As prisons are all different, there was no set style for the AMT to assume, but it was important that, where possible, the teams drew membership from the following disciplines:

- senior management – prisons have an overall manager called the 'governing governor', as well as several other governor grades, who are in charge of aspects of the life of the prison
- a medical officer – a prison doctor
- representation from the discipline staff – main grade, uniformed staff, who have the most daily contact with inmates.
- a hospital officer or prison nurse
- a member of the probation staff

- a member of the establishment's HIV counselling team, where possible
- a chaplain
- an appropriate professional from an outside agency.

Membership may also come from psychologists, education departments, works departments, and physical education instructors, depending on local factors. AMTs were intended to fulfil several functions in the management of HIV and AIDS:

- the facilitation of training and education for staff
- the organisation of sexual health and risk reduction training programmes for prisoners
- confidential liaison with health care teams
- contacting outside agencies
- promoting the work of the pre- and post-test counsellors
- setting up special events, such as World AIDS Day activities
- incident response – taking control of a crisis
- creation of a local policy.

Many local health promotion units feel that they are under-resourced to work in a consistent way with prisons, and there is the persistent problem of the funding of work to be undertaken with inmates who may not originally be local residents. This has become an issue of public health, and must be resolved elsewhere. Where it has not been possible to provide a regular service, some health authorities have supported successful short-term or one-off projects, such as prison art competitions connected with World AIDS Day, calendar projects – every prisoner is interested in the passage of time – and HIV theatre projects. A co-operative scheme was run at a YOI which involved the young people with writing a theatre piece, workshop sessions run by a local theatre education officer and a prison health promotion officer, and finally a performance by professional actors.

PROBLEMS ASSOCIATED WITH HIV PREVENTION IN CUSTODIAL SETTINGS

As yet, there are no comprehensive figures about HIV and AIDS in prisons in this prison system. Epidemiologically, in the community transmission of HIV occurs more often through sexual contact, rather than transmission through blood to blood contact in injecting drug use. However, prison populations by their very nature contain a greater number of 'rule breakers' than outside communities. It is acknowledged by the prison service that there is a serious illicit drug problem in prison establishments, and the drug prevention strategy 'Tackling Drugs Together' outlined in 1996 by the then Home Secretary underlined the importance of the mandatory drugs testing policy discussed above. The difference between drug and HIV prevention work in the community and in prison is marked:

In a prison	In the community
Possession of illicit drugs carries severe penalties, including further loss of liberty	Possession of illicit drugs may carry severe penalties, depending on the circumstances
Help from a drugs counsellor may be available, if the prison has access to one	Help from a drugs counsellor is available from a variety of locations, including community drug teams
Prison service prevention workers may feel compromised: does risk reduction training somehow give the nod of approval to drug taking?	Prevention workers do not have a dual role as health promoters/discipline staff
Prisons do not offer needle exchange facilities or free access to condoms	Needle exchange and free condoms are accessible at a wide variety of venues in the community
Anonymous testing for HIV is available to prisoners after contact with medical staff	Anonymous testing is available from a variety of centres

PRISON STAFF AND OUTSIDE AGENCIES: A GUIDE TO CO-OPERATIVE WORK

The formation of alliances and co-operative work between the prison service and external agencies is a logical step towards building healthy communities. In North-Western England, a regional AIDS Forum is one of several groups established which attract and support members from a large number of organisations, including the prison service. The National AIDS and Prisons Forum, which was established in 1989, continues to bring people together from the statutory and voluntary sectors to discuss and share information about HIV and prisons, and carries out policy work and research. Many of the members are prison service employees.

Traditionally, there has been an uneasy relationship between 'outsiders' and prison staff, with stereotyped and old-fashioned ideas causing some gaps in communication. This is not so much the case as we approach the millennium, and need not exist at all, if joint work is undertaken with a little research and understanding. Not all prison staff are 'dinosaurs' whose main agenda is to keep prisoners locked up for 23 hours a day; and not all community agency staff are of the belief that all prisoners are innocent, misguided wretches. One of the keys to a successful partnership is to behave appropriately.

For outside agencies:

- Fit in with the regime, rather than expecting it to fit around you
- Find out what the rules are and obey them
- Always keep appointments

- Remember that the security of the prison cannot be compromised
- If you don't know the meaning of something, ask an officer
- Wear appropriate clothing for the meeting you are attending
- Don't stereotype people.

For prison staff:

- Explain what the rules are, and why they are in place
- Do not expect newcomers to prison work to understand prison service jargon and acronyms – explain what they mean
- Keep appointments, or if possible, give notice of cancellations. Explain at the outset of a working relationship that in a prison incidents might upset the normal routine
- Be aware that 'voluntary' (as in voluntary sector) does not imply unpaid voluntary work – a high standard of professionalism is required of voluntary sector staff
- Don't stereotype people

REFERENCES

AIDS Advisory Committee (1995) Review of HIV and AIDS in prisons. London: HM Prison Service.
Department of Health (1992) The Health of the Nation. London: HMSO.
Director of Health Care (1995) Dear Doctor letter. London: HM Prison Service.
Directorate of Prison Medical Services (1991) Circular Instruction 30/91 – HIV and AIDS: Prison Service policy and practice in England and Wales. London: HM Prison Service.
Perkins S (1996) HIV and custody. London: The HIV Project.
Perkins S (1997) Prisons. In: K Alcorn (Ed), AIDS reference manual. London: NAM Publications.
Perkins S (1998) Access to condoms for prisoners in the EU. London: National AIDS and Prisons Forum, supported by the European Commission.
Perkins S & Robinson B (1995a) AIDS inside and out. London: HM Prison Service.
Perkins S & Robinson B (1995b) Talking about AIDS. London: HM Prison Service.
Shapiro H (1994) Druglink factsheet 6: Drug testing. London: ISDD.
WHO Global Programme on AIDS (1993) WHO guidelines on HIV infection and AIDS in prisons. Geneva: WHO.

USEFUL ADDRESSES

The National AIDS and Prisons Forum
c/o 169 Clapham Road
London SW9 0BU
Tel: 0171 582 6500

HM Prison Service
Directorate of Health Care
Cleland House
Page Street
London SW1P 4LN
Tel: 0171 217 3000

Body Positive
51b Philbeach Gardens
London SW5 9EB
Tel: 0171 835 1045

Health Education Authority
Trevelyan House
30 Great Peter Street
London SW1P 2HW
Tel: 0171 222 5300

National AIDS Helpline
PO Box 5000
Glasgow G12 8BR
Tel: 0800 567123

Positively Women
City Road
London EC1V 1LR
Tel: 0171 713 1020

The UK Coalition of People Living with HIV & AIDS
Kennington Lane
London SE11 5RD
Tel: 0171 820 8877

Chapter 11

Working in Hospital and Community Settings

Ina Simnett

INTRODUCTION

This chapter discusses what works and doesn't work through interventions in hospital settings and in the community (the word 'community' is used here to mean anywhere outside a hospital). It illustrates the importance of understanding how a setting works before taking action – especially the importance of understanding the culture, how to gain entry, designing the intervention to meet local needs and auditing (checking) what actually happens. It provides advice for 'outsiders' who are seeking to penetrate and work in settings other than their own. It will be particularly helpful to those who are seeking to work with NHS staff in hospitals or in the community, and to NHS staff who are intending to work in unfamiliar settings.

The first section, *Working in Hospital*, reflects on experience gained through a study of the health promotion work of hospital cardiologists in order to help them to help their patients towards healthier lifestyles.

The second section, *Child Accident Prevention*, examines undertaking a community-based child accident prevention strategy and describes specific examples of accident prevention work undertaken by Strelley Nursing Development Unit in a disadvantaged community in Nottingham. It will be useful to those working in, or aiming to work in, inter-agency healthy alliances and to those undertaking an assessment of local needs. It illustrates the importance of the beliefs of local people as a source of evidence for health promotion interventions.

The final section, *Breast Health Awareness*, discusses how evidence was gained about local women's breast health knowledge, views and perceptions and how, once acquired, it was used to develop a community health promotion initiative. It will be useful to those concerned with all stages of project development from the initial idea, to planning, implementation, evaluation methods and presentation of findings.

Evidence-based Health Promotion. Edited by Elizabeth R. Perkins, Ina Simnett and Linda Wright.
© 1999 John Wiley & Sons Ltd.

Section 11.1

Working in Hospital

Lesley Jones, Elizabeth R. Perkins, Ina Simnett and David Wall

WHY INVOLVE HOSPITAL DOCTORS?

Involving hospital doctors in health promotion is important for two reasons. They have a major influence on patient care, both directly, in what they do and say to patients, and indirectly, in how they encourage, discourage or permit other professional groups to behave. They also, more broadly, play a major part in the culture of the institution in which they work; if the concept of the Health Promoting Hospital (NHS Executive, 1994) is to become reality, more than paper commitment is required from organisations, and a variety of professional groups will have to integrate health promotion into their everyday practice. In the case of hospital doctors, this is recognised to be a difficult task. Weare's survey of teachers of undergraduate medical students (1986) commented that:

> Most defined health promotion as the primary prevention of disease . . . through patient instruction. . . . Many had reservations about this model, finding it unproven, negative, simple, repetitive boring, authoritarian and not a task for doctors, especially hospital doctors.

More recent work (Meakin and Lloyd, 1996; Weare, in press) suggests that some progress has been made in undergraduate education and that more is achievable, given changing attitudes; it is, of course, important that what is learnt in theory can be applied in practice when medical students start clinical work.

In this section we reflect on the experience gained in the course of working with hospital doctors in two main ways – a research study of a sample of cardiologists in the West Midlands, and the development of a resource pack called *Helping patients change their behaviour* (Simnett et al., 1997), aimed at junior hospital doctors in all specialties in the context of their postgraduate education. The discussion will consider relevant theory on organisational culture and the implications for

Evidence-based Health Promotion. Edited by Elizabeth R. Perkins, Ina Simnett and Linda Wright.
© 1999 John Wiley & Sons Ltd.

gaining access and selecting acceptable and effective methods to work with this professional group.

THE EFFECT OF CULTURE

It is hard to define culture; any definition is constrained by the culture of the definer! Hofstede (1981) sees culture as 'a system of collectively held values'. He sees it as a broad tendency to prefer certain states of affairs over others. Lambert (1996) emphasises the behavioural aspect of culture by suggesting that 'culture is by definition, learned behaviour'. This is an attractive definition, because the real (as opposed to stated) values of an organisation can be deduced by observation of behavioural norms. Hofstede (1981) makes the point that we cannot observe mental processes. What we can observe is behaviour, words and deeds.

Many writers have offered categorisations of culture (Handy, 1985; Hofstede, 1983; Robbins, 1990). Robbins' is the most helpful here because he suggests ten key characteristics along which cultures differ, providing an easily used checklist to describe a culture. This task is important for anyone attempting to work within a culture which is not their own (for example health promotion specialists seeking to work in the hospital setting). It is also important in the context of someone attempting to use a model of health promotion and behaviour change whose philosophical basis does not reflect the culture in which they want to use it. It is vital to recognise the tensions between the prevailing culture and the one which would naturally support the intervention you have chosen and make it effective. We suggest that during the initial phase in which any worker is 'gaining entry', they should also be seeking to assess the culture of that particular setting.

A useful amendment of Robbins' (1990) characteristics of culture in looking at hospital practice and health promotion might be:

- degree of control over patient management
- level of consultant control over junior doctors' initiative
- level of recognition of the need to integrate health care into a team approach
- support of the efforts of members of the health care team
- tolerance of initiative by other health care professionals
- type of training culture in existence in the workplace
- types and use of patient information record systems
- communication patterns between health care workers
- use of any reward system by 'managers' with more junior staff
- level of involvement of the patient in their own treatment and care
- tolerance of 'outsiders' within the health care team.

Clearly you cannot ask direct questions about these issues, since you are likely to get the answers people think are 'right'. However, careful observation and gentle discussion should elicit the information. Unless you have a lot of time and an explicit brief to do so, do not attempt to try and change the culture. Culture change is complex, takes time, and needs a strong lead from within an organisation. Identify what problems might arise because of the clash of cultures and do your best to minimise them. This may mean compromising your approach and your material, but it is best to start from where they are, not from where you want them to be.

GAINING ENTRY AND WHO TO WORK WITH

At first sight this might seem fairly straightforward, particularly to outsiders who are used to telephoning, making an appointment, and visiting to discuss the business in hand. Even though, as experienced health promoters and researchers, we knew that gaining entry would take careful preparation, flexibility and persistence, we found setting up research and pilot sites for our work much more difficult than we had expected. We were supported by our funders, the West Midland Region's Board for Postgraduate Medical and Dental Education and (for the survey only) the former West Midlands Regional Health Authority. Our credentials were thus excellent and we had considerable help from our funders in identifying local networks and potentially interested doctors. Nevertheless, we discovered that it takes a great deal of patience and perseverance to track down and talk on the telephone to a consultant. Letters sometimes appeared to drop into a void, although the fax was sometimes effective in at least establishing that we wanted to talk.

Once we had obtained permission to work in the departments – and no one refused research access, despite our concerns in the early stages – we developed a clearer understanding of why it had been so difficult to achieve the first contact. Our research required interviewing, and we started by asking the departmental secretary to make appointments for us. We found, however, that a lot were altered on site. We also found that interviews were impossible to time. The range was unusually wide, between two hours (two consultants), and 20 minutes (a registrar extracted from his work by the departmental secretary). We learnt early that effective work in most departments required two researchers who were prepared to spend the day there and interview junior doctors at random; working to any prearranged timetable was clearly impracticable. This is not because their consultants were unco-operative; they were willing in principle to help us. Hospital doctors are not only very busy; they can be randomly busy, working not only with regular commitments like clinics and ward rounds, but also with unpredictable clinical workloads.

What implications does our experience have for others? If you want to work with a team or department, you need to start with the consultant(s). The consultant's secretary is your best guide to making contact in the initial stages, and may well be the lynch-pin in future organisation of events. Have *concise* written explanations of what you want to do, and what it will achieve, ready to send or fax. It is as well to be able to back up your approach with information which is acceptable to doctors; references from medical journals carry most weight, and we found it useful that the *British Medical Journal* had recently covered the type of qualitative work which we wished to carry out (e.g. Mays & Pope, 1996). However, it is a mistake to assume that hospital doctors will automatically want a long academic discussion, either on paper or in person – we found that even with consultants the appetite for this varied enormously, and juniors had on the whole far more practical matters on their minds.

MODELS AND METHODS

Theories of health behaviour are inextricably linked with models of health and health promotion. The model of health used in a particular culture may emphasise and focus on disease management, health care, disease prevention, or health promotion, or a combination of any of these. Doctors traditionally tend to focus on the individual, disease management, and health care, nearly all of their training being in these areas. When this is considered alongside the tendency for most hospital patients to assume the 'sick role' with its attendant loss of control and power over self, it is not surprising that there can be some difficulty when introducing models of health, health promotion and behaviour change which stress empowerment. However, it would be a mistake to assume that all firms or departments are alike in this respect. Indeed the fact that the junior doctors are no longer always organised around one consultant testifies to the fact that ways of organising things in hospitals are changing.

During our research into cardiologists' understanding and practice of patient education and health promotion (Perkins et al., 1996), we found a wide variation in knowledge of, and use of, models of behaviour change and health promotion. These doctors as a group had very little familiarity with research on behaviour change and the appropriate practical strategies for health promotion which can be drawn from it. Only one doctor (out of a sample of 52), for example, had come across Prochaska and DiClemente's Stages of Change (1994). Some had doubts that a body of research on these issues even existed!

Whilst most doctors said they raised lifestyle issues with patients, the difficulties posed by lack of time were stressed. Written checklists for use on wards were not routine, and nor was the practice of recording, in the patients' notes, or in separate nurse records, which lifestyle issues had been raised and what progress had been made. Various strategies to help patients remember information were in use, as was enlisting the help and support of relatives and friends. However, the urge to use scare tactics or haranguing as an attempt to push the patient into medically approved behaviour were in use, and doctors were not aware of the limitations of these approaches.

Since we chose cardiologists as a group likely to be sympathetic to secondary prevention, these findings were salutary in thinking about the development of material for specialties where patient education could be expected to have a lower profile.

The pilot stage of the development of these materials was also salutary. We discovered that the materials were too long, and involved too much background explanation. What junior doctors really wanted was to be told how to do it and what to say. The case studies, checked by senior clinicians before pilot, used a blend of clinical and preventive input, and proved both credible and popular, fitting as they did into more familiar models of medical education. In our revised version we retained the case studies and restructured the theoretical input, relegating much of the academic justification to appendices for background reading, and changing our selection of models of working to suit the responses we received.

The Stages of Change model developed by Prochaska and DiClemente (1994) was felt to be easy to understand and to apply in thinking about individual patients. We therefore used this as the theoretical basis within which other techniques of behaviour change can be applied, Motivational Interviewing (Miller & Rollnick, 1991), particularly for the undecided and motivated stages, and Brief Interventions (Effective Healthcare, 1993; Rollnick et al., 1992), particularly for the unmotivated stage.

We recognised from the survey that many junior doctors, in particular, would be likely to know little about local resources which might help their health promotion activities, and the pilot confirmed this problem was widespread. Since SHOs rotate specialties every six months, and registrars have a commitment to the specialty but not necessarily to the local hospital where they are training, this is hardly surprising. As educational consultants with no local base, this was not a problem we could tackle directly, though in case studies we encouraged thought about local community services inside and outside the NHS, self-help groups, and the provision of written information.

WORKING WITH DOCTORS IN GROUPS

We designed the pack to be used either on an individual basis or as the basis for discussion within the department as part of educational input for juniors; we also recognised that some departments might wish to treat prevention as a team matter and include nurses or members of the professionals allied to medicine. The pilot gave us experience of a range of group situations, and confirmed many of our expectations after the research phase. On the basis of this, we would suggest the following as useful advice for 'outsiders':

• *Hospital doctors are very busy.* They will not take kindly to a philosophical exploration of the meaning of health and health promotion. They need short bursts of easily read and digested information. Practical examples and guidelines as to what they should do are desirable. Do not be misled into giving the underlying academic basis of what you are doing without checking out that they want it. It is enough that you have this available for those who want to dig deeper.

- *Be very clear about what they are expected to do in the session you are running.* Consultants vary in their teaching and training skills with their juniors, and within medical education attention is being paid to this difficult problem (SCOPME, 1994). It sounds a good idea to attempt to get a consultant to run a session, but what you mean by group discussion could develop into a monologue. Try to gauge the experience of the consultant in running a small group session before you commit them to exercising a skill they may not have.
- *Be ready for the unexpected.* Doctors turn up late, get bleeped in the middle of a session, leave early and may well not have read what you have sent. Do not take this personally – it is a consequence of the demands on doctors in the hospital culture. Ensure that the organisation of the session leaves nothing to chance. For example, if it is across the lunch period, you will either need to tell people to bring sandwiches, or provide them. If you want a room set out in a certain way, get there early and do it yourself.

WORKING THROUGH OTHER PEOPLE

Given the difficulties outlined above, it may well seem easier initially to make contact with nursing staff or other professions supplementary to medicine such as dietitians and physiotherapists. They will also have more time than doctors to spend on health promotion with patients. Specialist or rehabilitation nurses will have education and prevention as part of their remit and will be supportive of further health promotion input. In the survey, we explored the extent to which cardiologists sought support from other health care professionals within the hospital. In the interviews, rehabilitation classes and nurses were mentioned frequently as well as dietitians, physiotherapists and others. This suggests a level of comfort with handing over a major role in health promotion and behaviour change to others, and would ease the attempts of an 'insider' to initiate and co ordinate a more active programme.

However, this may not be true for all specialties, and even within cardiology the attitude of the consultant to the raising of lifestyle issues with patients was crucial. Where the consultant actively promoted the raising of lifestyle issues this happened in a wider variety of ways, and both cardiac rehabilitation programmes, and working as a co-ordinated multi-disciplinary team seemed to be better developed. Checking out the local culture according to the criteria listed earlier would certainly seem advisable before assuming other professionals could take a lead.

In any case, any health promotion attempt with patients really needs a team approach to ensure that all members of the team are supporting, and not sabotaging, the work of those who are taking the lead. For this reason an outsider must either start with the consultant or approach another person familiar with this hospital setting to carry out all the face-to-face work for them, including persuading the consultant to support it.

There will be advantages in using someone within the hospital setting to do this, since they will already have the contacts and know the culture. If this way is chosen, it will be important to ensure that insiders have up-to-date information on health promotion and behaviour change, training in facilitation skills, access to resources and support in their efforts. They will also need to know whether the materials and models they wish to use have been evaluated and in what circumstances they have been shown to be effective – this is essential information to have 'up one's sleeve'. Health promotion or public health support could be very useful here.

AUDIT AND EVALUATION

If the techniques and materials which you are using are already proven to be effective, there should be no need to run an on-going evaluation of their effectiveness. If you are transferring models or knowledge developed in another field, then it may be necessary to check that they can be transferred. We strongly recommend that anyone wishing to evaluate health promotion *effectiveness* seeks expert advice and help. During our research we came across attempts to prove effectiveness which were little more than satisfaction surveys. It is important that an evaluation focuses on the primary objectives of the intervention. Do you wish to give knowledge, change behaviour or improve health outcomes? (See Chapter 16.)

It is, however, very important to devise a means of regularly *auditing* the intervention which has been chosen. This is really about checking what you planned has happened, and the techniques and materials agreed on are being used. This will also be a useful record of activity if it is required by funders or by health authorities as purchasers. It is naïve to assume that somehow, presented with the evidence, doctors will inevitably use proven behaviour change methods effectively with their patients. Williams and Macintosh (1996), chronicling the fate of materials on cervical screening produced for use in general practice, showed that even when presented with evidence-based materials, doctors then proceed to make their own judgements about these materials and often not use them. This is not surprising when you consider that little has yet been done to bring the teaching and practice of preventive medicine into the mainstream of medical education (Cimino, 1996). It is helpful to remember that doctors themselves will be somewhere on the change cycle in the context of believing that prevention and health promotion are worthwhile and effective.

REFERENCES

Cimino J A (1996) Why can't we educate doctors to practise preventive medicine? *Preventive Medicine*, 25, 63–65.
Effective Healthcare (1993) Brief interventions and alcohol use, Bulletin No 7.
Handy C (1985) Understanding organisations. Third edition. Harmondsworth: Penguin Books.

Hofstede G (1981) Culture and organisations. *International Studies of Management and Organisation*, X(4), 15–41.

Hofstede G (1983) The cultural relativity of organisational practices and theories. *Journal of International Business Studies*, Fall, 75–89.

Lambert T (1996) The power of influence: intensive influencing skills at work. London: Nicholas Brealey Publishing.

Mays N & Pope C (1996) Qualitative research in health care. London: BMJ Publishing Group.

Meakin R P & Lloyd M H (1996) Disease prevention and health promotion: a study of medical students and teachers. *Medical Education*, 30, 97–104.

Miller W R & Rollnick S (Eds) (1991) Motivational Interviewing. London: Guildford Press.

NHS Executive (1994) Health promoting hospitals. London: Department of Health.

Perkins E R, Jones L & Simnett I (1996) Hospital doctors and prevention: a study of the views of cardiologists in the West Midlands (unpublished).

Prochaska J O & DiClemente C C (1994) The transtheoretical approach; crossing traditional boundaries of therapy. Malabar, FL: Kreiger Publishing.

Robbins S P (1990) Organisation theory, structure, design and applications. Englewood Cliffs, NJ: Prentice Hall.

Rollnick S, Heather N & Bell A (1992) Negotiating behaviour change in medical settings: the development of brief motivational interviewing. *Journal of Mental Health*, 1, 25–37.

Simnett I, Jones L, Perkins E R & Wall D (1997) Helping patients change their behaviour: a resource pack for hospital doctors. Birmingham: West Midlands Board of Postgraduate Medical and Dental Education. University of Birmingham, Medical School.

Standing Committee on Postgraduate Medical and Dental Education (SCOPME) (1994) Teaching hospital doctors to teach. SCOPME, 1 Park Square West, London NW1 4AJ, 0171 413 1943.

Weare K (1986) What do medical teachers understand by health promotion? *Health Education Journal*, 45(4), 235–238.

Weare K (in press) What kinds of medical education are needed to promote health? To what extent are we achieving them? In: N Temple & H Diehl (Eds), Prevention of disease in the western world. Athabasca, Canada: Humana Press.

Williams S & Macintosh J (1996) Problems in implementing evidence-based health promotion material in general practice. *Health Education Journal*, 55, 24–30.

Section 11.2

Child Accident Prevention

Kathy Brummell

INTRODUCTION

Accidental injuries to children are common, and the prevention of these has become an important target in health promotion. Accidents are the biggest killer of children aged over one year. Each year in Britain one in five children requires hospital or GP treatment for an accident. The morbidity from these accidents is high, with many children being permanently disabled or disfigured. The emotional and financial costs of these accidents are paid by the children and families involved in such accidents. Costs are also paid by the health services, and by society as a whole. Accidents to children happen most frequently in the setting in which they live: their home, and their local community (Avery & Jackson, 1993). The seriousness of children's accidents has been acknowledged by the government, and accident prevention has become a national target for health promotion (Department of Health, 1992). Until recently, little research has taken place into children's accidents. Some examples of effective interventions have been identified, but there has been relatively little research into the effectiveness of community wide interventions (Towner et al., 1993).

The aim of this section is to examine accident prevention work in the settings in which they occur. We first examine undertaking a community-based child accident prevention strategy in relation to the assessment of local needs, the resources available within the community, the resources available outside the community, the process of undertaking the strategy, and the dissemination of information. Secondly, we describe an example of accident prevention work undertaken within a community. Finally, evidence-based health promotion will be examined in relation to need, to the effectiveness of interventions, and to the example based on practice.

Evidence-based Health Promotion. Edited by Elizabeth R. Perkins, Ina Simnett and Linda Wright.
© 1999 John Wiley & Sons Ltd.

UNDERTAKING A COMMUNITY-BASED CHILD ACCIDENT PREVENTION STRATEGY

Forming a Healthy Alliance

A child accident prevention strategy is more likely to be successful if it is undertaken as a healthy alliance between a number of individuals and organisations (Towner et al., 1993). A joint initiative can bring together and utilise the knowledge, skills and resources of all these people. It is likely that one person, or a small group of people, will decide that 'something should be done' about children's accidents. This decision may be precipitated by a particular incident or a general increase in awareness of accidents as an issue locally. This person or group may identify other people locally, whom they think are likely to support an initiative, and will need to consider how to invite them to participate. One strategy may be to undertake a joint training day on accident prevention, as an awareness raising strategy, or potential participants could be invited to an exploratory meeting.

A joint training day may be of use if it is thought that an increased knowledge base of potential participants may be required. Useful topics for the day may include updating information about the epidemiology of accidents, exploring attitudes towards accidents, and examining models of accident prevention. Trainers will need to have a sufficiently detailed knowledge of children's accidents, as well as having the skills to facilitate groupwork. This day would also bring together people who may not otherwise meet, although they work or live in the same community. Participants may agree to arrange further meetings where a co-ordinated local accident prevention strategy could be discussed.

An exploratory or initial meeting will need to be arranged and facilitated by those who raised accidents as a local issue. It will need to have a clear agenda, but be flexible enough to meet the needs of all the participants. The group will need to identify what the key issues are, locally, in child accident prevention, and what actions are most likely to address local needs. They should decide exactly what they are going to do, who will do them, and propose a time-scale for these actions. They may also need to identify, and contact, further sources of support as outlined above. Co-ordination of the strategy may be delegated by the group to one individual, or undertaken by the group as a whole.

Carrying out any strategy will require detailed planning and commitment from all those involved. Communication between those involved will need to be clear, and regular meetings are important in ensuring that the strategy progresses effectively. Individuals need to be clear about the action that they will undertake in order to carry out the strategy. Evaluation of the strategy needs to be built into any plans, so that the effectiveness of the strategy can be assessed.

Any local child accident prevention strategy should be tailored to meet the needs of the setting within which it is implemented. Although preventing accidents to children is a national target, community-based interventions are most successful when they are tailored to meet local needs, and when they are implemented by an inter-agency healthy alliance. This is important as the numbers and types of accidents to children vary in relation to a number of local factors, and any local strategy will be most effective if these factors are taken into consideration (Towner et al., 1993). Therefore, the first step in planning any intervention is a local needs assessment.

Assessment of Local Need

A needs assessment of a community is based on information relating to the community. This assessment can be based on information that is already available, for example, information from the census, or information can be specifically collected by those undertaking the strategy. Decisions made about what information to collect will depend on a number of factors, for example, resources available to those undertaking the strategy and the time available in which to collect this information (Robinson & Elkan, 1996).

A local needs assessment can be based on a number of readily available sources of information. Useful sources include those listed below.

USEFUL SOURCES FOR A LOCAL NEEDS ASSESSMENT

- people who live in the community
- agencies who work with the community
- the local commissioning body of health services
- services that collect area wide information
- nationally collected data

Specific information may also be collected by those undertaking the strategy. There may be gaps in information from more readily accessed sources which those undertaking the strategy may wish to collect. For example, the numbers and types of accidents which occur to children living in homeless accommodation, or to children living in disadvantaged households.

Accessing sources of information will need to be negotiated by those undertaking the strategy. Access to local people is unlikely to be problematic for those who work directly with the community. Those who do not have direct access to the community may find that they have to set up networks in the community, or work through agencies who do. Access to other sources of information, local and national agencies and documentary information, should be available through direct contact or from local libraries.

This needs assessment may reveal information relating to local child accident prevention needs. Data may demonstrate both the number and types of accidents in a community. For example, the numbers of accidents in the home or on the road, and the types of injuries which occur most commonly in that community. In addition, information may be gained from local people about their beliefs about the causes of accidents and how they think accidents should be addressed locally. Local people may point out the incongruity of a local play area being sited next to a busy dual carriageway with no safe way being available for children to cross the road. This information is likely to underpin any strategy that is set up. For example, if local people believe that the dual carriageway is dangerous for children to cross, this may provide an initial discussion point between agencies and local people.

The needs assessment may also reveal information about resources available to address children's accidents in the community. Resources may be available within the community, or they may be brought into the community from outside.

Resources in the Community

Resources within the community include the people who live in the community, local agencies who work in the community, and the material resources already available in the community. These resources can be mobilised by those planning any intervention so that the strategy belongs to the community, and is undertaken by them, rather than done to them.

People who live in the community have the most intimate knowledge of the community and are a huge potential resource for change. Local people have a wealth of knowledge about the issues pertinent to the community of which those living outside the community may have little awareness. It is likely that any strategy initiated and implemented by them would be based on the perceived needs of the community as a whole, and would address these needs more effectively than those devised by outside agencies. They are more readily able to form networks of local people who are willing to work on any strategy, and have a vested interest in carrying the strategy through. Local people often have the knowledge and skills required to initiate change within their community. They may also use the strategy as a way of sharing and developing these skills within the community.

Agencies who work in the community are also a resource to the community. Agencies from many sectors may see accident prevention as a valid concern into which they can invest the resources available from their agency. Statutory agencies may include health services, social services, environmental health, police, fire, education, and road traffic accident departments. Voluntary agencies already working in the community may also feel that accidents are an issue that they should address. The commercial sector may also support initiatives in the community, for example local shops and businesses. They may provide funds or premises as venues for planning or effecting the strategy. These agencies may not normally work together, but may welcome the opportunity to work as a healthy alliance in order to address local needs in a co-ordinated strategy.

Resources in the community are likely to be found when undertaking a needs assessment. Examples of resources include material resources, such as community centres, family centres, and funds. Information is a resource, the beliefs held by local people in relation to accidents in the community are of particular importance. Access to local people is also an important resource; local people may have readily available communication networks which are a major resource for the effective undertaking of any work in the community setting.

Resources Outside the Community

Support for a local child accident strategy may be brought into the area from outside the community setting. External support can provide resources not available within the community itself. Examples of support that may be provided are finance, power and information.

External financial support is often required for any initiative. The amount of finance that will be required to undertake any strategy will depend on the size and nature of the initiative. Money may be required for a project worker to co-ordinate the strategy, or for material resources such as stationery or safety equipment. Sources of funding include local and national organisations and charities.

Power is a resource which may be used to support any initiative. Sources of power include national organisations, such as the Department of Health, the Child Accident Prevention Trust and the King's Fund. Local organisations are likely to be interested in accident prevention, for example purchasers of health services, and local councils.

Information as a resource can be obtained from many sectors. The collation of this information may provide a firmer basis for the successful implementation of an initiative. Those outside the area may have information about similar initiatives, or further sources of funding.

Dissemination of Information

Information relating to any strategy needs to be disseminated to a number of interested parties. These parties include those immediately involved in the strategy, those affected by the work, and others outside the area. Individuals and groups who are part of the healthy alliance working on the strategy should receive all documentation detailing the strategy. This ensures that the work is undertaken as a joint effort, and that the work proceeds as planned. Those supporting the work should receive regular updates as agreed with them. Funding bodies need to know that the support they are providing is being used to best effect. The wider community needs to know of any work that is affecting them. Communication with the community may use existing channels, for example community newspapers or forums. Those outside the immediate community may also need to know about any work being undertaken. National bodies would benefit from information relating to examples of good practice so that this can be shared for the benefit of others.

CASE STUDY: STRELLEY NURSING DEVELOPMENT UNIT (NDU) CHILD ACCIDENT PREVENTION WORK

Child accident prevention was a major focus for the work undertaken within the Nursing Development Unit (NDU) at Strelley Health Centre (Boyd et al., 1993; Brummell & Perkins, 1995). This section will describe this work as an example of a strategy undertaken to prevent accidents to children within a community setting. I begin by briefly describing the community itself, and the aim of the nursing development unit. I then go on to outline the assessment of need, and the under-taking of the projects aimed at preventing accidents to children within the community.

Strelley NDU was set up to explore a model of health visiting working in a disadvantaged community. The area covered by the health visitors working in the community consists mainly of five local authority housing estates. Chronic unemployment was a major disadvantage to those living on these estates. In 1991, in Strelley ward the unemployment rate was 16.7%. The degree of deprivation experienced on the estates in this ward was masked by the presence of some more prosperous housing. Serious inequalities were found in the community. For example, in 1992, on one health visitor's caseload, 80% of households with children under five had a head of the household who was unemployed, and 95% were receiving benefits (Boyd et al., 1993). Inequalities in health were also evident in the community. High standardised mortality ratios from diseases with avoidable causes of death were found. For example, in Bilborough ward the standardised mortality ratio for lung cancer was 162.92 (at that time the highest in Nottingham).

A number of projects were set up to target the social and health inequalities experienced within the community, and child accident prevention became one of the targets of the NDU. The health visitors set up four projects to address accidents to children.

1. First Aid

Basic first aid training courses were arranged for people living in the community. The courses were taught by a health visitor and a community worker. Funding for room hire and creche facilities was provided by the Public Health Department of Nottingham Health Authority. Pre-existing groups, for example at family centres and parent and toddler groups, were targeted, as well as inviting individuals to come to groups specifically to teach first aid.

2. Safety Equipment Scheme

A low-cost safety equipment scheme was set up to enable people to buy this equipment. The cost of such equipment may be a deterrent to people living on a low income and the lack of such equipment is a risk factor in children's accidents. Funding was made available by Nottingham Dispensary Fund and by Nottingham Health authority to purchase this equipment.

3. Strelley Accident Prevention Group

This was a community group made up of local people and agencies working with the community. The aim of the group was to raise awareness of children's accidents in the community. The group organised displays and presentations at community events, lobbied for improved facilities in the area, and raised funds for more safety equipment.

4. Traffic Calming

Road traffic accidents, caused by cars being driven at excess speed, was a concern of local people, and of statutory agencies. Local estates were to have traffic calming measures introduced, and the health visitors co-ordinated and facilitated communication between the community and the statutory agencies involved.

EVIDENCE-BASED PRACTICE POINTS

- Child accident prevention is an important concern for families and for services involved in promoting health. The size of the problem, and the effects of accidents, have resulted in accident prevention becoming a national health promotion target.
- Accident prevention strategies are most effective if they are planned to meet the health needs of the communities in which they are to be implemented.
- A collaborative approach between those who live in the community and those who work with the community will ensure that evidence can be gathered so that the strategy is planned and implemented more successfully.
- All those involved can mobilise the resources inside and outside the community to develop and implement a strategy tailored to meet local needs.

REFERENCES

Avery J & Jackson R (1993) Children and their accidents. London: Edward Arnold.
Boyd M et al. (1993) The public health post at Strelley: an interim report. Nottingham: Nottingham Community Health NHS Trust.

Brummell K & Perkins E R (1995) Public health at Strelley: a model in action. Nottingham: Nottingham Community Health NHS Trust.

Department of Health (1992) The Health of the Nation: a strategy for health in England. London: HMSO.

Robinson J & Elkan R (1996) Health needs assessment: theory and practice. London: Churchill Livingstone.

Towner E, Dowswell T & Jarvis S (1993) Reducing childhood accidents. The effectiveness of health promotion interventions: a literature review. London: Health Education Authority.

Section 11.3

Breast Health Awareness

Alison Mitchell

INTRODUCTION

Raising breast awareness within my local community has always been a key priority. Working as a clinical nurse specialist within the field of breast care has provided me with the opportunity to actively participate and develop health promotion initiatives within this field of health, my role being very much 'dual', working as a nurse/health promoter. I often use this dual aspect opportunistically, particularly when involved in training and education, using my body of knowledge, skills and expertise gained from the clinical aspect of my role to enable the delivery of accurate, reflective information. The dual role affords me a broad overview of breast care and health promotion, combining clinical experiences with those of the community, and encouraging transfer of knowledge and skills.

Sometimes, however, as a nurse health promoter working with a dual role, expectations and perceptions from others can be varied and conflicting. I can feel that I am fighting against the 'nurse' perceptions when acting as a health promoter, and I feel similar to Bridges (1990), who identified that nurses are stereotypically seen as 'ministering angels', 'battle-axes' or 'naughty nurses'. I have even been referred to as 'the cancer nurse'. However, on the positive side, being a nurse has provided me with the opportunity to discover how many women cope with and feel about breast and associated problems, whether it be about fear of cancer, level of knowledge and understanding, barriers to screening attendance, myths, anxieties and many other social and cultural aspects.

This piece of work hopes to reveal to you an example of how we gained our evidence about local women's breast health knowledge, views and perceptions and how, once acquired, it was used to develop a comprehensive health promotion initiative.

Evidence-based Health Promotion. Edited by Elizabeth R. Perkins, Ina Simnett and Linda Wright.
© 1999 John Wiley & Sons Ltd.

LOCAL HISTORY

Dudley is a town immersed in 'Black Country' culture and history. A variety of cultural views co-exist and cultural differences are equally apparent within both the white and ethnic social groups. Such multivariant, cultural lifestyles and influences need to be considered when planning health promotion interventions.

With a female population of approximately 157 000, breast health promotion has been high on the agenda of local health promotion personnel for many years. Breast screening was introduced in Dudley under the directive of the National Health Service Breast Screening Programme (NHSBSP) in 1988. The aim of the NHSBSP is to reduce the number of deaths from breast cancer by 25% by the year 2000 (Department of Health, 1992) through early detection. The success of this aim is, however, dependent upon at least a 70% service uptake.

In Dudley, we had struggled for many years to obtain the elusive 70%. Many health promotion initiatives were undertaken between 1992 and 1995 aimed specifically at increasing local knowledge of breast screening in the hope of increased uptake and service compliance. Our uptake rate did rise substantially from 55.8% in 1992/93 to 79% in 1994/95, which we like to attribute to our intensive health promotion initiatives, examples of which are given below.

PREVIOUS BREAST SCREENING HEALTH PROMOTION INITIATIVES IN DUDLEY

- Development of local information leaflets/posters
- Local advertising in press
- Breast screening talks to community groups
- Staff training – study days for primary health care staff
- Development of picture story boards for display
- GP surgery visits – training and education
- 'Open days' on mobile units, specifically aimed at Asian women
- Direct client involvement encouraging compliance:
    - production of newspaper articles with client involvement
    - client with husband involvement/partner support
    - interviews with clients on local radio
    - interviews with clients on local television

THE NEED FOR A NEW APPROACH

The initiatives described above were confined to medical/behaviour change approaches to health promotion (Ewles & Simnett, 1995), specifically aimed at increasing breast screening uptake. Having achieved local uptake levels in excess of the once elusive 70%, a breathing space now emerged to consider ideas to incorporate a 'broader', more holistic, and hopefully effective, approach. We looked to devise a breast health initiative for women of *all* ages to cross as many cultural and ethnic boundaries as possible. My clinical experience had made me aware of the large number of women, of all ages, who regularly attended breast clinics and were extremely frightened, anxious and concerned about wide-ranging breast problems. Problems such as breast pain and tenderness, breast asymmetry, nipple discharge, breasts they consider to be too big or too small or different sizes, breasts with lumps, bumps, thickenings, family history and women who intensely fear breast cancer – all common presentations at hospital breast clinics. It was obvious that women have great concerns and fears surrounding breast health issues and therefore an approach which could reach women of all ages, cross cultural and social boundaries, *not be* exclusive to women and could attempt to tackle *breast awareness* in its widest context was sought.

Proposals for Using Drama

The idea of using drama as an educational tool within the context of breast health was acknowledged and discussed. Why drama? The use of drama and/or theatre in delivering and portraying health messages has been increasingly popular in recent years. Theatre in Education has been acknowledged as a powerful method for exploring a wide range of social issues and problems in a controlled and supportive environment (Dunne, 1994) and has been used frequently within the areas of sexual health and HIV and AIDS (Blakey, 1991; Dunne, 1994; McEwan et al., 1991). Theatre in Education was also being developed within the field of breast screening, unknown to us, at the time of our initial project development (Cannon, 1995; Whyman, 1996). This highlights that in order to have more evidence-based health education taking place in practice, we need wider dissemination of current interventions, as already pointed out by other authors (for example, Meredith et al., 1995). A further justification is that links between art and health have been understood by many societies throughout the centuries, as has drama's superior qualities in its ability to affect cognitive and affective development at a number of different levels (Wright, 1993).

Developing a Healthy Alliance

Multi-agency working has long been recognised as the best way to achieve real and lasting changes to improve the health of communities. The *Health of the Nation* (Department of Health, 1992), which stresses the importance of bringing together many different sectors in the quest for improved public health, describes 'healthy alliances', stating that they provide a vital framework for meeting its targets. Joint working is also a fundamental principle for achieving goals of the WHO initiative, *Health for All by the year 2000* (Furrell et al., 1995).

Cross-agency boundary projects such as ours centre heavily on joint working, aiming to address breast health holistically. The alliance within our project is outlined below.

COLLABORATIVE ALLIANCE

- Clinical nurse specialist (Breast Screening Service)
- Women's health adviser (Health Promotion Service)
- Department of Public Health
- Primary health care staff
- Theatre company
- Local Sainsbury's store
- Local college
- Local Asian Women's Group

THE 'DUDLEY BREAST HEALTH CARE' PROJECT

Funding was obtained from Dudley Health, the local purchasing authority, for a small pilot project. The aim was to assess the effectiveness of theatre and theatre education techniques in raising issues pertinent to breast health, whilst using these approaches to reveal information about lay and professional perceptions and beliefs concerning breast health and screening. We saw the latter as a 'needs assessment' to provide us with detailed qualitative data from the women involved in the project, on all aspects of breast health. We intended to use the findings of the project to develop appropriate health promotion initiatives in the future, acknowledging that it is important that health promotion interventions are designed and developed based on previously gained evidence (Meredith et al., 1995).

Funding was obtained easily by applying to the Health of the Nation Special Projects Monies, providing data on local and national breast cancer rates, highlighting that early detection leading to early treatment has been shown to reduce the death rate from breast cancer. It was helpful that our local Public Health Report (Hamilton, 1995) had stated that 'appropriate action must be taken to detect cancer at an early stage through public awareness'. Indeed, it was a recommendation of this report to raise public awareness of the signs and symptoms of cancer to allow for earlier diagnosis and treatment.

Funding gained for this initial project amounted to £3,000. Some would regard this as a highly expensive research method to use for needs assessment work, due to a high unit cost per participant. We saw the positive benefits, however, of gaining local women's thoughts, feelings and interpretations of breast health, as being paramount to the development of future health promotion initiatives, acknowledging Dunne's (1994) recognition that such an approach can create a powerful exercise in community development.

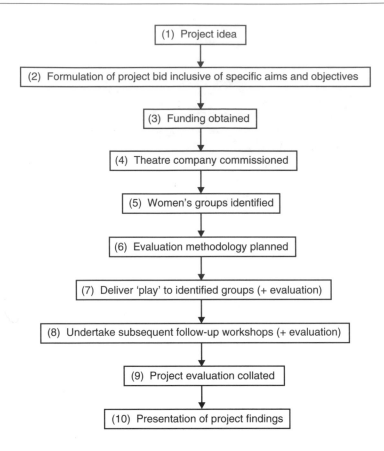

Figure 11.3.1 Stages of planning, delivering and evaluating a breast awareness project

Project Development

Figure 11.3.1 shows how we developed our project.

Stage 1   At this stage the project idea was identified and collaborative joint working (the 'healthy alliance') was developed. A literature search into 'arts and health' was undertaken. Project leaders were identified.

Stage 2   The project bid was formulated with great consideration given to aims and objectives (especially to ensure that these were achievable and realistic).

Stage 3   The bid was submitted for funding from an appropriate source (Health of the Nation Monies).

Stage 4   A theatre company ('Women and Theatre' from Birmingham) was commissioned. These are an experienced, well respected company renowned for previous arts and health work. We met with the company to discuss project content, structure and methodology.

Stage 5   We identified women's groups to be involved in the project through networking and developing links with ethnic community workers, meetings with personnel management of a local retail company, a project explanation to community service managers and establishing a link with a local college.
Four women's groups were identified:
- local Asian women
- staff from a local supermarket
- students from a local college (hair and beauty)
- a mixed group of health professionals (health visitors, nurses).

Stage 6   We explored evaluation methodology with Women and Theatre. It was agreed that qualitative and quantitative data would be obtained via questionnaires and video-taped workshops. Back-up material, i.e. information leaflets and answer sheets were developed.

Stage 7   All four groups were invited to see a play called 'Christine goes to the Doctors', one evening at the local town hall. The play tells the story of a relationship between an ordinary woman and her doctor and the lack of communication between them. A crisis point is reached where 'Christine' finds a breast lump. The play was followed by a session in which the audience interacts with the characters and the issues are reflected upon in discussion. Evaluation questionnaires were issued at the end of the session

Stage 8   Separate workshops were undertaken with the groups within 2–3 weeks of the initial performance. The participants were asked to:
- Brainstorm their perceptions of breasts and breast health.
- Identify any specific experiences from their childhood which influenced their feelings about their breasts.
- Create characters whom they felt *would* and *would not* attend breast screening.
- Role play these characters to explore reasons for their actions and to reflect upon ways in which screening and educational services could be adapted to encourage attendance.
- A health professional was present at *all* workshops and time was allocated at the end of each session to allow discussion and for clarification of any breast health care information which was raised.

Stage 9   The project evaluation was collated and a report of the project was written (Wright, 1996).

Stage 10   The project report was presented back to the initial funders with recommendations for further development.

Evidence Gained

This project provided us with extensive, valuable data on which to build and develop future health promotion initiatives. It revealed evidence of *local* women's knowledge and perceptions of breast health and explored the use of theatre as an effective method of breast health education.

A review of the data concerning the participant's perceptions of breast health led the report's author (Wright, 1996) to draw the following conclusions:

- That women perceived their breasts to be inextricably linked to their sense of femininity, resulting in fear of their loss because of what they represent to themselves and their partners.
- Women expressed reluctance to examine their breasts for fear of what they might discover and for lack of information regarding the procedure involved.
- Cancer was referred to euphemistically in terms of 'lumps'.
- Early, humiliating experiences were remembered light-heartedly, but were believed to have led to inhibited behaviour with health professionals in later life.
- Women identified emotional and social factors as crucial factors in determining breast screening uptake, as were economic and personality factors.
- Low levels of knowledge concerning breast awareness, causative factors of breast cancer and screening were revealed amongst the non-professional participants.
- Women's recommendations for adjustments to presently available breast screening services focused on improving educational input at all levels, from puberty onwards, plus increasing opportunities for communication between healthcare professionals and the general public around breast health issues.
- With regard to the use of 'drama', a high proportion of the study group considered both the theatre and the workshops to be very effective methods of communication of health messages, with a significant number of women (70%) stating that they felt they would change their behaviour as a direct result of the input.

Subsequent Developments

The project report was submitted back to the initial funders and on the basis of this research a subsequent bid for funding for our present project 'Play Safe – Be Breast Aware', was sought and obtained, enabling this initiative to be taken forward and developed. Women and Theatre, the company involved in the original research, were commissioned to develop a play based on the evidence gained, making it pertinent and relevant to women in the local borough. The play 'The Learning Curve' is a humorous and moving play, developed to encourage breast awareness in an interesting, enjoyable and non-threatening way. It was performed, with associated workshops, to 850 people, over 18 days between June 1997 and November 1998, with more performances planned for 1999. The experience has shown us that people *enjoy* watching the play and feel *encouraged* to talk about and question issues surrounding breast health.

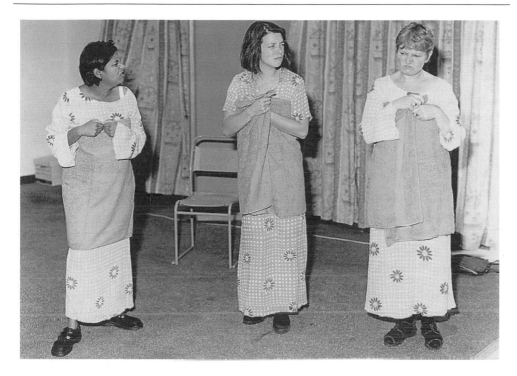

Figure 11.3.2   Women and Theatre performing 'The Learning Curve'

So . . . we in Dudley have found that 'drama' is a powerful medium in which to explore this specific health-related topic. We consider its use positive in aiming to strengthen the impact of breast awareness throughout our local borough and feel confident in its delivery as evidence-based health promotion.

REFERENCES

Blakey V (1991) You don't have to say you love me. An evaluation of a drama-based sex education project for schools. *Health Education Journal*, 50(4), 161–165.

Bridges J M (1990) Literature review on the images of the nurse and nursing in the media. *Journal of Advanced Nursing*, 15(7), 850–854.

Cannon N (1995) Lifescreen – calling all women. A breast screening theatre in health education project. Evaluation report commissioned by Kensington and Chelsea and Westminster Health Commissioning Agency.

Department of Health (1992) The Health of the Nation: a summary of the strategy for health in England. London: HMSO.

Dunne N (1994) Acting for Health, acting against HIV. A report on the effectiveness of theatre in health education in HIV and AIDS education. Birmingham: The Theatre in Health Education Trust.

Ewles L & Simnett I (1995) Promoting health: a practical guide. London: Baillière Tindall.

Furrell R, Oldfield K & Speller V (1995) Towards healthier alliances. London: Health Education Authority.

Hamilton A (1995) Dudley 1995 Health File. The Annual Report of the Director of Public Health. Dudley: Dudley Health Authority.

McEwan R T, Bhopal R & Patton W (1991) Drama on HIV and AIDS: an evaluation of a theatre in education programme. *Health Education Journal*, 50(4), 155–160.

Meredith P, Emberton M & Wood C (1995) New directions in information for patients. *British Medical Journal*, 311, 4–5.

Whyman R (1996) Screen For Your Life. A report of a theatre in health education project used to improve breast screening uptake (unpublished). Walsall: Walsall Community Arts Team.

Wright P (1993) An illuminative appraisal of the uses of drama in health promotion. Unpublished MSc dissertation. Birmingham: University of Central England.

Wright P (1996) A qualitative study of lay and professional perceptions of breast health and the use of theatre as an effective method of health education (unpublished). Dudley: Dudley Health Authority.

Part III

Gathering, Assessing and Using Evidence

Edited by Linda Wright

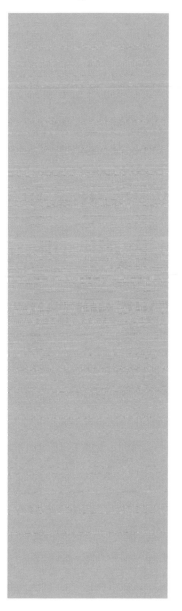

Chapter 12

Doing Things Right

Linda Wright

The first two parts of this book are concerned with thinking about what evidence means in health promotion and the social contexts for gathering evidence. The focus of Part III is on the constraints, challenges and realities of assessing and gathering evidence in health promotion contexts. It is not a comprehensive description of research and evaluation methods, nor is it a 'how to' guide; textbooks and manuals already exist in abundance. Our interest is mainly in exploring the issues involved in health promoters' choice and use of research methods and techniques – on doing things right, within the resources you have available to you.

Most health promoters are not research specialists. Your main responsibilities may not be doing research or even reading other people's research. Working in an evidence-based way is only one element in the range of health promotion competencies (see Liz Rolls' discussion of national occupational standards for health promotion in Chapter 5, Section 5.3). You are likely to have limited time, skills and resources to assess and gather evidence, which immediately limits your choice of research methods and techniques, by ruling out those that are beyond your technical competence, too time consuming or too expensive. The gap between what the textbooks say you should do and your skills and available resources can be so huge that you may be left feeling powerless to do anything at all. As one health promotion specialist put it:

> In Scotland we have a two-tier research world. At one level there are the Universities, big teaching hospitals and clinicians that can attract big money to do things properly. Then there's the rest of us who are doing what we can with very little money, no dedicated staff and pressure to get on and deliver the goods (Perkins & Wright, 1998, p 40).

Given these very real limitations, and the perceived gulf between the academic world and health promotion practice, how can health promoters embrace evidence-based practice? The general principles proposed in Chapter 1 can be translated into personal activity at three levels:

Evidence-based Health Promotion. Edited by Elizabeth R. Perkins, Ina Simnett and Linda Wright.

- reflective practice
- looking for, assessing and using existing evidence
- gathering and using new evidence.

REFLECTIVE PRACTICE

In Chapter 1, we suggested that reflective practice is one of the roots of evidence-based health promotion. Being a reflective practitioner involves both 'thinking on your feet' (reflection-in-action) and taking the time to think about how you could have done things better (reflection-on-action). Both processes involve problem identification, generating solutions, testing solutions and learning from your experience. As noted in Chapter 1, by reflecting in and on action you are actively gathering, assessing and using evidence – the evidence from your personal experience. Developing your skills in reflective practice will therefore not only improve the quality of your work, it will also improve your ability to assess and use other forms of evidence. For example, in Chapter 13, Margaret MacVicar describes how her own reflective practice, coupled with her use of other forms of evidence, are enabling her to change the way she teaches research to student nurses and midwives.

Individuals differ in their abilities to be reflective practitioners. Like any skill, it requires practice; some acquire the skill rapidly during childhood, while others may need a lot of help and coaching to develop it. The good news is that reflective practice skills can be developed. One way to start is by setting aside some time to reflect-on-action; the exercise below offers a framework for doing this.

DEVELOPING YOUR SKILLS IN REFLECTION

You can do this exercise in your head, but it may help you to reflect if you write down your responses to the questions.

1. Think back over your most recent health promotion activities and pick out something that was problematic, or did not work out as well as you had hoped.
2. Recall the event or situation:
   - Where and when did it happen?
   - Who was involved?
   - What happened?
   - What did you do?
   - What were the outcomes?
3. What did you want or expect to happen (your goals)? How did the outcomes differ from your expectations?

Now Define the Problem

4. Think about how you felt before, during and immediately after the situation, e.g. relaxed, tense, playful, tired, angry, stressed, overworked, bored, happy.

5. Why did you experience these feelings and how did they affect the situation? Identify any feelings that were particularly helpful or unhelpful in managing the situation.

Generate Solutions

6. Make a list of as many solutions as possible to the situation you have described. The solutions should be personal – things you could have said or done. Include all solutions you can think of, including the bizarre, extreme and unusual, e.g. 'I could have done nothing', 'I could have written to the Prime Minister', 'I could have walked out'.
7. Now pick out the solutions that seem worth trying.

Test Solutions

8. What have you learned from the experience that will improve your health promotion practice?
9. Now complete the following sentences.
   Next time this situation occurs:
   I will (do) . . . and avoid doing . . .
   I will say . . . and avoid saying . . .
   I will feel . . . and avoid or control feelings of . . .

You could also try:

- Keeping a diary of your work and using it to help you to focus and structure your reflections.
- Setting aside a specific time of the day for private reflection on your work.
- Finding a colleague who can act as a 'critical friend' – someone who understands your work and will help you to reflect on it (not someone who will tell you what to do!).
- Setting up a development group with like-minded colleagues (see Anne McClelland's account of a health visitor development group in Chapter 14, Section 14.3).
- Ensuring that your health promotion practice is adequately supervised – and using your supervisor to facilitate your reflections.

LOOKING FOR, ASSESSING AND USING EXISTING EVIDENCE

Working in an evidence-based way means more than being a reflective practitioner. It also means being aware of and using existing evidence to inform your health promotion practice. As Margaret MacVicar points out (Chapter 13, Section 13.2), being professional about your work means basing it on the evidence that is currently available. To do this, you need both to develop critical appraisal skills and to set up a practical system for retrieving and reading new evidence and reflecting on its implications for your own role and the setting in which you work. After completing studies for initial qualification training, health promoters may discover that finding the time and structures to locate, retrieve and review evidence can be more difficult than developing the skills to do it.

Elizabeth Perkins in Chapter 13 (Section 13.1) provides practical advice on doing (and surviving) literature searches. In addition to special searches, you also need to set up a system for ensuring that you receive regular information about new evidence relevant to your work. This usually involves some work and money to set it up. Once you have it organised, you will at least have made sure that important new evidence (or a reference to it) arrives on your desk – but you still have to read it!

One important strength of health promotion is the informal and formal networks that exist between groups of health promoters. You can use these as part of your structure for keeping up to date with evidence. One of the findings of a recent survey of health promotion specialists in Scotland (Perkins & Wright, 1998) was that looking for evidence often started with a telephone call or conversation with a colleague who had done recent work on the issue being explored. This approach is important because it can save you a lot of time. Explain your interest and ask what research is good or recent. Get hold of these. If you find a piece of research that seems relevant, contact the authors if you want more information than the published report provides. Usually they will want to help, to ensure that their work influences practice.

SETTING UP A SYSTEM FOR KEEPING UP TO DATE WITH NEW EVIDENCE

- Subscribe to bulletins that list newly published material in your field. For example, the Health Promotion Authority and the Health Education Board for Scotland publish regular bulletins of journal articles of interest to health promoters. Alcohol Concern publishes a quarterly 'Current Awareness Bulletin' of journal articles and books on all aspects of alcohol.
- Subscribe to professional journals.
- Subscribe to a journal abstracts service in your field.
- Find out if there are any local or national networks of health promoters working in your field and if there is, join it.
  The national health promotion agencies and charities operate many networks based on settings (see Chapter 7) or topics, e.g. 'Drug and Alcohol Findings' is a new network set up to promote evidence-based progress in the drug and alcohol fields (see Useful Address at the end of this section).
- Set aside a regular time, at least once a month, to read your pile of journals and bulletins.
- If you have access to the internet, you can access research information electronically. Many journals can now be accessed on-line. Take a look at the thousands of news groups; there may be one, or several, that are worth joining.

- If you have access to e-mail, find out if there are any research mailing groups you can join, to extend your network. Why not set one up yourself, made up of people who have similar health promotion interests?
- Share your reactions to new or challenging evidence with your colleagues.
- Negotiate with your manager a strategy for your continuing professional development, which includes attending important courses and conferences.

Critical reading of evidence is necessary to appraise of its strengths and weaknesses. In appraising a research report, your goal is not to place the researcher 'on trial', but to identify the contribution it makes to new understanding (Parahoo & Reid, 1988). Worries about producing research that is good enough to go 'on trial' is one reason why health promoters do not publish their work. Consequently many small-scale local studies receive a restricted distribution, which limits their contribution to health promotion's evidence base.

Reading any material, whether it is a newspaper article or a paper in 'Health Education Research, Theory and Practice', involves making value judgements about its merit or worth. However, to critically review a piece of research, you do need to have a basic understanding of research – its language, meaning and methodologies. Short 'research appreciation' courses have been found to be useful as an introduction to critical reading of research (Hicks, 1994); while doing small-scale research yourself will both help you to understand the difficulties involved in doing research and bridge the gap between academic research and health promotion practice. Critical reading is a skill, which will improve with practice; it may also help you to develop your skills in gathering evidence yourself (French, 1998).

The level of criticism used when reading research evidence depends on your purpose. You will need to take a systematic approach and evaluate all aspects of the material if you are reading:

- with a view to implementing the findings in your practice
- as part of a literature review for your own research study
- to learn more about research methods.

If you are reading for general professional interest, then a more superficial review will be appropriate. Using a checklist of questions can be helpful in developing a systematic approach to assessing evidence, particularly for novice readers of research reports. Elizabeth Perkins' advice in Chapter 13 or guidelines such as those given by Parahoo and Reid (1998) and Ewles and Simnett (1998) are good starting points; although you are strongly encouraged to develop your own checklist guided by criteria relevant to your own health promotion practice. More experienced literature reviewers will have built up their own system for making judgements about the quality of the evidence and its relevance to their work. Remember that no research study is perfect, so it is better to read research for its positive contributions and to view it as generating further questions, rather than producing solutions.

Reading and comparing a variety of research studies will enable you to draw conclusions about the variations in quality of the available evidence. Critiquing an individual study tends to emphasise its weaknesses, whereas comparison of several studies encourages a focus on both strengths and weaknesses (French, 1998). Effective use of existing evidence implies that you have an overall picture of what all of the evidence means. This involves bringing together interpretations of research reports from a variety of sources to achieve a synthesis of its meaning and concepts. The skills involved are *not* the same as those used to appraise individual pieces of research and novice practitioners may find this difficult at first. See Elizabeth Perkins in Chapter 13, French (1998) and Cooper (1989) for practical advice. For example, it can help to draw a web diagram of the key relationships between the concepts contained in individual studies (Owens & Nease, 1993). Taking a tip from qualitative researchers, having a 'long soak' in your bath of evidence can also help you to interpret it. This might include taking a break of several days after reading the evidence, to enable your brain to have time to reflect on its meaning and relevance.

An essential element of your synthesis will be specifically identifying the implications of the literature review for health promotion practice. For those working at local, rather than national, level this will mean interpretation of the evidence in relation to priorities and plans for local services and health promotion programmes. If you think your review might be useful to others, then do consider writing it up for publication.

GATHERING AND USING NEW EVIDENCE

Not all health promoters are in a position to do research to gather new evidence. When faced with situations where the available evidence to guide health promotion practice is thin or even non-existent, it can be tempting to decide to go ahead and gather some evidence yourself – but when is it appropriate to do this and what exactly should you, or could you, do? Practitioners' concerns about gathering new evidence by doing health promotion research fall into four groups: competence, time and resources, quality, and implementation of findings.

COMMON CONCERNS ABOUT DOING HEALTH PROMOTION RESEARCH

Concerns About Competence

'I am not an academic'
'I am not clever enough'
'I don't know the language'
'I don't understand statistics'

'People will criticise me'
'I hate computers'

Concerns About Quality

'What is good enough research?'
'What level should I be working at?'
'It will be boring'

Concerns About Time and Resources

'How can I fit it all in?'
'I don't have time'
'It is too expensive'
'I don't have a computer'
'I don't know who can help'
'I can't be bothered with all this detail'
'I have to get on with *doing* health promotion'

Concerns About Dissemination and Implementation

'If I do this research, will anyone take any notice?'
'I could not produce anything that is worth publishing'
'Will the results be useful?'
'Will it have any impact on practice?'

Achieving Research Competence

Research skills are developed by health promotion practitioners in the same way as any other skills through practice and feedback on that practice (Perkins & Wright, 1998). This is the main method used for teaching students research skills. Hands-on experience continues to be the way that practitioners will develop research competence after qualification. While the principle of learning through doing applies strongly to the development of research competence, ethical and cost considerations mean that this learning demands appropriate support, supervision and management. Managers themselves may feel inexperienced in supporting their staff's research activities, and few services, even specialist health promotion services, employ research specialists. Based on a needs assessment study (Perkins & Wright, 1998), the Health Education Board for Scotland's strategy for developing the research skills of health promotion practitioners is built around a variety of initiatives that will support learning through doing. These include a toolbox of practical guidance on research and evaluation, a research support network, research dissemination and secondments to enable practitioners to develop research experience (Wimbush, 1998). Ways that you might develop your own research competence are suggested below.

WAYS TO DEVELOP YOUR RESEARCH COMPETENCE

- Keep a diary and reflect on what you do
- Shadow an experienced researcher (*i.e. observation only*)
- Work with a more experienced researcher (*sharing the tasks and the responsibility*)
- Negotiate supervision by an experienced researcher (*payment may be required; you would be expected to conduct the work yourself*)
- Negotiate an apprenticeship to an experienced researcher (*with agreed learning goals for your improved competencies*)
- Join or form a team of practitioner researchers
- Find a mentor
- Read a book (or two)
- Training courses
- Open learning programmes
- Distance learning programmes (*particularly if local courses do not meet your needs, or you work in a remote area. Learning via the internet has hugely extended your choice of training course*)
- Join or form a development group (see Anne McClelland, Chapter 14)
- Join or form a network (*contact the National Health Promotion agencies for information on existing networks*)
- Start small (*remember small successes are more valuable that heroic failures*)
- Work within the time and resources you have available
- Always negotiate support from your manager

Time and Resources

Busy health promotion practitioners may well be justified in saying they have no time to do research. Before confirming this assumption, it is worth assessing the cost of *not* gathering new evidence for your health promotion practice:

- How much of your work is based on belief, superstition, received wisdom, the need to be seen to be doing something, or political whim, rather than evidence? For examples, see Margaret MacVicar's comments on nursing practice in Chapter 13.
- Could gathering new evidence actually save you or your organisation time and money, e.g. by scrapping ineffective services or working more efficiently?
- Does any of your health promotion activity carry any risk to your clients/patients/community? If so, how certain are you that it is supported by sound evidence?
- How vulnerable are you to criticism from stakeholders ('Does it work?', 'Is it value for money?', 'Why should I purchase or fund your work as opposed to X's?').

Selecting your research questions to link with your service priorities is an important stage in defining your scope for doing research, as is reviewing the literature to ensure that you will not be reinventing the wheel by repeating work already done elsewhere. It may be more cost-effective to commission the gathering of new evidence from an outside research agency or consultant, particularly if time or skills are not available in-house. Building in, or bidding for, funding for research as a component of all new work (as needs assessment, evaluation or both) will also help to secure future resources and develop evidence-based practice. For example, Glasgow Health Promotion Service routinely allocates 10% of every project's funding to research and evaluation.

Investment in setting up modest monitoring systems, possibly involving only small changes in the way a health promotion activity is recorded, can greatly enhance your service's capacity to gather new evidence about need and outcomes. For example, the Bridgwater project, by adopting a systematic approach to planning, recording and review, has challenged the myth that detached youth work to prevent crime and drug misuse cannot be measured or evaluated (Bowen, 1997). Also see Jane Powell's account of monitoring patient progress in cardiac care rehabilitation in Chapter 16 (Section 16.1).

Purchasers and commissioners of services may have unrealistic views of what kinds of research can be achieved within limited resources; this is where making a case for 'doing things right' becomes a professional and political necessity. It is clearly not possible to do an outcomes evaluation on a project set up six months ago, to analyse and report on 500 questionnaires in two days or conduct a community-based needs assessment for £1,000. Unfortunately, useful advice such as how long research takes and how much it costs is not usually found in research textbooks. Here, local networks, the national health promotion agencies and commercial research outfits are likely to provide more practical guidance.

Quality Assurance in Practitioner Research

Chapter 1 suggests some general principles for collecting evidence yourself, in the context of 'good enough' research. Despite the proliferation of research textbooks, there is very little published guidance on what 'good enough' might be for health promotion practice. Indeed, this was one of the reasons for this book!

All of the contributors to Part III have addressed this issue in relation to their own accounts of gathering evidence. Most of them are health promotion practitioners themselves. Several have explicitly acknowledged the difficulties in ensuring quality in their research, e.g. Anne McClelland (Section 14.3) and Heather Roberts (Section 14.2) in relation to needs assessment in Chapter 14, John Balding and colleagues in relation to their schools survey data in Chapter 13 (Section 13.3), and in Chapter 16, Jane Powell on monitoring cardiac rehabilitation (Section 16.1) and Graham Simmonds in relation to a practitioner-led evaluation study (Section 16.2).

Alison McCamley-Finney and Majella McFadden suggest quality criteria for doing qualitative studies in Chapter 15 (Section 15.1), and further advice is found in Secker et al. (1995) and Rogers et al. (1997).

As with the development of research competence, asking for and receiving feedback will improve the quality of health promotion practitioner research. This is traditionally achieved through publication, and peer review. The bulk of health promotion practitioner research is, at best, 'grey' literature, often not written up at all, or not disseminated. Practitioners will argue that their purpose is only to inform local practice – yet as emphasised in Chapter 1, how can evidence be good enough to inform action, yet not good enough to publish? Many of the sources of information listed under 'Setting up a system for keeping up to date with new evidence' (p 280) may be alternative vehicles for obtaining feedback on your own research. So are discussions with colleagues or managers, a lunch time seminar, or a workshop at a locally organised conference.

Dissemination and Implementation of Findings

Practitioner research is practical research. The findings should be used, otherwise your efforts will be wasted. When planning to gather new evidence of any kind, it is worth thinking strategically about how this evidence will be used and by whom. Will the results be used solely within your department or team? Which other services could/should/might use the results? Do purchasers of your service want the results or do you just hope they might be interested? Which people do you feel *should* use the results but might not take any notice? This is the point where negotiation with all potential stakeholders is important, to gain a commitment to act on the results. If you suspect that, despite your best efforts, the research you do will be ignored, then this is a very sound reason for not doing it. I discuss this issue in relation to evaluation in Chapter 16.

In needs assessment studies one of the greatest challenges for health promotion is ensuring that the evidence is utilised by local services (see the discussion of the tension between evidence and practice in Chapter 1). There is also a huge imbalance between the extensive available evidence on health promotion programme impact and the limited evidence on dissemination and implementation. All too often, funding for research does not adequately cover its dissemination, let alone implementation. Moreover, the lack of recognition of change as a process places yet another set of unrealistic expectations on practitioners in relation to making a new project work.

READING PART III

Part III is divided into five chapters, each of which considers a different feature of gathering, assessing and using health promotion evidence. Chapter 13 examines issues related to getting research evidence into practice, from the perspectives of literature searches, research training and using data. Chapters 14 and 16 feature the two main types of research done by health promotion practitioners – needs assessment (Chapter 14) and evaluation studies (Chapter 16). Qualitative research is an important, but contentious source of evidence for health promotion practice, which is why we have devoted a chapter to these methods (Chapter 15) and not to quantitative research methodologies, although John Balding and colleagues' contribution to Chapter 13 considers the uses of quantitative data.

This part of the book is perhaps best read with a particular practical purpose in mind; so for example, if you are interested in doing or commissioning a needs assessment, read Chapter 14. All of the chapters aim to expose and debate the difficulties and challenges involved in gathering evidence, particularly in relation to the much recorded theory–practice gap.

REFERENCES

Bowen C (1997) The Bridgwater Detached (Street) Youth Work team. Somerset: Somerset County Youth Service.

Cooper H M (1989) Integrating research: a guide for literature reviews. Second Edition. London: Sage.

Ewles L & Simnett I (1998) Promoting health: a practical guide. Fourth edition. London: Baillière Tindall.

French B (1998) Developing the skills for evidence-based practice. *Nurse Education Today*, 18, 46–51.

Hicks C (1994) Bridging the gap between research and practice in assessments of the value of a study day in developing critical research reading skills in midwives *Midwifery*, 10, 18–25.

Owens D K & Nease R F (1993) Development of outcome-based practice guidelines – a method for structuring problems and synthesising evidence. *Journal of Quality Improvement*, 19(7), 249–263.

Parahoo K & Reid N (1988) Research skills: 5. Critical reading of research. *Nursing Times*, 84(43), 69–72.

Perkins E R and Wright L (1998) Developing research awareness, knowledge and skills amongst health education/promotion specialists and health promoters in Scotland. Final report of Phase 1: Training needs analysis. Edinburgh: Health Promotion Board for Scotland.

Rogers A, Popay J, Williams G & Latham M (1997) Inequalities in health promotion; insights from the qualitative research literature. London: Health Education Authority.

Secker J, Wimbush E, Watson J & Milburn K (1995) Qualitative methods in health promotion research: some criteria for quality. *Health Education Journal*, 54(1), 74–87.

Wimbush E (1998) The research training needs of health promotion practitioners (conference paper). Second Nordic Health Promotion Research Conference, Stockholm, 9–11 September 1998.

USEFUL ADDRESS

SCODA
Waterbridge House
32–36 Loman Street
London SE1 0EE
Tel: 0171 928 9500

Chapter 13

Evidence into Practice

Linda Wright

INTRODUCTION

The focus of this chapter is on bridging the gaps between health promotion evidence and practice. In Chapter 1, we referred to the challenges of implementing research-based practice, and noted that, in contrast to the extensive range of studies of health promotion programmes, there are still relatively few studies that address their dissemination, adoption and implementation. This chapter suggests three different types of bridges between evidence and practice by offering help with locating and interpreting existing evidence, an analysis of the process of developing research skills and some practical examples of how basic descriptive data can be used to inform local health promotion action.

Section 13.1, *How to Survive Literature Searches*, acknowledges that health promotion practitioners will have limited time and resources to access and interpret existing evidence and therefore need a different approach to the purely academic researcher. It offers practical guidelines on doing literature searches, including finding relevant evidence and making sense of it.

Section 13.2, *Integrating Research into Nursing Practice*, considers the research–practice gap as experienced by nurses and midwives, from the perspective of a nurse trainer. It considers the application of health promotion evidence within the broader context of nursing and midwifery practice. It considers the different types of evidence that nurses and midwives draw on to inform their practice, including their personal experience, scientific evidence and aesthetic evidence. It also reflects on the process of learning to use evidence and suggests ways in which this can be developed through training.

In complete contrast, Section 13.3 takes an intensely practical focus, by providing five different examples of how basic quantitative descriptive data can be used in health promotion practice. *From Evidence to Action Using Health Behaviour Surveys* describes a questionnaire to measure the health-related behaviour of schoolchildren and illustrates

Evidence-based Health Promotion. Edited by Elizabeth R. Perkins, Ina Simnett and Linda Wright.
© 1999 John Wiley & Sons Ltd.

some of the ways in which it has been used by schools. It gives examples of how the data collected using this standardised instrument can be used to identify differences between schools or communities and indicate priorities for health promotion within the school curriculum and for programmes with parents.

Section 13.1

How to Survive Literature Searches

Elizabeth R. Perkins

FACING THE PROBLEMS

Taking evidence-based health promotion seriously implies a commitment to finding out what evidence other people have collected, preferably before you start work yourself. The arguments are obvious:

- the evidence may show what works well and what doesn't, so you can save yourself and others a lot of work and possible embarrassment
- someone may have done something very similar to what you had in mind, in which case you can build on their experience.

The problems are also obvious:

- time
- access
- making sense of what you find
- (rarely mentioned, this) boredom.

I read a lot of literature reviews in articles submitted to the academic journal for which I review. Many of them bore me, because they lack any spark of personal interest from their writers – almost certainly, the writers were bored too. For many people, the requirement to review the literature has become a deadly chore rather than a voyage of discovery. If literature searches in pursuit of evidence-based health promotion are going to justify the time they will take to do, there needs to be a focus for interest, and a different approach is needed from the purely academic.

Evidence-based Health Promotion. Edited by Elizabeth R. Perkins, Ina Simnett and Linda Wright.
© 1999 John Wiley & Sons Ltd.

COLLECTING MATERIAL

People faced with the need to read round a subject are likely to see this as a requirement to spend days in a library. This in itself may be daunting – not everyone shares the natural academic's sense of a library as a gigantic toybox stuffed with good things, in which they can play for hours. Instead it may seem more like a maze, with the high shelves blocking any clear vision of the way out, or a bog into which the unwary can sink beneath piles of papers, never to be seen again. Even if their image of libraries is relatively benign, many professionals find it hard to envisage being able to spend much time there, and therefore need to use such time as they can find to the best possible effect.

Use What You Have

You probably have something on the topic in question on your desk. Look at the references and see what seems worth following up. This is the start of your shopping list for the library.

Use Your Network

If the library is some distance away, it is possible to make a useful start on a literature search without leaving your place of work. All you need is a telephone. Ringing up colleagues or friends who have an interest in this area will extend your knowledge of individual authorities or institutions. The network can also lead you to the so called 'grey' literature, on new projects not yet published. You can follow up contacts like this from the office – often university departments have lists of publications relating to particular projects, departmental interests, or the work of senior members of staff. Institutions also commission reviews – try the publications lists from the national health education bodies and the York University Centre for Reviews and Dissemination (CRD).

Specialist libraries may also be able to provide you with good starting points; they may have lists of publications covering your subject area or be willing to do a more specific literature search for you. In the UK the national health education institutions have libraries with outreach functions; depending on your professional affiliations and your topic area, there will be others to try also, like the King's Fund for health issues, the Institute for the Study of Drug Dependence for drugs issues, and the various nursing and midwifery professional institutions. Ring up and see what they can do on the phone and by post; policies on charging vary, but photocopying specific articles is likely to cost, and individually tailored searches do take the librarian's time (as opposed to yours) and may not always be available, or available for free.

If you make a start in this way, you will be better briefed before you get to a library, and have a list of things to find on your first visit. It may then be easier to reframe the library as an extension of existing networks – a source of new colleagues you would never otherwise meet.

In your local academic or professional library there will be specialist staff who are there to help readers make the best use of the library's facilities. They will be able to advise you on the catalogues and databases on site and how to use them. These resources are designed according to a logic which is consistent but which may not be identical with your own: 'If you want to retrieve library materials, you must think in the terms used by the cataloguer, not the subject specialist' (Mann, 1986, p 52).

It is therefore sensible to ask for help in using these resources, particularly since the facilities available can change quite a lot in a few years. If you are returning to an institution where you trained a few years back, don't expect yourself to know the ropes. A local specialist librarian is a crucial element in your network for this kind of purpose – if you don't already have contacts with such a valuable person, develop some now!

Use Your Abilities to Focus and Plan

In order to help specialists to help you, you will need to be able to explain what you are interested in and translate it into the kind of keywords they have in their various databases. In identifying useful books, you can start with the catalogue; this, of course, will be restricted to what is on site. For journal articles, you will need to be able to use indexes and abstracts. The kind of databases you will need depends on the topic you have in mind; see Mann (1986), Lee (1996) and Martindale (1997) to give an idea of the range, or better still, ask a librarian!

Both catalogues and indexes are likely to give you a number of references which are no use to you. This is a particular problem with indexes, and if you have access to computerised versions it can be reduced by using more than one keyword – *stress* in *midwives*, for example. Martindale (1997) has a series of excellent worked examples from a health service perspective on using library resources.

- Be prepared to work in stages – if you get a flood of material, narrow the focus; if a dribble, try broadening it.
- Look for key references that keep appearing in other people's work and see that you read these.
- If you tend to have trouble getting focused, find someone to help you talk the project through before you start.

Use the Internet

If you have access to the internet, you can use it as a way of extending your network. As with libraries and bookshops, you can spend a lot of time wandering around exploring, and enjoy yourself in the process. To make productive use of the web, you will need both to put in some time building up knowledge about how to use it and where to go, and to be focused about your project itself. Finding the right user-groups and web sites will depend very much on your topic and slant. You cannot use search engines to track them down without keywords, so the issues are in many ways similar to using libraries effectively! If you are a novice on the web, invest in one of the numerous introductory books and remember that many of the skills you need will actually be old favourites, transferred to a new setting.

Use Your Imagination

Be prepared to think laterally. Databases, while very useful, can get you into a clinical rut in health promotion. If this is happening, try a variety of ways of freeing up your thinking. Drawing a 'mind map' of possible connections between your problem and other issues might help (Buzan, 1989). Wander round the shelves in a good bookshop or library, surf the net, see what's been written for the intelligent lay person and see what their references are, think of something in another clinical area which might be similar. The single most useful reference I found for my PhD was a book I found in a second-hand collection in my local university bookshop. It was on abortion in the USA; my research was on breastfeeding and whooping cough immunisation in the UK. The link was in their key concepts – decision-making.

WORKING ON THE MATERIAL

Assessing It

Once you have collected your mass of material, you will need to sort it. Some papers will inevitably be better than others for your purpose. An early division to make is to distinguish opinion pieces from research studies. The research studies will need assessment to see how far you can safely rely on the conclusions for your own purposes. Firstly, it is important to identify what the authors were trying to do – many qualitative studies provide excellent descriptive material on clients' perspectives or on the detailed problems of changing practice, and are subjected to criticism for not being something they were never intended to be, like a randomised controlled trial (see Dale Webb, Chapter 3). Good studies normally discuss the strengths and weaknesses of the methods used, as well as snags which developed in this particular application of the method, so that readers can have some idea of how the authors see the significance of what they have found. If this is not included, in a short article, for example, this work may have to be done by the reader, drawing on knowledge of the uses of the methods concerned (see the rest of this part of the book for examples).

Many of the questions which researchers should ask of themselves are well within the competence of professionals without a research background. For example, it takes no specialist training to ask the following:

- When was the study done and how relevant are the findings to your problem now?
- What is said about the size of the sample and how was it obtained?
- What kind of built-in bias is there in the collection process?
- How typical is the sample likely to be of the wider population it is supposed to represent?
- How similar is the study area to your own?

You can also think about the risks of collecting misleading information:

- If questionnaires or interviews are used, what attempts have been made to make it easy for respondents to tell the truth as they see it?
- If this is an observation study, what might the observer not see − or not have thought to record?
- If it is a study which makes use of statistical tests, what do these statistics show about the likelihood that the results happened by chance?

Given all this, you can consider whether the conclusions seem to be supported by the evidence. Would you pull out the same issues for emphasis, or would you read the data differently?

Thinking About It

Once you have assembled your material, and sorted out anything which seems seriously unreliable or in other ways unsuitable, you will need to make some combined sense of what is left. Most introductions to research concentrate on assessing single papers, and this is not the same as producing an overview (French, 1998). It helps to hold two different approaches in tension:

- Does this answer my questions?
- What does this tell me that I never thought to ask?

Reading for evidence-based practice involves using a practical focus. Remember your starting point − does this mass of paper tell you anything you can use? Does it give insights into clients' perspectives? Does it describe techniques which work, or don't work? Does it tell you how long a process took to set up, or to undertake? Does it give you ideas on how to proceed with colleagues, or what to avoid?

In the course of your networking you may well find, or be offered, literature searches done by someone else. These can look like a heaven sent solution to your problem, particularly if they are recent and directly related to your interests. They may indeed cover the ground admirably and save you a lot of work, but it is important to check why they were done, and to be prepared to collect at least some of their key references to read yourself. Everyone reads differently for a different purpose and their purpose may not be yours. The CRD reviews, for example, are highly reputable; they work to precise criteria (NHS CRD, 1996) and are concerned with clinical effectiveness. If you want to know how to set up a project, rather than which method to use for it, their selection of studies may not do what you want.

Feeling Around It

If what you have collected is boring you, don't just abandon the work, or write it up and bore other people! Instead, use the boredom. What is it about? Given what you wanted to know in the first place, what is the nature of the disappointment you're suffering? This may give you a framework to write it up critically, or it may tell you that you need to think more broadly (see Use your Imagination, p 294). If your focus is evidence-based practice, it is important to bear in mind the value of saying that, within the time available, you have found nothing that advances your work – if this is indeed the case. Local experiments can then proceed with suitable caution, and you can continue to look out for anything really useful in the professional press or in your contacts with other people.

KNOWING WHEN TO STOP

Think about your own learning style, strengths and weaknesses. Are you a person who likes to get on with the job, or one who prefers to see that it is all carefully thought out first, even if it does take a bit longer? Do your colleagues see you as a source of lots of bright ideas which need sifting, or as the person who sticks to the point? The problem of when to call a halt and how wide to throw the net will become inextricably entangled with your own characteristics, and here it pays to try to counteract your natural tendencies – slow down and spend a bit more time if you are an action person, don't chase those final references which just might be useful if you are meticulous. If you are full of bright ideas you will need to focus; if you have a very sure grip on the point you may not be looking broadly enough to find the really helpful material. As a rule of thumb, it is either time to stop or time to change your approach radically when you are learning nothing new about the problem you are investigating, or nothing you can use.

Within a framework of evidence-based practice, the deadline for the completion of your main literature search may well be set by practice, not by theory. You cannot emulate university departments or the CRD if you only have a week available. It is worth keeping notes of the way you have worked as well as what you have found, so that if you have time to revisit the issue later you can avoid repetition of effort – and so that if necessary you can explain to enquirers what you have been able to do in the time. There will always be something you've missed, and something new you can learn!

REFERENCES

Buzan T (1989) Use your head. Third edition. London: BBC Books.

French B (1998) Developing the skills required for evidence-based practice. *Nurse Education Today*, 18, 46–51.

Lee R (1996) How to find information: medicine and biology: a guide to searching the sources. London: British Library Science Reference and Information Service.

Mann T (1986) A guide to library research methods. New York: Oxford University Press.

Martindale K (1997) Using the library. In: S Maslin-Prothero (Ed), Study skills for nurses. London: Ballière Tindall.

NHS Centre for Research and Dissemination (1996) Undertaking systematic reviews of research on effectiveness: CDR guidelines for those carrying out or commissioning reviews. NHS Centre for Research and Dissemination, University of York.

Integrating Research into Nursing Practice

Margaret MacVicar

APPLYING RESEARCH TO PRACTICE

The Educational Gap

Integrating research into nursing practice is a complex challenge for education and practice alike. This discussion is based on the experience both of teaching research to pre-registration student nurses and midwives on diploma courses, and of under-taking research on this process. My experience in research education has confirmed my expectations that teaching can be enhanced by exploring and then taking account of the way in which students learn and understand the subject. My own research has contributed enormously to my appreciation of these processes, and also suggests that the level of understanding an individual student has about research and their commitment to it impacts crucially on their student practice (MacVicar, 1998).

My observations led me to think that many of the difficulties which nursing has encountered in its promotion of research in practice could have been avoided, and rest with the failure of the profession to invest sufficiently in education in *using* research for practice. The opportunity for pre-registration students to learn about research for practice, which arose due to the reforms in nurse education, has resulted in some students being more comfortable with research in practice and keener to use it than many practising nurses, for whom research may be unfamiliar and unwelcome. Naturally the implementation of research findings has been difficult in these circumstances.

Many writers in this field such as Kitson et al. (1996) and Rolfe (1994) advocate models of implementation or ways that research can more easily become part of practice. While these may contribute, they are insufficient in themselves. The education of individuals in research is the first and essential requirement for the integration of research into practice. Whether formally educated or self-taught, nurses in practice have to believe in the worth and value of research. This belief is

Evidence-based Health Promotion. Edited by Elizabeth R. Perkins, Ina Simnett and Linda Wright.

not easily acquired and cannot be commanded. It involves the individual being willing to take on a perspective which includes knowing and seeing that research, as a way of building scientific knowledge, does indeed provide us with sound evidence which can contribute to practice. Such a position will not be fully effective without support from elsewhere, but it is the first essential to research becoming part of practice. Help in developing such an understanding has been a major deficit to date in the education of most nurses (Chambers & Coates, 1993; Perkins, 1992).

Research into Practice – a Problem or an Opportunity for Nurses?

Students entering nursing and midwifery often have difficulty in seeing the relevance of research to practice. They also have varied notions about what research means, and this may also be the case for experienced practitioners (Hicks et al., 1996). For the purposes of this discussion the word research is being used to mean either an activity to discover, develop and test knowledge (i.e. doing research), or as a source of scientific knowledge accessed through research reports for use in practice (i.e. reading and critiquing).

While there is considerable educational overlap in subject content and skills required for both of these aspects of research, it would appear that reading research for practice is seen as a lesser activity, given the rewards which doing research can command in degrees, career progression and status. In the process, the not inconsiderable preparation required for critical reading is both played down in theory and neglected in practice. Being viewed as a reader of research, rather than a researcher, may be one of the many undermining influences for practitioners attempting to become conversant with research for practice.

At the simplest level, access to libraries and other information sources to find evidence for good practice have been found to be a practical difficulty in many NHS Trusts (Walshe & Ham, 1997). Swanson et al. (1992) report efforts to provide nursing units with information by allowing nurses to select articles of interest to them and by encouraging nursing units to subscribe to journals. Some attempts were also made to produce recommendations for clinical questions and to facilitate meetings between unit staff and researchers. The new quarterly journal *Evidence-based Nursing* may prove to be of help, as were some initiatives previously in networking (Leighton-Beck, 1997).

When research has been accessed and shows indisputable findings which can be accommodated into existing knowledge and practices, then few would argue with implementation. However, even some simple factual knowledge is not accessed or incorporated easily without much debate and delay, and students frequently question why there is such a lack of uptake. For example, there is considerable evidence that pre-operative fasting times do not need to be the 12 hours commonly experienced by patients (Chapman, 1996; Hung, 1992). Yet to reduce fasting times is a complex task, given the team of people it affects, and given factors such as the perceived uncertainty of operating times. Thus there are competing demands which may take priority, even though it is clear that starving patients for so long may be detrimental to them. In such situations supportive and effective management is vital to successful implementation of research findings. It is here that policies and protocols are important, but such strategies are empty without the research perspective and will to action of the practitioners involved.

Findings from qualitative research are of a different nature in the sense that they may inform the individual's understanding and perspective rather than the implementation of an intervention which can be measured by outcomes. For example, understanding how adolescents and young adults experience ulcerative colitis (Brydolf & Segesten, 1996) demands reflective consideration; nurses who understand the restrictive effects of this condition on the normal lifestyle of this age group will be able to be more sensitive in the care they offer.

WAYS OF KNOWING: THE PLACE OF SCIENTIFIC KNOWLEDGE IN NURSING

Having drawn on the research findings of other disciplines for decades, nursing is now giving priority to developing its own scientific thinking and this demands from nurses an understanding of the nature of scientific knowledge and its strengths and weaknesses. Otherwise nurses are faced with the options of uncritical acceptance or total rejection, neither of which are acceptable for thinking practitioners. Referring to research knowledge in practice, Luker and Kenrick (1992) talk of 'reclassified knowledge' which they see as knowledge being used for practice where its source has been lost. This corruption of scientific knowledge is problematic, because unless we are aware of the source of knowledge we use and its limitations, we may use it inappropriately. Facts may then be treated as absolutes rather than deriving their status from human reasoning. Consider this example:

> Patient   Nurse, I've got really bad pain.
> Nurse   You can't have, I gave you something for it and you can't get another injection for two hours.

The fact of the patient having stated she is in pain counts for less in this reply than the fact that an injection of analgesia *may* provide pain relief for about four hours.

While science is an essential feature of good and professional care it is quite evident that nursing cannot be practised with science alone. There are many ways in which nursing knowledge can be categorised. Burnard (1987) classifies it as experiential, propositional and practical, but the one which I find most useful is Carper's (1978). She delineates ways of knowing as empirical (including science), aesthetic, ethical and personal, and I see this as a categorisation which does away with the theory–practice dichotomy in knowledge and the notion that the art of nursing is the manual delivery of care. Science need not devalue other ways of knowing; the task for us is to embrace non-scientific scholarship as well, rather than allow our other ways of knowing to remain unacknowledged, unexamined and considered lacking in scholarly rigour. There is a need to be confident with them. Thus research for nursing can also encompass the development of the non-empirical, the aesthetic, the ethical and intuitive and the wholeness of nursing activity. Nurses need to understand the scientific perspective as one way of knowing amongst many. At times scientific knowledge is of such certainty that it has to take priority. At other times the novelist may have more to say to us.

Aesthetic knowledge in nursing appears to hold little sway. It contrasts with science as far as structure and generalisability are concerned (Phenix, 1964). The aesthetic has to do with perceptions of beauty, harmony and wholeness and particular instances or scenarios. Its cultivation appears to be of crucial importance. I have used stories, poetry and paintings in my teaching and have offered short options on the arts and nursing and the arts and midwifery. This is the traditional way to source aesthetic understanding in non-nursing fields but it is a marginalised knowledge source in nursing. I think it is barely discerned as a knowledge source by many.

AN EXAMPLE OF AESTHETIC KNOWLEDGE IN PRACTICE

As a midwife in the 1960s, when I practised in various parts of the world, I realised that I just took a far gentler approach to the second stage of labour than other midwives. Very directed pushing seemed gross and unacceptable and I tended not to use it. I allowed women to push spontaneously and simply be in touch with the ebb and flow of their contractions. This was not informed by research (though this practice could be justified in this way in the 1990s) but simply because heavily directed pushing just seemed so ugly and distorting unless in an emergency or other clinical considerations. Being aware of balance and harmony and the integrity in things in relation to care is at present an uneducated potential which we need to use.

By contrast, *science* is concerned with facts to do with the actual world experienced through reasoning and the senses. It has a structure which consists of concepts, theories and laws, each connecting in a hierarchical form to the observable and verifiable. Its soundness is such that it can be predictive and is open to scrutiny and replication. Nursing science pertains to nursing phenomena and aspires to harnessing the strengths of the traditional sciences as a way of providing for sound, systematic care. Given this, it is a little shocking that nursing practice is not better informed by science. Here is a story which serves as a reminder to us of the need to scrutinise our practice.

A LACK OF SCIENCE IN PRACTICE

Some years ago, when expecting my second child, my membranes ruptured spontaneously at 36 weeks as I lifted my two-year-old back to his own bed. I was admitted to a labour bed in a large maternity hospital as dawn broke on an August morning. The midwife was examining me. Suddenly she became tense and started semi-dancing back and forth round my bed and looking out the window to the grass below. She was muttering 'Oh, one for sorrow, one for sorrow. Oh, where is the other one?' At this point, already worried about my pregnancy and about leaving my other child at home I felt a sudden fear for my baby. This sudden change in the demeanour of the midwife who was examining me was alarming. Then, realising that neither I nor my pregnancy was the focus since I was really unattended, I elicited from her that it was the presence of a single magpie in the grounds which concerned her and she was desperately searching for a second one to say 'Two for joy'.

I was not amused at such superstitious behaviour which had caused me deep fear, however momentary this had been. The fact that she broke off to indulge in a piece of superstition gave me little reassurance that my care would be based on good science and not peppered with omens.

One of the characteristics of science is that it strips away such superstitions and provides logical, rational and empirical knowledge on which to base our practice. Superstitions are highly inappropriate if they hinder care. Our patients or clients can reasonably expect that our knowledge is not just the same as theirs but is beyond theirs in rigour and legitimacy.

BUILDING KNOWLEDGE ABOUT STUDENT LEARNING

Doing Research as Part of the Job

When my own research project started in September 1992, I estimated that it would take three-and-a-half years. I am still trying to finalise it. While its status has been as an extra, since it is not a requirement of the job, in reality it is not an extra since it has been a crucial influence in the way I have taught. I am reminded of the story from a Church of Scotland minister (probably a fairly common sentiment) when he told how a young boy who was carrying a younger sibling replied to the remark 'That's a heavy burden you're carrying', by saying, 'That's no burden, that's my wee brother'.

This research is no burden to me, but is a way and means of being creative. And this feeling is well-known amongst those who discover the pleasure of doing research – finding things out for themselves (Roe, 1952).

It was as subject leader in a small team teaching research to student nurses and midwives that I needed to discover more about teaching research and its outcomes. It was quite evident after a literature search that we were entering the unknown of research teaching (Clark & Sleep, 1991) and the most concrete guide we had was 'not to turn students off research' given the many difficulties of the subject and to 'engender a positive attitude' given that this may be related to research utilisation (Champion & Leach, 1989). I needed to know more.

In order to discover, to explore and to add to the knowledge base I adopted an ethnographic approach which has been rewarding and exciting, and has influenced my practice:

- I was able to build in some changes for the students who were my informants and for future intakes of students.
- The very challenge of the subject was such that we adopted very supportive strategies which frequently involved one-to-one tutorials for preparation of assignments and seminar papers.
- Teaching strategies such as seminars were important and appreciated and this strengthened the emphasis on these.
- By adopting a research methodology of in-depth interviews and participant observation where the students were fully knowledgeable and agreeable the research in itself became a teaching/learning strategy.

All the time I was developing a theoretical understanding of the process of learning about research and the outcomes and could test this out with subsequent intakes. It was encouraging to find that students could recognise others' experiences as akin to their own. This meant that the findings reached from one group of students had some relevance for other groups. My research provided me with a sureness to my work which I had seldom experienced before. It was the creation of useful knowledge (however modest) which could be communicated to others and which stands as a record of my work which was so rewarding.

Students' Accounts of Their Own Experience

There are many little things which help or hinder students in their learning. Some of the students I taught were prepared to tell me how they saw the formal aspects of the research component of their courses and to share some very personal experiences from both practice and theory. They provided me with invaluable information and through a selection of quotes I hope to give some encouragement to readers who are hesitant about research as a subject. For others it may provide some understanding of the little breakthroughs in learning which require to be nurtured.

In the Beginning

I came out of the first lectures totally lost, mystified. I didn'ae understand most of it . . .

. . . it's as if we're looking at what researchers are researching. . . . We're looking at the researchers, rather than gathering information ourselves.

I didn't really understand data either, you know data collection. I didn't realise that it's not just written down information churning out of computers.

What is Research?

Medical research, I never imagined it would be research as it is.

. . . for a lot of us research was either market research or just men in white coats in laboratories.

Research was just something out on its own and it was a subject with great emphasis put on it.

Reading and Putting in the Effort

I think it started off for me as a necessity, to read, to understand and then when I started reading I started to enjoy it, so I carried on reading because then I could understand.

I didn't really have a clue until the seminars came along, and understanding how everyone else felt at understanding research . . .

On Seminars and Moving On

Had to look up in the dictionary to see what a seminar was.

Your mind is made up in a certain area and then you hear other people . . .

Doing the actual seminar paper, I think I just suddenly realised and understood the whole thing. . . . It actually made me understand all the lectures, it's taken me all this time.

You also pick up good points and adapt them for your own.

I actually read my paper again, the actual report and found things in it I hadn't seen the first time . . .

Ethnography was the first research style which the students were introduced to. It was used to help students enter a research/scientific perspective by portraying the personal, the everyday and the subjective as legitimate concerns of science. Smith (1992) was a popular text which many students could relate to from their own nursing experiences.

It [Smith, 1992] was something you could pick up from any point where you left off and it was the actual reading of that that changed my views on research. There was something that immediately struck me as something almost I could apply to myself – personal experience.

Being Accountable with Research

I think you have such a responsibility on you. You are going to be a midwife and the responsibility is on you. I need to be sure that what I am doing isn'ae just what one person says.

On Becoming Different Personally

Well my husband says that I've totally changed like in my thinking since I started . . . you tend to think a lot more, you know making him feel dumb . . .

On Being Different in Practice and Theory

I felt when I was bringing up any ideas there, they were being thwarted.

People were sort of thinking, 'well you know we've been doing this for such a long time, and here's this student coming along'.

In general I don't think research is really in the minds of people.

Just even the slight insight that we have got lets you question what other people have written . . .

Even results you read in the press you consider; before you would have said 'that's fact' but now you know it's not so black and white.

The Hard Hard Facts and Their Analysis

I found . . . the quantitative research, particularly the statistical analysis, very difficult.

I think it is one of the most difficult subjects. During the lectures I would have as well no been there. I sat and laughed. I just cannae believe that.

You'd be as well taught in a foreign language, but we all got through it because we can come up and ask.

I read something that said 'If it's too difficult to read, that isnae my problem trying to read it, that is their problem the people that have written it'.

As far as the tests, the statistical tests, I don't really understand them. But I think if you've got sort of half an idea, you can go to the textbooks.

Making Vital Connections

The only way that I can see that nurses can move forward is by research . . . now I see them as intertwined . . . at the beginning I just saw research as 'Oh God I'll never get the hang of this and I don't understand why it's here'. But now I do, I know that it's necessary to nursing . . . I see them together.

More an Outlook

I was surprised when I went in and was working and I felt some people just see midwifery as a job. I don't see it as a job, I see it as an outlook sort of. I think it's up to you if you want to stay up to date, because I've heard a few midwives say 'If I hear another word about research, I'll go off ma heid'.

Questioning

The questionable practices hold fast, like you always take a patient out of the room head first. . . . The extreme lengths one particular midwife went to get a woman out of the room head first, rather than feet first . . . the woman was in labour, she was in a lot of pain, being taken down to theatre for section. The midwife was trying to negotiate head first . . . she actually moved up so that we could turn her head first because I had a slightly stronger pull . . . and I said 'why?' And she said 'We always take them out head first'. So I asked a few midwives and they just started to laugh and said 'Oh that's right, they only go feet first if they are dead'.

RESEARCH IN PRACTICE, PERSONAL AND APPROPRIATE

. . . and I said to her 'You know I read something . . . give me a wee minute and I'll go and check, but I'm sure there's other ways that you can get close to your baby and bond with your baby' and I went away. I had read it in the nursery about three weeks before, the first time I had been there, and I went back and read the same article and there were other articles on bonding, what parents could do, it was different forms of care and it was to do with massage and things like that . . .

I said, 'Would you like to read them?' This sounds awful prejudiced of me but she was a schoolteacher and . . . obviously it would have been as beneficial to everybody but I thought she might like to read them for herself, so I said to the other members of staff 'would it be okay'. . . . There was one on Kangaroo care and there was one on massage to stimulate natural endorphins in the baby and it cuts down on the amount of pain relief the babies require and it initiates bonding and there was another article and she took the three of them away and she came back the next day and she said, 'They were great, they were really excellent, have you any more?' I said I hadn't, but I spoke to the sister in the special care nursery and she said, 'Well I can arrange for other articles to be made available if she wants.' But I said about initiating some of this the Mum had read. Obviously you've got to treat it tentatively but the Mum's quite keen to get skin to skin contact with the baby and from then as the baby got better they did incorporate it into the baby's care and the Mum got involved.

Practitioner Education

Research is a way for practitioners to establish practice knowledge as more than the personal and idiosyncratic. We once depended on a strong oral tradition but this has gone and our knowledge must now be recorded differently. Practitioners owe it to themselves to become conversant with research and there is a formal requirement for this. The students I taught have, through time and effort, found research useful, both for understanding and participating in practice. Those who are new to nursing and direct entry midwifery can be so caught up in antici-pating the activities that they associate with the work that it is a surprise to discover that those very activities are under a scientific scrutiny unknown in earlier times. The motivation to enter nursing is often fuelled by wanting to help others and novices often perceive themselves as well able to do so. As a result the introduction to a scientific perspective with its questioning and sceptical characteristics demands a profound change in ways of thinking and doing.

Research textbooks quite rightly place an emphasis on nurses being able to critique research reports, but this is difficult for students and for some practitioners not least because reports are polished and edited for publication and are in themselves artefacts of a special type. So when it comes to reading research for practice, the aim needs to be much more exploratory in the early days, with notions of critical appraisal coming later. For practitioners who have a good knowledge of their subject area they may be able to judge the findings for fit and feasibility before they are able to be discerning about the methodology which produced the findings. Experience needs to be used as a strength when learning about research, but it does not automatically confer understanding in other ways.

Knowledge needs to be shared by all of us in an egalitarian manner. The importance of serious dedicated education in the use of research in practice as a worthy pursuit in itself cannot be overstated. Part of the development of a science requires agreement between those who are contributing. If practitioners do not become involved in the debate about what constitutes our science then it will be decided by outsiders. It is up to practitioners to carve out the new and create, in our learning and practice, ways of and approaches to knowledge development which are pertinent to the requirements of the health of our patients and clients. To do this there are few teachers but ourselves and our clients. My own perspective is to encourage students to enter into ways of seeing but not to say 'now copy'.

IN CONCLUSION

Student nurses and midwives are required to learn about research for practice and this dovetails well with the current focus on evidence-based health care across the professions. The emphasis that I and my colleagues in one college of nursing placed on it was in requiring that the students learn to read research in a discerning way. I have argued from my experience and my research on the matter that students can learn to value and see the relevance of research for good practice. Some will go further and take the initiative to introduce research into their practice even before registration. Such progress in learning, however, is cognitively challenging, and the ensuing difficulties require strategies in teaching which are supportive and encouraging.

Elitist expectations of students' understanding about research can compound the problems for them and cause fear in the students that they are unable to understand. Research learning in particular can benefit from a realistic assessment of students' level of knowledge and from generous sharing of knowledge and explanations with them. Even small 'helps' can allow for realisations and progress. Student effort in learning about methodology, in reading research reports and in writing for discussions in small groups also needs encouragement and time.

Those who use research findings in practice are not operatives at the end of research production by others. They have to be creative with others' research within the milieu in which they practise. For many nurses and midwives who are well educated in research, doing research will not be a choice but for others, doing research becomes an attractive step, to answer questions, and to 'find out for yourself', within your own practice.

REFERENCES

Brydolf M & Segesten K (1996) Living with ulcerative colitis: experiences of adolescents and young adults. *Journal of Advanced Nursing*, 23, 39–47.
Burnard P (1987) Towards an epistemological basis for experiential learning in nurse education. *Journal of Advanced Nursing*, 12, 189–193.
Carper B A (1978) Fundamental patterns of knowing in nursing. *Advances in Nursing Science*, 1, 13–23.
Chambers M & Coates V (1993) Research in nursing, Part 2. *Senior Nurse*, 13, 1.
Champion V L & Leach A (1989) Variables related to research utilization in nursing: an empirical investigation. *Journal of Advanced Nursing*, 14, 705–710.
Chapman A (1996) Current theory and practice: a study of pre-operative fasting. *Nursing Standard*, 10(18), 33–36.
Clark E & Sleep J (1991) The what and how of teaching research. *Nurse Education Today*, 11, 172–178.
Hicks C, Hennessy D, Cooper J & Barwell F (1996) Investigating attitudes to research in primary health care teams. *Journal of Advanced Nursing*, 24, 1033–1041.
Hung P (1992) Pre-operative fasting. *Nursing Times*, 88(48), 57–60.
Kitson A, Ahmed L B, Harvey G, Seers K & Thompson D R (1996) From research to practice: one organisational model for promoting research-based practice. *Journal of Advanced Nursing*, 23, 430–440.
Leighton-Beck L (1997) Networking: putting research at the heart of professional practice. *British Journal of Nursing*, 6(2), 120–122.
Luker K & Kenrick M (1992) An exploratory study of the sources of influence on the clinical decisions of community nurses. *Journal of Advanced Nursing*, 17, 457–466.
MacVicar M H (1998) Intellectual development and research: student nurses' and student midwives' accounts. *Journal of Advanced Nursing*, 27, 1305–1316.
Perkins, E R (1992) Teaching research to nurses: issues for tutor training. *Nurse Education Today*, 12, 252–257.
Phenix P (1964) Realms of meaning. New York: McGraw-Hill.
Roe A (1952) A psychologist examines sixty-four eminent scientists. In: P Vernon (Ed), Creativity. Harmondsworth: Penguin.
Rolfe G (1994) Towards a new model of nursing research. *Journal of Advanced Nursing*, 19, 969–975.
Smith P (1992) The emotional labour of nursing. Basingstoke: Macmillan.
Swanson J M, Albright J, Steirn C, Schaffner A & Costa L (1992) Strategies for teaching nursing research. Program efforts for creating a research environment in a clinical setting. *Western Journal of Nursing Research*, 14(2), 241–245.
Walshe K & Ham C (1997) Who's acting on the evidence. *Health Service Journal*, 107(5547), 22–25.

Section 13.3

From Evidence to Action Using Health Behaviour Surveys

John Balding, Anne Wise and David Regis

INTRODUCTION

There are difficulties with evidence-based health promotion if we are looking for something analogous to evidence-based primary care. For example, we have been much engaged by recent concern about the consumption of 'alcopops' by young people. One difficulty here is that there are no guidelines about young people's intake as there are for adults, as there are no comparable studies of the effects of alcohol on their physical health.

Here we will describe some of the ways we collect and use other types of evidence to support health promotion with young people in schools and communities.

Our work began with an approach to health education which might be described now as *evidence-based curriculum development*. We occasionally witness heated exchanges about the health of young people; such exchanges are often fuelled by differences in our perceptions of young people. These differences may be based on our own striking personal experiences, or on colourful anecdotes recounted in the staffroom (or reported by the media). However, misjudgements and misrepresentation of young people's lifestyles may lead to misguided interventions.

This led to the development of our *Health-Related Behaviour Questionnaire* (HRBQ) (see e.g. Balding, 1997), to make some progress towards a more objective picture of young people than the anecdotal. Pupils in a given year group are asked to complete anonymously a survey booklet which takes a broad inventory of their current or recent health-related behaviour. This gives everyone involved in the debate, including the pupils, a more objective picture of the behaviour of the whole year group.

This evidence collected from young people is not only used in the planning of health promotion/education in schools, but is often prominent in the *content* of the

Evidence-based Health Promotion. Edited by Elizabeth R. Perkins, Ina Simnett and Linda Wright.
© 1999 John Wiley & Sons Ltd.

education. We have collected many examples over the years where the levels and patterns of young people's behaviour is used as stimulus material in the class-room. Not every survey exercise encourages those who provide the data, and those who help to collect it, to work with the results. Quite apart from the enhanced sense of involvement and relevance, the opportunity to discover problems with interpretation or memory, and other sources of unreliability, is unrivalled.

More recently health authorities have become interested in the data as a way of informing and monitoring their own local planning, and this is now a main focus and motivation for our work.

HOW TO COLLECT GOOD DATA

Our approach to collecting reliable evidence in a school setting has a number of distinct features.

A Collaborative Approach

We have throughout the development of our work with schools *consulted* teachers and health professionals over the questionnaire content. Our key criterion is not academic (is this question interesting?) but practical (how will these data be used?).

The involvement of teachers in the content of the questionnaire has always been a feature in the development of the HRBQ since its conception in 1975, in which the views of 50 secondary school teachers were sought on the first draft.

Since these early days, the HRBQ has evolved and developed under continuous scrutiny, and much revision has taken place. Professions other than teaching have continued to be drawn in to influence the content, and the teachers' concept of health behaviour has had to be balanced against other professional views. One might expect a temptation to concentrate on behaviours that suit a medical perspective. However, health personnel are usually very keen to adopt the per-spective of the 'whole person' and can always see the value of personal and social aspects of the questionnaire (e.g. self-esteem, perceptions of local environment).

This bottom-up approach evident in the development of the HRBQ is an under-lying theme throughout the survey process. We have known other pieces of research where those collecting the information from respondents then disappear with it, publishing only in academic journals. We try to foster a sense of a pro-ductive collaboration with schools (as opposed to having the work done to them by a health authority). With their commitment enhanced we also see a positive effect on the pupils' co-operation; often those concerned can't wait to get the data back!

Although we consult, the content of the questionnaire is still our responsibility. There are always pressures to include new topics, and to include more detailed questions on the existing topics. These exhortations must be balanced against the time and effort required for the pupils to complete the survey. The survey can provide evidence only for the topics covered, and attention will be called to them whether or not the data are exceptional. Moreover, the content of the questionnaire may be seen to represent a view of what 'health' is, so that excluded topics may slip down the list of priorities.

The Collection of Data in the Classroom

The key question for us in the collection of good data is: Are the teachers and pupils convinced of the value of the survey and of its potential benefits to all concerned?

The quality of the information returned to the school reflects the manner and atmosphere in which the data were collected. In each school, supervisors can be found who can generate an atmosphere of importance for the task, can inspire trust in the confidentiality and anonymity of the exercise, and provide support for the completion of the questionnaire. Our guidelines for the collection of data are clearly laid down and rehearsed with the supervisors, who are experienced teachers, well-known to the pupils. Those with difficulties in reading or writing can be separately catered for using the usual practices of the school. Strong commitment and careful preparation by schools is the norm, particularly when good and sympathetic local support is available from health authorities.

EXAMPLES OF EVIDENCE-BASED HEALTH PROMOTION

Use of Research Data in Classroom and Staffroom

Review of Questionnaire Content by Staff

The Schools Health Education Unit has developed a Questionnaire Content Exercise (Balding, 1992) which enables information relating to the health and lifestyle behaviours of the pupils to be shared with teachers of all subjects. This gives the school a unique opportunity to work across the curriculum with relevant and realistic material supplied by the pupils themselves.

In this exercise, staff are asked to consider which of the survey questions would provide data of which their curriculum area could make positive and relevant use. Distributing these selected results to the curriculum areas enables further cross-curricular opportunities to be developed, as data from popular questions are used across several subject areas, thus bringing evidence from various aspects of health education into everyday and practical classroom use.

Return of Data on Disc

With the advances made in information technology during the last ten years, schools are now much better placed to work with the survey results at a 'hands-on' level. So, as well as working with the summary tables, schools can work with selected unaggregated results in a computer-readable format. Both pupils and staff are thus able to interrogate the data further, discovering, for example, whether there are links between any selection of lifestyle characteristics in the data, leading to the prediction of further links, discovering if their predictions are correct, and discussing the significance of their findings. The content is adaptable to many subject areas and the relevance of the data to the young people themselves makes it a particularly attractive way of introducing health topics.

We are careful to 'prune' the data so that key questions or extreme values, which could identify certain individuals, are excluded. (If individual pupils would like feedback on their own health risk scores in a survey we can return a printout via a confidential 'PIN'.)

Opportunities for Activity in the Community

A common observation made from the results relating specifically to active participation in sport and leisure activities is the decline in regular involvement with age, especially with the female respondents. However, what is also observed is the variety of physical activities in which the pupils are involved.

We have designed a a series of 'workshops' (Balding, 1992) to help teachers examine, and reflect upon, the evidence from their own survey, either as a group or in discussion with pupils and/or parents. The workshop, *A Balancing Act*, has as one of its aims the encouragement and promotion of pupils' activity levels, reflected in the Physical Education National Curriculum Programme of Study (Key Stage 3):

> Pupils should be given opportunities to engage in health-promoting physical activity,
> where possible within the local community.

In reviewing the results from their survey many questions are posed:

- What picture does it present?
- Is it satisfactory?
- What about any gender differences?
- To what extent does (or should) your PE programme complement the resources available outside school?
- Is there a strategy that could be devised to make outside activities more accessible to your current pupils?

Such questioning leads many schools to ask their pupils for fuller details of the sporting activities in which they were involved. In one such school, a large map of the catchment area was set up in the school lobby showing locations of activity, with threads leading to a label bearing club details. In particular, a contact person (usually a pupil) was identified as the link between school and the club, as it was observed that the most difficult step to take was going to a new club on your own.

Differences Between Schools or Communities

Following an approach by a paediatrician we have included some questions related to asthma in our surveys. We currently ask two questions:

1. On how many days have you taken any medication for asthma in the last week?
2. When you run, do you 'wheeze' and have trouble breathing (not just feel out of breath)?

Each year we collect together all the data from all the school surveys throughout the calendar year and publish the results in a series of books. From the data set used for the *Young People in 1993* book (Balding, 1994) we have 14 511 males and 14 149 females who answered both of the asthma questions. These numbers exclude 414 pupils in the surveys whose replies to one or both of these questions were missing or uncodable. Let us call those who report *any days at all* for the first question the *dosers*, and those who reply *quite often* or *very often* to the second question the *wheezers*. Taking these samples as the base (100%), what percentages of these boys and girls are wheezers or dosers? (Table 13.3.1 and Figure 13.3.1.)

Now, clearly the wheezers and dosers overlap to some extent (Table 13.3.2). From this we can see that there is a proportion of some 7–8% of children who report some breathing difficulty and did not medicate during the previous week. A natural interpretation of these data is to say that these unmedicated wheezers are in fact likely to be untreated asthmatics whose quality of life may well be improved by referral to health care professionals. (We might also label the wheezing dosers as *children with asthma that is being treated*, and the non-wheezing dosers as *well-managed asthmatic children*.)

We have also examined the rates of wheezing and dosing in different schools. In this example, we find that the school with the most *dosers* (School C) is not the school with the most *wheezers* (School A); the school with potentially the most *undosed wheezers* need not be either of these (Figure 13.3.2). This unevenness is very interesting, and suggests a strategy for targeting schools for screening programmes. (Which school's health care contacts would you approach first?) The reports returned to each school now routinely include an individual analysis of any disparity between wheezing and dosing.

Table 13.3.1 Percentage of young people aged 11–16 years in 1993 sample reporting asthma symptoms (*wheezers*) and asthma medication (*dosers*) (14 511 males, 14 149 females) (Balding, 1994)

	Males		Females	
Dosers	1723	(12%)	1459	(10%)
Wheezers	2344	(16%)	2889	(20%)
Total in sample	14 511	(100%)	14 149	(100%)

This example shows how evidence from the survey method can prompt action in schools and communities. Moreover, one of our 'workshops' (Balding, 1992) on the asthma data explores a number of issues, including:

- parental attitudes to asthma
- peer reactions
- changing medical practice around asthma.

Geographical Analysis of Data

Schools are often keen to know how they match up to other schools in the area, although they are not responsible for the behaviour of their pupils in the community; we can generate a comparison of a school's data with the collection of data from a given region, but these are only returned to the schools, so that if health authorities want access to this information they have to work through the schools.

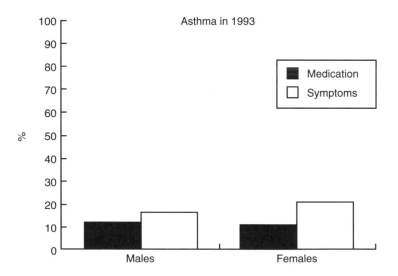

Figure 13.3.1 Percentage of young people aged 11–16 years in the 1993 sample reporting asthma symptoms (*wheezers*) and asthma medication (*dosers*) (14 511 males, 14 149 females) (Balding, 1994)

Table 13.3.2 Overlap between percentages of young people aged 11–16 years in 1993 sample reporting asthma symptoms (*wheezers*) and/or asthma medication (*dosers*) (14 511 males, 14 149 females) (Balding, 1994)

	Males		Females	
No wheeze, no dose	11 404	(79%)	10 857	(77%)
No wheeze, doser	1384	(10%)	1833	(13%)
Wheezer, doser	763	(5%)	403	(3%)
Wheezer, no dose	960	(7%)	1056	(8%)
		[100]		[100]

(Typically schools are keen to work with health authorities, and are happy to share the data as long as they feel in control.)

In many authority-based surveys we have also collected ward and enumeration district information from pupils. This means that data collected in schools can later be organised by location (Figure 13.3.3), which takes some of the focus away from schools and back to communities.

It is also possible to relate such differences to census and other demographic data which health authorities have available, including indices of deprivation. Also, the health authority will be able to relate the sample in each area to numbers known to be living there. This detailed analysis is most valuable to planners, since health care and promotion is often best delivered at community level (Figure 13.3.4).

More recently, as the profile of GPs has risen in the health service, we have started collecting data about the young person's family doctor. Data about their health-related practices, broken down by 'GP code', can then be analysed.

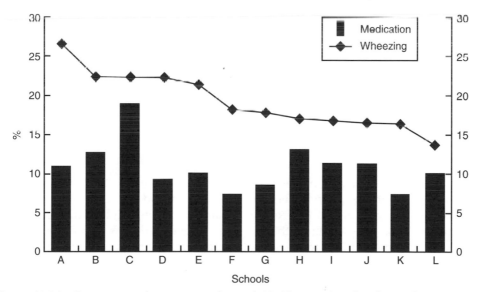

Figure 13.3.2 Percentage of young people aged 12–15 years in a local sample reporting asthma symptoms and asthma medication (Balding, 1994)

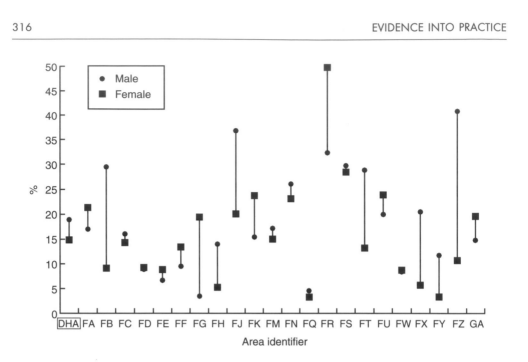

Figure 13.3.3 Percentage of young people aged 14–15 years in a local sample reporting 'ever tried' illegal drugs: figures for whole sample (DHA) and by area (Balding, 1994)

Another route for working with communities is to publish the survey data for public and professional use. The map shown in Figure 13.3.4 is from one of a whole host of reports across the country which have been produced by local health authorities to publicise the results of their survey, and to prompt action by various parties and partners concerned with young people.

Working with Parents and Other Adults Through Schools

Here are two out of many examples that show the potential for using HRBQ data with parents.

Information About Sex

Typically there is a contrast between where young people say their main source of information about sex is and where they say it should be. The main source is different for different ages and sexes, with parents scoring highest in the younger age groups. Also interesting is the disparity between the two assertions (Table 13.3.3). How can we interpret these data? Our first concern was that the young people were being critical of their parents, but in fact they were much more generous than that – when interviewed the usual response was that *in an ideal world* parents would be the main source, but they accepted that this was in fact unlikely, due to embarrassment on both sides.

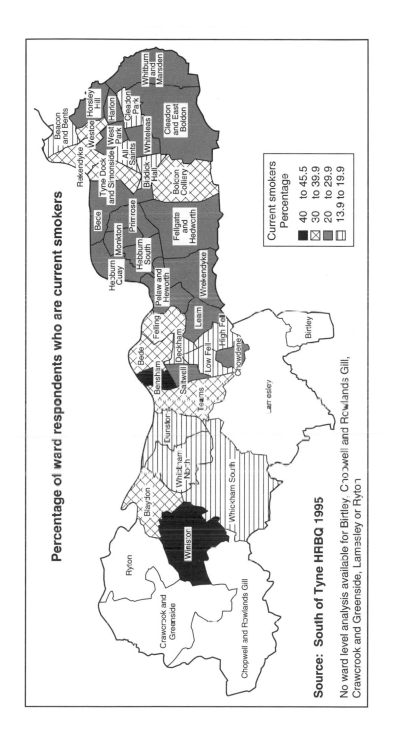

Percentage of ward respondents who are current smokers

Source: South of Tyne HRBQ 1995

No ward level analysis available for Birtley, Chopwell and Rowlands Gill, Crawcrook and Greenside, Lamesley or Ryton

Figure 13.3.4 Percentage of young people aged 14–15 years in a local sample reporting current smoking, by ward (Loggie et al., 1996) (Reproduced by permission of Gateshead and South Tyneside Health Promotion)

Table 13.3.3 Percentages among 14–15-year-old males and females reporting actual and preferred main sources of sex information (3703 males, 3569 females) (Balding, 1997)

	Males (%)	Females (%)
Main source is:		
Parents	15	20
School lessons	27	14
Friends	28	26
Main source should be:		
Parents	42	49
School lessons	37	31
Friends	7	5

We were also concerned about the teachers: how were they feeling? We know from many studies, including our own (Regis, 1996), that most parents and children welcome schools' involvement in sex education. Moreover, if the question were 'What is your most accurate source of information?' or 'What is your main source of information on contraception?' we should expect that the votes for lessons as the actual and desired main source of information would be very much higher.

How can schools help parents (and vice versa) over this issue? In our view, in an ideal sex education world both parents and teachers would play a role and would also work together on it. We have a 'workshop' for use in schools to promote this contact (Balding, 1992) which uses the model of a school's successful parents' evening.

In this way the evidence furthers both our understanding of each group's point of view and, hopefully, a better service for young people.

Drinking Alcohol at Home

This topic illustrates three stages in the evolution of the questionnaire content. The first stage revealed what seemed to be high levels of consumption of alcohol by young people (Table 13.3.4), including some reports of intake exceeding adult guidelines. In any one school, of course, these figures may be higher or lower, and may be higher or lower than the school originally thought.

When we first presented data like these, in around 1980, to teachers, and particularly parents, there was often concern but also a caution: could we be sure of the figures? A question was often put: *where are they supposed to be getting all this drink from?* At a parents' evening this can be discussed at the time, but we can also refine the survey content to cater for this query in the future. So we devised a further question, which included the *home* among other possible drinking venues (Table 13.3.5).

Table 13.3.4 Percentages among 12–15-year-old males and females reporting numbers of units of alcohol consumed last week (Balding, 1997)

Units	Year 8 males	Year 8 females	Year 9 males	Year 9 females	Year 10 males	Year 10 females
None	62.1	67.4	49.1	52.5	42.7	44.6
1	6.2	9.1	7.4	8.9	4.3	7.1
2	6.9	6.6	6.5	7.6	6.8	7.9
3	4.6	3.6	4.5	4.4	3.3	4.9
4–6	8.9	6.6	12.3	11.5	12.3	12.8
7–10	5.3	3.6	6.9	7.2	10.7	9.8
11–14	2.5	1.4	5.4	3.1	6.5	5.2
15–20*	1.6	0.8	4.1	2.5	6.3	4.3
21–28	1.2	0.5	1.8	1.5	3.9	2.2
28 or more units	0.8	0.3	2.0	0.8	3.2	1.1
	[100]	[100]	[100]	[100]	[100]	[100]
Valid responses (count)	5079	5092	1333	1308	4253	4215

1 unit = alcohol contained in half pint standard strength beer, lager or cider
* Up to December 1995 the recommendations were: 14 units (women) and 21 units (men)

Table 13.3.5 Percentages among 12–15-year-old males and females reporting places where alcohol was consumed last week (Balding, 1997)

	Year 8 males	Year 8 females	Year 9 males	Year 9 females	Year 10 males	Year 10 females
At home	23.6	20.2	33.4	31.4	35.8	30.5
At a friend's or relation's home	12.0	11.0	20.3	18.6	25.9	24.7
At a disco, club or party	7.5	5.9	13.2	12.2	13.9	15.5
At a pub or bar	4.3	2.9	9.5	7.4	11.5	13.3
Outside in a public place	9.5	7.6	16.8	15.9	24.5	19.9
None of the above (or missing data)	66.1	70.1	51.1	53.9	44.1	45.8

The top-line data point the finger rather firmly at parents: *are we, at home, encouraging our children to drink?* As well as perhaps causing further disquiet at a parents' evening this may also produce some confessions: yes, we do give our children alcohol at home. And with the confessions we may also have some justifications. For example, it is often suggested that it is out of a feeling of responsibility that parents will introduce their children to alcohol at home.

However, we have been asked a further question: *if these young people are drinking at home, do their parents always know about it?* This prompted the next addition to this part of the questionnaire: an enquiry an to parental awareness of drinking at home (Table 13.3.6).

Table 13.3.6 Percentages among 12–15-year-old males and females reporting parental awareness of alcohol being consumed at home (Balding, 1997)

	Year 8 males	Year 8 females	Year 9 males	Year 9 females	Year 10 males	Year 10 females
I do not drink alcohol at home	33.9	32.9	23.7	19.8	23.7	21.9
My parents always know	42.3	42.4	41.3	43.2	36.9	34.5
My parents usually know	11.2	11.3	18.9	20.6	20.3	21.2
My parents sometimes know	7.3	7.8	10.3	11.7	12.9	14.1
My parents never know	5.3	5.6	5.8	4.6	6.3	8.2
	[100]	[100]	[100]	[100]	[100]	[100]
Valid responses	5133	5103	1357	1313	4348	4313

Table 13.3.6 shows that some children drink at home only with parental knowledge, while a substantial proportion do drink at home on occasion without their parents knowing anything about it. Discussing the implications with parents is the next stage in the process: in the context of this chapter, we are simply using this sequence to illustrate how the content of the questionnaire has evolved under challenge and debate with parents in the communities served by the schools in which we work. Answers are notorious for generating further questions, but these questions can be addressed!

SUMMARY AND CONCLUSIONS

In conclusion, our practice over the years has demonstrated that the collection of survey data has a number of outcomes:

1. A body of evidence which provides a basis for debate, rather than a heated head-to-head exchange of views. Community data can be used to promote links between parents and schools, and between schools and health authorities.
2. Evidence from surveys provides a more objective perspective on issues. A picture of the whole population can be used as the basis for planning, rather than colourful anecdotes and media reports. The size of any problem can be assessed and plans and resources can be targeted appropriately; health promotion activities in the community can be put into place alongside curriculum review in schools. The data are significant for governors, parents, GPs, community health workers, social services, environmental health and other professionals. The end of the survey is the starting point of the 'real work'!
3. As well as providing a picture at one moment in young people's lives, many health authorities have used the service to track 'cohorts', re-surveying year groups after an interval, thus providing information about the effects of local changes or intervention programmes.

REFERENCES

Balding J W (1992) After the survey: nine workshops using the Health-Related Behaviour Questionnaire. Exeter: Schools Health Education Unit.

Balding J W (1994) Young people in 1993: the Health-Related Behaviour Questionnaire results for 29,074 pupils between the ages of 11 and 16. Exeter: Schools Health Education Unit.

Balding J W (1997) Young people in 1996: the Health-Related Behaviour Questionnaire results for 22,067 pupils between the ages of 12 and 15. Exeter: Schools Health Education Unit.

Loggie J, Jordan C & Dicks A (1996) Signposts to health: findings from the health-related behaviour survey. Jarrow: South Tyneside Health Commission.

Regis D (1996) The voice of children in health education: use of the Just a Tick method to consult children over curriculum content. In: M John (Ed), Children in our charge: the child's right to resources. London: Jessica Kingsley.

Chapter 14

Health Promotion Needs Assessment

Linda Wright

INTRODUCTION

A need is the gap between what currently exists and what people could benefit from. Needs assessment involves gathering evidence to identify, describe and analyse these gaps and using this evidence to make decisions about priorities and programmes. In health promotion, needs assessment is the starting point for planned interventions at all levels; whatever your role is, you will require evidence about health needs. If you plan, purchase or commission services, you will require evidence of health need to make strategic decisions at a group, community or neighbourhood level about the basic direction for local health promotion programmes, e.g. coronary heart disease prevention. If you manage health promotion services, you will use the evidence from needs assessment at an operational level, to inform the development of a particular programme such as promotion of exercise and physical activity with low income groups. If you are mainly involved in delivering health promotion, you will use the evidence from needs assessment to work in a client-centred way, by tailoring your activities to the needs of your client groups.

This chapter explores some of the problems and tensions involved in doing needs assessment in health promotion contexts and in relation to core health promotion values such as individual and community participation. As with the other chapters in this part of the book, it is not a 'how to' manual, although practical advice is included, particularly in relation to doing lifestyle surveys in Section 16.2 and assessing family health needs in Section 16.3. The chapter aims to enable you to consider your own role and remit in relation to needs assessment and the issues you might need to consider in gathering this kind of evidence. Most importantly, the chapter considers how needs assessment evidence is *used* in health promotion and the factors that might limit or hinder its use.

The first section of this chapter, *Approaches to Needs Assessment*, highlights many of the tensions discussed in Chapter 1. It considers what is meant by 'need' and different approaches to needs assessment. Some of the ethical and political issues that relate

Evidence-based Health Promotion. Edited by Elizabeth R. Perkins, Ina Simnett and Linda Wright.
© 1999 John Wiley & Sons Ltd.

to doing needs assessment are discussed. The current NHS perspective on needs assessment and the impact of consumers are debated in relation to health promotion values.

Despite their expense, *Lifestyle surveys* are a fashionable method of collecting evidence of the health promotion needs of communities. Section 16.2 explores the relevance of these approaches to health promotion, their characteristics, their uses and limitations.

Sections 16.2 and 16.3 both propose a model of needs assessment based on community participation. Section 16.3, *A bottom-up approach to family health needs assessment*, is an account of how a group of health visitors attempted to bridge the gaps between their assessment of need at individual, family and community level.

Section 14.1

Approaches to Needs Assessment

Linda Lawton

INTRODUCTION

Assessment of need is the necessary starting point for any planned health promotion intervention with a group or within a community. The assessment process requires as much attention to detail as does the planning of any subsequent intervention. This overview begins with a consideration of the issues surrounding needs assessment. It looks at what is meant by 'need' and at who decides on needs and on priorities. It raises a number of ethical, social and political issues for those working on the promotion of health. The section provides a description of different approaches to needs assessment and a discussion of their strengths and weaknesses. It concludes with a consideration of the issues involved in putting the information obtained through needs assessment into practical use.

DEFINING NEED

The starting point for any discussion of approaches to need assessment is to define what is meant by 'need' before moving on to describe the approaches that can be employed to assess that need. There are a number of texts that have discussed these concepts in detail. Those used here are put forward by Ewles and Simnett (1992), drawing on the work of Bradshaw (1972), who identified four kinds of need.

Normative Need

This is need as defined by professionals or experts. Standards are set against which some kind of measure is made. Any gap identified is judged to be the need of that individual or group. No account is taken of the opinions or values of those being assessed which may not accord with those undertaking the assessment; who may frequently make value judgements as well as drawing on research or information from other locations.

Evidence-based Health Promotion. Edited by Elizabeth R. Perkins, Ina Simnett and Linda Wright.

Felt Need

This is need where individuals have identified what they want. Felt needs are shaped by the circumstances of the individual; their experiences, their knowledge and their understanding. People cannot have a felt need for things that they do not know exist. If an individual is not aware that a service is available, say large print leaflets for those whose vision is impaired, they will not have a felt need for such things.

Expressed Need

This is where people say what they need. That is, they turn a felt need into a request or demand. Not all felt need will be turned into an expressed need. Groups and individuals may be prevented from doing so by lack of access to those who would respond to such a need. There may be other barriers to expressing needs such as a lack of motivation, particularly if there is no opportunity or there are barriers perceived, either real or imagined. Also, there may be a lack of communication skills or of assertiveness. In the past, a lack of demand has sometimes been taken by service providers as an absence of need for a particular service.

Comparative Need

Here need is defined by comparing two similar groups or individuals, rather than making a judgement against normative standards. For example, in health promotion terms, a development worker may be appointed to work with one community but another community with similar characteristics may not have a community development worker. The second community would be seen as having a comparative need for health promotion input.

ISSUES AROUND THE ASSESSMENT OF NEED

An examination of the process of defining need in itself highlights some of the ethical and political issues that surround the process of needs assessment. It has already been shown that it is possible to identify different kinds of need and, in the minds of those involved in the promotion of health, this should lead automatically to the question of who defines need and who sets priorities. It has to be acknowledged that no one involved in health promotion can possibly tackle every need in every community. What is required is a clear perspective of the process of needs assessment and an awareness of the issues surrounding that process.

The NHS and Needs Assessment

The focus of needs assessment within the NHS shifted explicitly during the early 1990s. Health needs assessment became defined as the need for health services and was described as 'the first step towards health care' (Brambely, 1995). Although this situation had existed in practice for a number of years, it was only around that time that it was stated explicitly in NHS official documents, for example as this extract shows:

> health needs assessment should strictly be taken to mean the known ability to benefit from health care (From: EL(91)40 March 1991).

It is possible to postulate the reasons for this open acknowledgement of a narrowing in focus; one was undoubtedly the introduction of the internal market; another was the growing acceptance, not least by the NHS, that there is no direct relationship between health services and health status, and that the determinants of health and thus the greatest capacity to enhance health status lie outside the remit of the NHS. This is by no means a new concept but superficially it has been maintained that the NHS has this role, although this has not followed through in the allocation of resources. The focus has been on allocation of resources to secondary care and high tech medicine rather than into preventative and health promotion programmes.

This situation has complicated matters for those in health promotion who have sought to broaden the debate to look at health needs within a social model of health. This is particularly true for those operating within the NHS where the focus is on services for ill-health and a medical model of health.

Consumerism

Another issue to consider is the political climate in which needs assessment is carried out. There has been a sharp rise in consumerism over the last ten years. People have been encouraged to think of themselves as consumers of services, rather than passive recipients of services. The launch of the Patients' Charter within the NHS brought into the health care arena the notion of patients as consumers with certain rights. All services had to have in place mechanisms for dealing with complaints from users and most now actively seek the views of users or potential users. In this there is a need to ensure that those who in the past did not put forward their views are not further disadvantaged. For those already assertive and articulate, these new procedures may serve to make it easier for them to put forward their opinions and concerns and may increase the volume of such comments. They will not necessarily increase the spectrum of the population engaging in a dialogue over needs within the community. Those intent on undertaking needs assessment need to guard against this by careful planning of the approach and methods to be used.

Ethical Issues

A further issue to be addressed is one that is both political and ethical, namely that of deciding priorities: political because of the power relationships involved and obviously ethical because in deciding who receives health promotion the decision on who is not receiving such interventions is also being made. In a community development project, the members of the community would be involved in ranking needs in order of priority, but how are communities able to influence the decisions that identify their community as the one to be awarded the development project? Who influences the decision? How can those engaged in health promotion seek to ensure that as clear a picture as possible of the needs of different groups is presented? From a list of competing needs to be addressed, who decides which is to receive the health promotion interventions and which are to be deferred until this year, next year, sometime, never? Those engaged in health promotion need to be aware of power relationships and be prepared to challenge during the decision-making process. Part of the health promoting role is about raising the level of awareness amongst colleagues and organisations of these political aspects.

Having identified that there are different aspects of need, the question then moves on to how can this need be identified?

APPROACHES TO NEEDS ASSESSMENT

An Epidemiological Approach

Epidemiology is the study of the patterns of disease within a population or a community. It draws its information from mortality and morbidity statistics. Thus its focus is on ill-health and on the determinants of disease. Its underlying definition of health is therefore centred on the absence of disease.

One of the strengths of an epidemiological approach is that it relies on data that is quantifiable. And whilst there are problems with classifying the cause of some deaths the event to be counted is in itself clearly identifiable. A further strength is that mortality data is readily available through departments of public health within district health authorities. This obviates the need for those involved in the promotion of health to set up mechanisms to collect the raw data, since this type of data is collected routinely in the UK at a national level and it is possible to analyse the data at a district health authority level. Further manipulation allows the data to be presented at electoral ward level, thus it is possible to undertake statistical analysis and look at the determinants of disease. It is also possible to make comparisons between areas. For example, two areas of a town that are geographically close may show very different patterns of disease. One may have a very much higher rate of death from coronary heart disease which would not be picked up simply by looking at the epidemiological data for the town as a whole.

Morbidity data is also collected nationally through such mechanism as general practice records, returns on notifiable diseases, child health records and the government's General Household Survey. The fourth National Morbidity Survey was carried out in 1997. Morbidity data is less complete than mortality data and suffers from the drawback that it sheds no light on why there is a particular pattern of disease within a particular community. For example, sickness absence certificates will identify individuals suffering from back pain but only in those individuals in employment. In one sense the data generates more questions than it provides answers to those questions originally posed and other sources of data are then needed to shed light on why a particular pattern exists, the epidemiological data having provided the 'what'.

An epidemiological approach is a quantitative one that works on data collected indirectly. It does not involve any dialogue with the population under scrutiny. From a health promotion perspective it also has too narrow a focus: on disease and on health as the absence of disease. There have been many discussions of the inadequacy of this as a definition of health and it is not intended to discuss those arguments here. Rather the aim is to highlight the constraints of this approach, particularly in constraining the thinking of those using the data. Starting a piece of health promotion work with a disease focused needs assessment makes broadening the debate to a holistic approach to health that much more difficult.

A Socio-economic Approach

This approach focuses on the social and economic characteristics of a community or population such as the numbers in employment, the types of housing or the numbers of elderly people or the rate of teenage pregnancies in the area. An advantage of this type of approach is that there is already a wide variety of data collected by a whole range of organisations at both local and national level. This makes it possible to undertake comparisons between different areas and to highlight inequalities between different communities and between different groups within the same area. This approach is professionally led. The assessment of need is based on a picture of a community built up of quantitative data that is essentially a view about a community rather than from a community, although it is possible to obtain the opinions of the community as well. The information gained by this approach does begin to identify some of the factors that influence the health status of the people within a community, although its interpretation needs more than a professional perspective. The resources required to collect socio-economic data are mainly those of staff time to identify and track down data already held by different organisations and then to collate that data. This process can also prove useful in bringing people from different organisations together to work in alliance on firstly identifying needs and then moving on to develop work to address those needs.

A Behavioural Approach

The focus of this approach is on the individual. Data is collected directly from the community involved, to generate information on their lifestyles, their knowledge of disease risk factors or their attitudes to factors that influence their health.

Personal details such as age, sex, education and employment status are also included. The focus is very much on surveying a sample of the community to build up a picture of what it does and thinks. An advantage of data of this type is that it is in the main quantitative and it is possible to make comparisons between groups and communities.

The main problem with this approach is that the focus is on individuals rather than on social and environmental factors. This in turn has led to the development of health promotion programmes that seek to modify behaviours that are known to be risk factors for the development of certain diseases and conditions. Whilst it is estimated that 25% of hospital beds are occupied by people suffering from preventable conditions, to simply strive to bring about individual behaviour change has resulted in limited success in the past. This has often led to criticism that health promotion does not work, rather than a realisation that behaviour cannot be addressed in a vacuum.

Health and lifestyle surveys were commonly carried out during the 1980s in the UK. Surveys were also being carried out to support coronary heart disease prevention programmes in countries such as the USA and Finland. Surveys were often carried out to establish a baseline, for example the number of smokers within a community, the percentage of people eating healthy food choices, etc. There are issues about obtaining representative responses. One drawback to this approach is the cost and time in obtaining the data and analysis and interpretation in order for needs to be assessed. Partly because of a questioning of the appropriateness of a behavioural approach to needs assessment and partly because of the sheer expense of gathering the information, the use of health behaviour surveys declined, but has come back into vogue as an approach to needs assessment has increased with the publication of national strategies that contain targets that again focus attention on individual lifestyles and behaviour change such as the *Health of the Nation* (Department of Health, 1992) strategy for England.

Again, it is the professional who decides, from the large amount of data usually generated, what the needs of the community are and how they are to be addressed. This may not accord with the community's view of its most pressing needs and may lead to the implementation of inappropriate interventions. One further problem with self-reported information on health behaviours is a phenomenon that is well documented by researchers in the social sciences (for example, Hughes, 1976), namely the existence of public and private accounts in which individuals respond at different levels to the same question. At the public level, individuals provide answers that they believe concur with the professionally held view or are the answers wanted. This may not be an accurate picture of their health behaviour nor accurately reflect their views on factors affecting their health. These would be gained by obtaining a private account – the views they express to friends or family. Superficial research into behaviour risks only accessing the public account. More careful research using different techniques such as group or individual interviews could render the information more accurate and a truer reflection of the community studied.

A Community Participation Approach

There are a number of terms in existence to describe this approach to needs assessment such as community involvement, empowerment and client-centred approach. What is implied is that the community is involved in the assessment of their own health needs. The degree of involvement may vary from seeking community views on local issues and needs through to involving the community in developing the needs assessment process and in decisions on priorities for action. The obvious strength of this approach is that it is not professionally dominated. At its best it results in fruitful partnerships between the community and the voluntary and statutory sectors. But there is a need for caution. Foremost is the need to avoid raising unrealistic expectation. At the outset, those involved in promoting health need to clearly state the boundaries of their work and the limits to their capacity to address identified need. Then there is the clear need to avoid 'data raids' (Wadsworth, 1984) following which the community never hear of the researcher again. In short, the needs assessment is done not *on* the community but *with* the community (Dam, 1996).

ISSUES FOR EVIDENCE-BASED HEALTH PROMOTION PRACTICE

There are a number of practical issues for health promotion in the areas covered in this section. Firstly, the main approaches to assessing health needs have been described in isolation but clearly it is possible and desirable to use more than one approach in assessing health promotion needs. The approach selected for assessing need will in turn influence the approach adopted in the subsequent health promotion intervention. For example, relying solely on lifestyle data as the basis for assessing need may make it hard to steer away from an intervention based solely on behaviour change. Thus the design of any research on health needs assessment is all important (Dam, 1996).

The approach to needs assessment will also determine the nature of the data collected. In a planning group, those working in health promotion may wish to work more widely than the traditional medical model but may find that they are restricted by the availability of data that is purely focused on behaviour. Also it is the case that much professional training places greater credence on quantitative than on qualitative data. An important role will be to influence the needs assessment process to include the collection of valuable qualitative data.

In needs assessment, as in any other activities involving information gathering, it is important to avoid 'analysis paralysis', by which is meant the tendency to undertake increasingly detailed analysis at the expense of any activity to act upon the information generated. Part of the planning of a needs assessment will include consideration of time-scale. The approach and the information gathering techniques adopted both influence the time-scale. Time can be a crucial factor both in ensuring the information is current and in holding the attention of the community involved in the needs assessment (Hunt, 1993).

Finally, although a needs assessment exercise is identified as the starting point of health promotion programme planning, it is not unknown for activity to stall at this stage. There may be a number of reasons for this and the lack of action may or may not be intentional. There is a responsibility on those in health promotion to seek to ensure that action does result, although this is not always easy given that health promotion usually involves working in multi-disciplinary or multi-agency groups where different organisational agendas may be in play. The result of needs assessment should be 'a dynamic community profile, blending quantitative health and illness statistics and demographic indicators with qualitative information, political and socio-cultural factors' (Haglund et al., 1990). This should then lead on to the development of aims to meet the needs identified.

CONCLUSION

The climate for demonstrating a sound evidence base for practice was strengthened by the publication in late 1997 of the government White Paper on the NHS (NHS Executive, 1997). In it the importance of needs assessment was emphasised, as was the need for partnership between health authorities and local authorities and local communities. Part of the role of those involved in promoting health will be to contribute to the widening of the debate on needs assessment away from the need for services to the need to address health and its determinants. The challenge will be to develop the needs assessment process and then to use the outcomes to address inequalities, bearing in mind that a health need is not the same as a health problem and that the real experts on the health needs of a particular community are the people who live in that community (Baum, 1993).

REFERENCES

Baum F (1993) Healthy cities and change: social movement or bureaucratic tool? *Health Promotion International*, 8, 31–40.
Bradshaw J (1992) The concept of social need. In: L Ewles & I Simnett (Eds), Promoting health: a practical guide. London: Scutari Press.
Brambleby P (1995) Tracking the financial shifts. In: C Riley, M Warner, A Pullen & C Semple Piggott (Eds), Releasing resources to achieve health gain. Oxford: Radcliffe Medical Press.
Dam J T (1996) Healthy research in cities: a case study on the translation of health research into action in the Netherlands. *Health Promotion International*, 11(4), 265–276.
Department of Health (1992) The Health of the Nation: a health strategy for England. London: HMSO.
Ewles L & Simnett I (1992) Promoting health: a practical guide. London: Scutari Press.
Haglund B, Weisbrod R R & Bracht N (1990) Assessing the community. Its services, needs, leadership and readiness. In N Bracht (Ed), Health promotion at the community level (pp 91–108).
Hughes J A (1976) Sociological analysis: methods of delivery. London: Nelson.
Hunt S M (1993) The relation between research and policy: translating knowledge into action. In: J K Davies and M P Kelly (Eds), Healthy cities; research and practice. London: Routledge.
NHS Executive (1997) The new NHS: modern and dependable. London: HMSO.
Stevens A & Raftery J (1990) Health care needs assessment. In: Moving forward – needs, services and contracts. A DHA Project Paper. Leeds: NHS Management Executive.
Wadsworth Y (1984) Do-it-yourself social research. Melbourne, Australia: Victoria Council of Social Services.

Section 14.2

Lifestyle Surveys

Heather Roberts

WHAT DOES 'LIFESTYLE' MEAN IN RELATION TO HEALTH?

'Lifestyle' is a very vague term, although most people have some concept of what it means. At its most basic, it means personal behaviour that has a direct impact on our individual health and well-being, such as cigarette smoking. However, theories of health promotion show that behaviour and consumption are conditioned by the contexts in which we are brought up and live, and so a broader definition of lifestyle recognises factors integral to health related behaviour and change models (see Chapter 4), such as people's knowledge, beliefs and attitudes, and their economic and cultural circumstances (Blaxter, 1990; Kickbusch, 1989). Smoking status, diet, exercise, alcohol consumption and use of health services are commonly studied, although sensitive subjects, such as sexual health and environmental issues may also be explored. These lifestyle factors, some of which have been studied as single topics in, for example, the General Household Survey and other Office of Population, Censuses and Survey reports, are seen as predictors of future health status, and are often referred to as indirect or intermediate indicators of health.

HISTORY OF LIFESTYLE SURVEYS

Using research designs from the social sciences, lifestyle surveys draw samples of people from a defined population and systematically study them to make inferences about that population. They became fashionable in the mid to late 1980s, and there are many examples of initiatives from around that time, some of which were reviewed at a conference by the Health Education Authority in 1989 (Leyden et al., 1990). Although some of the larger surveys have continued and national surveys have been established, as shown below, the initial flurry of local initiatives seems to have petered out. This could be due to a number of reasons, such as reorganisation of health authorities, lack of funding, or possibly that such surveys simply failed to be as useful as was originally envisaged in producing high quality local data for policy making and planning.

Evidence-based Health Promotion. Edited by Elizabeth R. Perkins, Ina Simnett and Linda Wright.
© 1999 John Wiley & Sons Ltd.

SOME MAJOR NATIONAL SURVEYS

Measuring Change Over Time

Health Survey for England

Social Survey Division of OPCS for the Department of Health's *Health of the Nation* initiative

Key publications: 'Health Survey for England' titles: contact HMSO bookshops for most recent titles

A Survey of the UK Population: Health and Lifestyles

Key publications: Contact the Health Education Authority, Hamilton House, Mabledon Place, London WC1H 9TX, for most recent titles

The Health and Lifestyle Survey

Key publications: Blaxter M (1990) Health and lifestyles. London: Tavistock/Routledge. Cox B D, Huppert F A & Whichelow M J (Eds) (1993) The Health and Lifestyle Survey: seven years on. Aldershot: Dartmouth Publishing Company Ltd

The Welsh Heart Health Survey

Key publications: Contact the Health Promotion Unit for Wales, Ffynnon-las, Ty Glas Avenue, Llanishen, Cardiff CF4 5DZ, for most recent titles

'One off' (to date) Population and Topic Based Surveys

Black and Minority Ethnic Groups in England: Health and Lifestyles

Key publications: Contact the Health Education Authority, Hamilton House, Mabledon Place, London WC1H 9TX, for most recent titles

Sexual Behaviour in Britain

Key publication: Wellings K, Field J, Johnson A M & Wadsworth J (1994) Sexual behaviour in Britain: The National Survey of Sexual Attitudes and Lifestyles. Harmondsworth: Penguin Books

WHY ARE LIFESTYLE SURVEYS RELEVANT TO HEALTH PROMOTION?

Interest and investment in obtaining lifestyle data was prompted in the 1980s by increasing recognition of health promotion as a speciality within public health. As such, it required its own information by which to inform policy, planning and practice. Further, and in the face of scepticism about the credibility of health promotion, it was essential for us to establish a means of assessing and monitoring the impact of health promotion. Both managers and practitioners were conscious that mechanisms to routinely produce population-based data, the 'bread and butter' of strategic planning in public health, were absent. The only practical solution by which to 'plug the gap' was to approach the local lay public directly for information.

Not surprisingly, there was some conflict over which data lifestyle surveys should collect, depending on professionals' definition of health promotion and practical constraints. Some considered it adequate to simply monitor some behaviours most closely related to health risk by obtaining quantitative data – such as finding out the percentages of smokers, those taking too little exercise, consuming a less healthy diet or drinking more than recommended levels of alcohol. They saw such data as having a role to play in population health needs assessments, particularly if able to make comparisons between localities to highlight priority areas. It should be noted that the capacity to do 'in-district' analyses of lifestyle from recent national surveys is limited by low numbers.

In contrast, many health promotion specialists were understandably concerned that behaviour measures alone would not reflect the full impact of their work. They wanted data to reflect shifts in knowledge, attitudes and beliefs, culture and context which, over perhaps protracted periods of time, would lead to the ultimate outcome of behaviour change. They also wanted surveys to be informed by a broad definition of 'health' to enable them to explore psycho-social aspects of health, such as stress and social support, and the wider context of people's lives. For example, in carrying out a 'healthy eating' project for women, survey data may show that those with the least healthy diet do not know what constitutes a healthy diet, cannot get to shops that sell appropriate foods at an affordable price, or state that they have no intention of changing because of family resistance. When such data are related to theories of behaviour change (see Chapter 4) they may pinpoint the stage of progress local people have reached and so have the potential to influence health promotion activities. Further, much health promotion activity takes place among target groups within a population and in specific settings and so health promotion specialists wanted survey questions that were relevant to populations within small areas, such as wards, a GP's practice or an identifiable neighbourhood. Thus health promotion staff saw a need for complementary quantitative and qualitative data to help them to not only measure but also understand healthy and unhealthy risk-related behaviour. This would enable them to target programmes tailored to meet the conditions and needs of specific communities known to them, and so avoid the broad-brush, often 'victim blaming' approach of some national agenda setting campaigns.

WHAT USE ARE LIFESTYLE SURVEYS TO HEALTH PROMOTION PRACTITIONERS?

In theory, therefore, lifestyle surveys have the potential for all or some of the following. To:

- set baseline measures
- monitor change over time
- inform local health promotion activities
- help us to interpret what characterises people's behaviour, and understand that behaviour.

My own experience and observations are that surveys have tended to be successful at the first two objectives, but only when programmes have been appropriately funded, sustained and samples are adequate, for example, the Welsh Heart Health Survey which started an ongoing rolling programme in 1985 (see above). Findings from surveys have often been used in 'in-house' reports and reviews of health status. They have also been systematically or opportunistically used in media awareness-raising activities. However, successfully addressing the more difficult third and fourth objectives has been much more problematic: bridging the gap between research and practice has not been easy. Many health promotion staff have been left half drowning in a sea of information. Making practical use of the wealth of information to be found in tables of data, and 'hidden' in computer files awaiting interrogation, has proved a major stumbling block to practitioners. In my experience, even those health promotion practitioners who have had the motivation to use local data have not had the research, computing and data interpretation experience to analyse and interpret data at anything other than superficial level, let alone the time to do so. Substantial support or specific training for practitioners following-on from the practical collection of data and initial reports has been needed, but seems to have been problematic. As a result, while there are many examples of lifestyle survey data being used in, for example, Director of Public Health annual reports and academic papers, there is little published evidence that health promotion staff have used local lifestyle survey data to inform their programmes. This comment is, of course, rather a crude generalisation. Practitioners often tend to get on with their work, and do not always write it up for dissemination. Sadly, some feel that because their work is small scale it is not important enough to share. Examples of health promoters successfully using data in practice are, I believe, the exception and far from the rule. The lesson seems to be that, before deciding to carry out a survey, it is essential to consider resources beyond the data collection and initial report stage.

CHARACTERISTICS OF LIFESTYLE SURVEYS

One of the key characteristics of lifestyle surveys is their variability, in terms of their scope, methods, sample size, age of population studied, cost and quality of data. These reflect both the survey brief given and the skills and resources available to those carrying out the survey: 'in-house' staff or those commissioned from, for example, commercial agencies and universities. Repeat surveys have tended to occur at gaps of between three and five years, with the latter probably more realistic, as confidence intervals on measures are often wide and change within the population is likely to be slow, for example, smoking has reduced at about 2% per year. Exceptionally, the Health and Lifestyle Survey (see above) had a seven-year gap between surveys. It is also unusual as it has followed up a cohort established in 1994/5, rather than taking new cross-sectional samples for each wave of data collection. Major surveys, such as the Health and Lifestyle Survey, have often taken objective measures as well as self-reported data, for example, height and blood pressure, but most others have not. Some survey methodologies have checked the validity and/or reliability of their questions by, for example, test/retest, but again this is not common as this requires additional skill and resources. The need to measure change and maintain comparability of data sets has meant that while improvements or variations in method may be thought desirable over time, they may be inadvisable. The result of all this fragmented activity has been a huge range of survey instruments, data of varying quality and results that are often not comparable across populations. The government attempted to overcome this in the early 1990s by establishing a National Survey Advice Centre, but it closed in the mid-1990s after pump-priming monies ran out.

SURVEY METHODS AND DATA QUALITY

Most often, lifestyle surveys are postal, face-to-face or occasionally a combination of these. Unusually, a survey among adults in Scotland which terminated in 1995, used an on-going system of collecting data using Computer Assisted Telephone Interviews, based on a random digit dialling. The generally recognised characteristics of each of these methods are shown in Table 14.2.1. Many texts give practical details of how to conduct surveys, including sampling techniques (e.g. de Vaus, 1991; Fink, 1995; Salant & Dillman, 1994). Among young people, school-based surveys using self-completion questionnaires are popular (See Chapter 13, Section 13.3), although the methodology of school-based surveys is less well documented other than in survey reports. Generally, good co-operation from school staff, high response rates from pupils and rapid data collection from large numbers have attracted increasing numbers of researchers to this approach. As the health promoting schools initiative has developed momentum, my experience is that survey fatigue is setting in. Schools seem less willing to participate in projects without a clear indication of the benefit to the school in doing so. Further, the ethics of using school classes, a 'captive sample', is increasingly being debated (Denscombe & Aubrook, 1992).

The quality of your data depends on using a sound methodology. For example, your sample must be large enough to give accurate population data, especially when target sub-groups within the population are studied – consult a text book to work out how many you need in your sample, bearing in mind likely non-response, or, better still, ask a friendly statistician to help you. The highest possible response rate needs to be achieved, with around 70% being high for a postal survey. Despite using every practical technique to maximise response, such as follow-ups and reply-paid envelopes, non-response is almost inevitably going to bias your data. Bear in mind that people give personal health information

Table 14.2.1 Characteristics of survey methods

Postal surveys	Telephone surveys	Face-to-face surveys
The most economic of population surveys	Moderately expensive	Expensive
Sampling frames of individuals may be badly out of date	Unless using CATI, only give access to those with listed phone numbers and so are biased	As postal surveys
Poorer response rates obtained, often below 70%, and reminders are needed	Reasonable response rates, but persistence needed	The best response rates, up to 90% or more, but persistence needed
Can cover large samples in widely spread geographical areas quickly	More time-consuming	The most time-consuming
Easy to repeat	Easy to repeat, but may require interviewer training	Easy to repeat, but may require interviewer training
Lends itself to closed questions	More suitable for open-ended questions	More suitable for open-ended questions

voluntarily and that some will choose not to do so no matter how hard you try to gain their co-operation. Excessive pressure can be counter-productive and lead to poor quality data.

Studies of non-responders show that they tend to be some of the groups that you, as a health promoter, are most interested in. For example, they will be those in lower socio-economic groups or the unemployed, males, especially younger males, from ethnic minority groups, the elderly and very elderly, and smokers (Roberts et al., 1996; Smith & Nutbeam, 1990). Low response, and so response bias, particularly from studies in so-called disadvantaged communities where the above characteristics dominate, is therefore a major headache. However, you may consider that the accuracy and completeness of data informing an epidemiological study and a community-based health risk assessment may be different: for example, I would argue that the accuracy of evidence epidemiologists need to show causal relationships is greater than the accuracy needed to demonstrate that something should be done to eliminate or reduce a real or perceived threat to local health.

COMMUNITY PARTICIPATION AND LIFESTYLE SURVEYS

One of the key characteristics of most surveys has been that their content, conduct, analysis and dissemination of results have been controlled by health professionals with the lay public seen as passive recipients of questionnaires and givers of data. This is, crudely, the normative approach to needs assessment. On the other hand, health promotion staff can take an alternative approach based on theories of community participation in health (Kroutil & Eng, 1989). These enable staff to see the surveying process as one in which professionals are resources facilitating members of the community, working with them and not for them, being supportive but non-directive. Here the ultimate objective is to stimulate well informed local people to work together for change. Arguably community capacity can be increased in the process by local people learning new skills in both planning a survey method, deciding on questions to be asked and carrying out the survey which provides them with information of direct relevance – and so potential power – in arguing for change. This may be a somewhat idealistic model. In reality, when there is no major health issue and no local lay leader creating spontaneous community participation, the process is probably more akin to 'facipulation' (Tones & Tilford, 1994), a mix of facilitation and manipulation, with professionals having an existing or hidden agenda.

One end of the spectrum of community participation has been the sensible strategy of feeding back health-related information to responders. This type of 'information giving' is a far less radical participatory approach than you might wish to implement, but it is also far less contentious. It is a very practical activity requiring little extra effort from those running the survey, although it does add to its costs. It could be argued that the promise of information is an incentive that increases response by a particular sub-group, and therefore biases results. If this is true, then this is an additional bias to those already outlined above: the possible benefits need to be weighed against this arguably slight disadvantage.

Health information related to surveys has been distributed in various ways, most usually immediately after a doorstep interview or requested through postal surveys and returned by post. Respondents usually choose leaflets they wish to receive from a preselected list covering topics related to the survey questions, such as diet, how to stop smoking and the details of local services. This is more practical than creating an open-ended demand for information which could be very time-consuming to satisfy. Studies demonstrate quite clearly that people from 'hard to reach' groups will ask for feedback. In my own work in an economically depressed area, over 60% of respondents requested at least one leaflet from a postal survey (Roberts & Beales, 1993), and even more have been shown to take leaflets after an interview (Liddiard, 1988). People who do want information are more likely to be women than men and younger rather than older. They are likely to be highly selective in the leaflets they opt to take; for example, in the survey that I conducted, an average of three leaflets was chosen out of the nine offered. Those selected were generally relevant to respondents' situations. The actual impact of health information distributed to respondents in terms of health-related change has not been studied in depth. Even so, it seems reasonable to suggest that at worst it does no harm and, at best, may do the cause of health promotion some good by targeting information on those who wish to receive it.

An offer to send the results of the lifestyle survey back to participants is likely to be very popular and, again, seems an ethically sound activity. In my own work more respondents asked for a printed leaflet about this than for any other piece of information: two out of five of all respondents. To achieve this step adequately, someone needs to be prepared to present information in a short and snappy format rather than a long and wordy report. Technology is making this an easier task once the content has been selected. Complementing a printed short report with one or more local meetings to present findings is another possible strategy. Going down this route needs careful forethought. Your credibility could be badly damaged if you don't have answers to reasonable questions that local lay leaders might ask. For example, 'Now you know, what are you going to do about it?' If the survey had been carried out within the framework of a more inclusive community participation project, rather than based on the professionally dominated normative model, then turning that question to, 'Now *we* know, what are *we* going to do about it?', might be more feasible and result in community action.

More inclusive and intensive participatory models have been taken from the developing world, and there is now a small but fascinating group of published and unpublished studies in education and health in the UK that have succeeded in involving local people both formally and informally and with varying degrees of power within the survey process (e.g. Carr-Hill, 1984; Liddiard, 1988; Snee, 1991). For example, lay people have been involved at one or more of these stages:

- deciding whether a survey needs to be carried out or not
- deciding on the survey content
- deciding on the survey method
- designing the survey instrument
- administering the survey using postal, telephone or face-to-face methods
- data entry and validation
- data analysis
- interpretation of data
- report writing, disseminating and presenting data in different ways for different purposes, such as for community groups, council meetings and the media.

For health promotion staff the attractions of this process should not obscure the difficulties of these steps, some of which are outlined below. Many are inherent in community participation of any kind.

- Staff can be caught in unresolvable conflict between their employers' and the community's interests. For example, 'I want to know about the smoking status of young people' versus 'We want to know about anxiety caused by crime and how it inhibits old people going out.'
- The option is not cheap. Teaching/learning time and effort is expensive in cash and emotional investment from both professionals and lay people.
- The time required to complete the task is protracted, for example, it took 18 months to complete the work instead of a few months (Snee, 1991).
- Questionnaires are unlikely to be transferable to another location.
- Community expectations of what can be done based on survey results may be raised, but not be realistic, and so threaten the credibility of health staff who engaged them in the work but who cannot respond to findings.

The implications of this review are that lifestyle surveys do not necessarily have to be conducted only to fulfil the information needs of health authorities. Located within theories of community participation they have the potential to make the community not only more knowledgeable about its own health, but also more willing and able to act on its own behalf.

REFERENCES

Blaxter M (1990) Health and lifestyles. London: Tavistock/Routledge.

Carr-Hill R (1984) Radicalising survey methodology. *Quality and Quantity*, 18: 275–292.

Cox B D, Huppert F A & Whichelow M J (Eds) (1993) The Health and Lifestyle Survey: seven years on. Aldershot: Dartmouth Publishing Company Ltd.

Denscombe M & Aubrook L (1992) 'It's just another piece of schoolwork': the ethics of questionnaire research on pupils in schools. *British Educational Research Journal*, 18, 113–131.

de Vaus D A (1991) Surveys in social research. London: George Allen and Unwin.

Fink A (Ed) (1995) The survey kit. London: Sage.

Kickbusch I (1989) Good planets are hard to find. WHO Healthy Cities Papers No. 5. Geneva: WHO.

Kroutil L A & Eng E (1989) Conceptualizing and assessing potential for community participation: a planning method. *Health Education Research*, 4, 305–319.

Leyden R, Gobel F & Killoran A (Eds) (1990) Health and lifestyle surveys: towards a common approach. London: Health Education Authority.

Liddiard P (1988) Milton Keynes Felt Needs project. Milton Keynes: Open University Press.

Roberts H & Beales J G (1993) Responding to the responders: feedback from a postal survey. In: Health Education and the Mass Media. How to communicate effectively (pp 197–201). Amsterdam: Dutch Centre for Health Promotion and Health Education.

Roberts H, Bali B & Rushton L (1996) Non-responders to a lifestyle survey: a study using telephone interviews. *Journal of the Institute of Health Education*, 34, 57–61.

Salant P & Dillman D A (1994) How to conduct your own survey. Chichester: John Wiley.

Smith C & Nutbeam D (1990) Assessing non-response bias: a case-study from the 1985 Welsh Heart Health Survey. *Health Education Research*, 5, 381–386.

Snee K (1991) Neighbourhood needs. *Community Outlook*, 1(2), 38–39.

Tones B K & Tilford S (1994) Health education: effectiveness, efficiency and equity. Second edition. London: Chapman & Hall.

Tones B K, Tilford S & Robinson Y K (1989) Health education: effectiveness and efficiency. London: Chapman & Hall.

Wellings K, Field J, Johnson A M & Wadsworth J (1994) Sexual behaviour in Britain: The National Survey of Sexual Attitudes and Lifestyles. Harmondsworth: Penguin Books.

Section 14.3

A Bottom-up Approach to Family Health Needs Assessment

Anne McClelland*

INTRODUCTION

The principal skill of health visiting is in needs assessment at three levels: the individual, the family and the community. Yet these levels have been fragmented in practice and theory. This is an account of a bottom-up approach to needs assessment which grew out of health visitors' concerns to implement an integrated approach to needs assessment that utilised information from all these levels.

In 1993 a number of health visitors in Rotherham formed a development group to examine the ordinary aspects of our practice. Membership of the group is fluid, according to individuals' commitments and enthusiasm, as most of the work undertaken is extra to the workload. We see ourselves as building on a tradition of development and research undertaken by others.

BACK TO BASICS

At an early stage in our group's development our discussions demonstrated a basic conflict – if we all shared the same beliefs, why couldn't we agree a way forward? We held a half-day workshop in order to re-examine basic practice and establish a common framework. We looked at four areas:

1. the meaning of health
2. what is health promotion?
3. our own values and beliefs
4, people power.

These topics naturally evolved as fundamental to our work and methods.

---

* On behalf of Rotherham Health Visitor Development Group.

Evidence-based Health Promotion. Edited by Elizabeth R. Perkins, Ina Simnett and Linda Wright.
© 1999 John Wiley & Sons Ltd.

Health

Health visitors have traditionally taken a social model of health rather than a medical model and everyone strongly endorsed this. However, when it came to the specifics dissent set in. Everyone recognised that the utopian ideal of the WHO (1946) definition was far from practical, but being pragmatic and accepting less also seemed defeatist. We felt more comfortable with the idea suggested by Seedhouse (1986), that health can be defined in positive and negative statements. This was certainly more practical and as one wit suggested, reflected the ups and downs of our working realities rather better.

Health Promotion

We felt concern that the positivist approach and goals of health promotion had been hijacked by the medical profession into disease prevention and victim blaming. We were also aware of Robinson's (1983) criticism of our practice, that by expanding into non-disease aspects of health we were solely engaged in pursuing professional ambitions and fencing off lay areas of health knowledge as our own area of expertise.

Values and Beliefs

Whether experienced or newly qualified, as health visitors we had all been trained in the four principles of health visiting as originally set out by the Council for the Education and Training of Health Visitors (CETHV) in 1977. This work had been re-visited by the then Health Visitors Association (HVA, now Community Practitioners and Health Visitors Association CPHVA), the principles of which are set out below:

1. The search for health needs.
2. The stimulation of an awareness of health needs.
3. The influence on policies affecting health
4. The facilitation of health enhancing activities (Health Visitors Association, 1992).

We agreed with their conclusions that the principles were still relevant to practise and needed a high degree of skill in implementation. We believed we had these skills and in particular the ability to work with a huge range of client groups and agencies.

People Power

This means working in partnership. It is fundamental to WHO's (1978) view that equal partnerships are an essential cornerstone to good practice in primary health care. It has been demonstrated that equal partnerships make health care more effective, accessible and acceptable (Rifkin, 1990). To the development group, it meant involving clients and communities in the decision-making processes and implementation of programmes of health care.

The workshop was a difficult half-day, with everyone having to come clean about how they practised health care. It is hard to do this without people feeling vulnerable and intimidated. We opted for a consensus view rather than identifying good and bad elements of practice.

MAKING PLANS

The prospect of deciding on a workplan for the development group was a much easier task than finding a common framework. We were effectively inarticulate, without the means to translate our work with individuals, families and communities to a broader audience. In consequence, we were being measured solely by individual assessments, usually for child health contacts, that ignored the bulk of our work, which was family and community orientated. We were struck by Jean Orr's comments (1992, p 126), 'As community health workers we make statements of our professional intent in such global terms as to be often meaningless. What do we mean by "assessing family health" or assessing the physical, social and emotional health of families and individuals? We simply do not have the tools at present to undertake such an exercise.' We needed to find a measure based on the family, that could encompass the individuals within that group and the community they lived in, in order to provide a holistic assessment that was relevant to people in their communities. We therefore wanted a means of assessing family health that could also feed into our community profiles and would be based on a partnership approach.

Some tools were already in the process of development and we knew of two distinct models for use in family assessment. The York family health assessment (York Community Health Services, 1992) used a bio-medical approach and mostly closed questions. It was A4 in size, well produced and looked attractive to complete. The Nottingham family health assessment (Nottingham Community Health, 1992) used a social health approach and more open-ended questions. It was A5 in size, on photocopied paper and did not look appealing. However, we opted for the Nottingham model because it better matched our own ideology. It covered four sections on physical, emotional, social and community health, on both an individual and family basis. We felt that the Nottingham model needed some improvement as it was too literate, especially in the social and emotional health section. We introduced pictorial representations and linear scales which could also explore family relationships. We changed the cover page which showed a mixed group of people, as such scenes are exclusive, i.e. if you don't see yourself there, then it can't be for you. We opted for symbolic representation that would have positive connotations across cultures and came up with a tree – the tree of life, the family tree.

TESTING, TESTING

It was important to pre-test the usability of this version of the family health assessment on as broad a basis as possible. We used the same evaluation tool as Nottingham in order to enhance reliability but also to save inventing another one. The evaluation looked at user-friendliness by health visitors and clients and not at the information gathered.

The usability testing involved 14 health visitor and 22 family evaluations. The families generally expressed positive views and thought they were useful. The health visitor evaluations were also mostly positive and people made comments that it actually felt like working in a partnership with clients. They also noted that families were able to share with them public health information that was new. On the negative side, two health visitors felt they gained no new information about the individuals and it was very time-consuming; at the least ten minutes and the most two hours, with the mean being one hour. The health visitors who were the most negative had worked in their areas for many years and knew their clients very well. They felt they had nothing to gain by adopting this tool.

A few minor changes were made to improve the focus of the open-ended questions. At this point we also pooled our experience to devise a small booklet of guidelines for health visitors to help them when using the family health assessment.

The next stage was developed much more opportunistically. We wanted to look at client views in more depth and as one member of the development group was looking for a research project for her thesis, we gratefully married the two. She was able to select families on the caseloads of two health visitors in the same area, on the basis of random sampling, and interview families after they had completed their family health assessments. She acquired the approval of the ethics committee and was supervised by the university. It gave us the advantage of getting the development work progressed on the cheap and with outside supervision that would offer constructive criticism. She used semi-structured interviews with eight families and a questionnaire with the two health visitors, abstracting from the data using thematic content analysis. Table 14.3.1 gives a summary of her results (Higginbottom, 1994).

Client satisfaction with the family health assessment was on a par with that noted by the York study (York Community Health Services, 1992) at 95%. Interestingly, some families felt it was completed in a few minutes, yet the health visitors recorded times of 45–90 minutes, with a mean of 50 minutes.

DEALING WITH THE UNEXPECTED

By now the health visitors in the group were starting to make some generalisations about the family health assessments. We found when it came to drawing up a health plan at the end of the assessment there was often nothing to do. Families

Table 14.3.1 Summary of results

Themes	Examples
Client rights	to professional time, someone to listen, focus on family not baby, open agenda
Partnership	work in non-directive way, empowerment, mutual respect
Community health	drugs, pollution, road safety
Client satisfaction	not intrusive, positive and therapeutic, family and community health, relationships

were practical when completing the assessments and showed that they understood the role they had to play in protecting and improving their health. They knew that smoking was bad for you, but was better than stress, violence or heroin. They made choices about the immediate options around them and few considered long-term goals that were years into the future. For us there were no big surprises amongst the families' health needs. We also noted a ripple effect amongst the families, as they discussed their assessments with their extended family and friends. Issues like heart disease and cancer and bereavement had an airing as individuals considered the effect their family was having on their health. The assessment also highlighted relationships within the family, for example learning that children have their own points of view, and recognising how they relate to others – who is the spokesperson, the public face of the family?

In contrast the community health needs generated by the assessment proved to be a revelation. It was like putting a jigsaw together, as each family contributed information that built up a picture of local health issues which was very different to the information previously available. Three important community health issues emerged from the data: drug-related problems, sale of cigarettes to children and road safety.

The Drugs Problem

Families identified specific problems in the community – speeding motorbikes using the pedestrian alleys, drug sales in the park, sale of cheap drugs outside the local comprehensive school, inability of the police to act, rise in local burglaries, private security firms being employed by residents and coercion brought to bear to encourage participation. The completed picture showed a deliberate targeting of the area as a new drugs base and centre. It later transpired that this was part of a very large criminal operation across South Yorkshire. The park was the initial 'drop' where users came to place their order and money; the goods would then be delivered by motorbike through the pedestrian alleys of the nearby estate to avoid detection and pursuit. The low price sale of drugs outside the comprehensive school was a deliberate promotional exercise and, needless to say, in a very short space of time a large number of under 25s in the area were addicts using and selling mainly heroin. The syndicate then moved into a block of maisonettes and the dealing from there proved unstoppable. Crime in the area rocketed as people needed money to feed their addiction. These effects were reflected in the local crime figures, reported in the local paper, were recounted at councillors' surgeries, had an impact on GP surgeries, and contributed to a decline in the local environment, fear of crime and mental health issues. The problem proved so intransigent that the local authority took the decision to demolish the blocks of maisonettes and deprive the dealers of a base. This largely appears to have worked as the 'big fish' have moved on, but at what cost! Drug addiction is so endemic that there are now many minor traders; the waiting list across South Yorkshire for drug rehabilitation has doubled; there is a housing shortage; environmental blight; fear of crime; a community under siege; and increased local poverty – devastating at any level, for the individual, the family and the community.

Sale of Cigarettes to Children

We already knew from the work of the school nurse that smoking amongst schoolchildren, especially girls, was above average at 14 years (25% of girls were regular smokers before they were 14). We were therefore horrified to discover from the family health assessments that the sale of single cigarettes to children was commonplace. One particular shop was identified, but most alarming was news that the ice cream van outside the comprehensive school was also doing this trade. Worse was to come when other local families informed us this was common knowledge and a widespread practice; in the neighbouring area the van actually went onto school premises to sell ice cream and cigarettes.

Speeding Traffic on Residential Roads

Parents were concerned for the safety of their children and felt action was needed to slow traffic. Cameras are now used on the main road to good effect but have been of little benefit for the side roads.

The local health information was so much richer, real and accurate than any of the professional health information we were accustomed to using locally. The family health assessment was the means to open up this source and illustrated how feeble our efforts were in dealing with community health on an individual basis.

WORK IN PROGRESS

The information obtained from the family health assessment environment page was piecemeal and fragmentary. The richness of the information was revealed by the deciphering skills of the health visitors who translated the single assessments into collective knowledge. This approach relied on the stability of the health visitor workforce. The development group approached a local women's group to ask for ideas as to how we could ensure this information was captured, even where there was a transient population and staff. It was interesting to note that the women's group had little awareness of the heroin dealing locally and were more aware of what every health visitor would consider the perennial community health issue – dog faeces in public places. It made us realise that communities are not unified or holistic places. We wanted a method of discovery within the family health assessment.

In their literature review of community needs assessment, Billings and Cowley (1995) look at the role of what they term the 'consumer perspective' and we call 'people information'. They present the local view as being the consumer feedback to a state enterprise developed and accepted as a means of 'bridging the gap between the "micro" and "macro" levels of health estimation' and also as a means of promoting the rationing debate. The development group felt that this philosophy was paternalistic in nature and liable to promote inequities. We wanted a more inclusive and partnership approach. We needed to use our current methods of family work, as well as work with a variety of community groups, to explore ways of re-designing the environment page of the family health assessment. We originally thought that we could ask the local women's group to start from a blank piece of paper, but now realise that we have to do the preparatory drafting work and design a range of options for the group to comment on. Partnership is after all about taking responsibility on a basis of equity.

The development group also considered what was the point in collecting information if it could not be used effectively? We did not have strategies to utilise the information generated by the family health assessments and that needed to be remedied. We needed better strategy networks within our own Trust, the local health authority, the local authority and other agencies. Individuals were willing, but the culture of our modern health service and organisational hierarchy make it particularly difficult for practitioners to raise issues on an on-going basis at policy and strategic level. The period since the publication of our community health information has been a time for consolidation and thought as to how this work might best be taken forward. We had originally intended at this time to test the family health assessment on a much grander scale. Now we realise we must re-work the environment page and put into place information strategies that can most effectively utilise the data that is collected. We, as practitioners, have an especial loathing for wasteful collection of irrelevant and unused information.

AND SO . . .

There are many issues we have yet to address – such as who doesn't it work for, does it work in translation, is it translatable? The time it has taken to progress this far makes development work seem more like a hobby than fundamental to our practice. We don't write research reports; we write notes, in order to keep pace with development, but also because we don't have the resources. The family health assessment fits alongside the other work done by the development group and has to be adaptable to a fluctuating group membership. Development work is about living life on the hoof and brings as many questions as it does answers; but that's how it should be – a reflection of life in practice.

REFERENCES

Billings J & Cowley S (1995) Approaches to community needs assessment: a literature review. *Journal of Advanced Nursing*, 22, 721–730.
Council for the Education and Training of Health Visitors (1977) An investigation into the principles of health visiting. London: CETHV.
Health Visitors Association (1992) The principles of health visiting: a re-examination. London: HVA.
Health Visitors Association (1992) Principles into practice. London: HVA.
Higginbottom G (1994) A preliminary study into the effects of using a family health assessment tool. Unpublished thesis. Sheffield: Sheffield Hallam University.
Nottingham Community Health (1992) Your family's health. Nottingham: Nottingham Community Health.
Orr J (1992) Assessing individual and family health needs. In: K Luker & J Orr (Eds), Health visiting: towards community health nursing. Oxford: Blackwell.
Rifkin S (1990) Community participation in maternal and child health/family planning programmes. Geneva: World Health Organisation.
Robinson K (1983) What is health? In: J Clark & J Henderson (Eds), Community health. Edinburgh: Churchill Livingstone.
Seedhouse D (1986) Health – the foundations of achievement. New York: John Wiley.
World Health Organisation (1946) Constitution. New York: WHO.
World Health Organisation (1978) Primary health care. A joint report by the Director-General of the World Health Organisation and the Executive Director of United Nations Children's Fund. Geneva: WHO.
York Community Health Services (1992) Family health matters. York: York Health Authority.

Chapter 15

Using Qualitative Studies

Linda Wright

INTRODUCTION

The use of qualitative methods for gathering and analysing evidence is important to health promotion researchers and practitioners, because many of the questions we ask cannot be answered using traditional, scientific, quantitative research methods. In health promotion we are not only interested in what people know, think and do in relation to their health, but also the place and meaning of such thinking and behaviour in their social worlds.

One of the current factors limiting our attempts to be evidence-based health promotion practitioners is the nature of the evidence available. All too often, the evidence derived from quantitative descriptive studies is sufficient to tell us that we should be doing something about a particular health problem, but insufficient to tailor an intervention to client needs at local level. For example, time-series national surveys have gathered considerable descriptive data on who drinks what, where and when; they indicate that young people are tending to drink more alcohol, more often. Analytical studies have provided extensive data on the alcohol-related risks and harms experienced by young people. This is ample evidence to justify a health promotion intervention aimed at young drinkers. However, when it comes to deciding what kind of intervention might meet young people's needs, the evidence is much thinner. We know considerably less about the place and meaning of drinking alcohol in young people's lives. We know little about what kind of drinking behaviour is considered acceptable or unacceptable to different groups of young people in different social settings, nor do we know much about the self-control strategies young people adopt (Wright, in press).

Qualitative studies can help to provide answers to these types of questions and thus inform an intervention which is credible, relevant and acceptable to the target group. Qualitative studies can also help health promoters to work more effectively in different settings (see Part II), by analysing the multiple meanings created by individuals' and

Evidence-based Health Promotion. Edited by Elizabeth R. Perkins, Ina Simnett and Linda Wright.
© 1999 John Wiley & Sons Ltd.

groups' interactions with their social environment. This type of qualitative evidence complements and extends the evidence from quantitative survey data.

This chapter considers the features of qualitative research and contrasts these approaches with those of traditional, scientific methods. It explains what qualitative research methods are, when they can be used and offers some criteria for quality. The latter consideration is important, in countering criticisms that evidence derived from qualitative studies is not valid or sufficient to inform health promotion action. The chapter concludes by discussing ways in which evidence from qualitative studies can be used in health promotion.

REFERENCE

Wright L (in press) Young people and alcohol: a literature review (provisional title). London: The Health Education Authority.

Section 15.1

Qualitative Studies in Health Promotion

Alison McCamley-Finney & Majella McFadden

INTRODUCTION

This section aims to provide the reader with a practical guide to using qualitative research methodologies in the field of health promotion. Many working in health-related fields are often hesitant about using such techniques given common presentations of qualitative approaches as unscientific and subjective. By providing information, tips and illustrations from field work carried out by the two authors, a critique of such portrayals will be offered and, as well, a case developed for the value and relevance of qualitative approaches for those working in health fields.

EXAMPLES IN THE SECTION ARE DRAWN FROM THREE STUDIES

- A study of young people and drug use, funded by Trent Regional Health Authority. The study was conducted with a colleague over a period of 12 months. It involved group and individual interviews with seven groups of young people about their perceptions and feelings of their own and others' drug use (AMF).
- An observational study of a group of friends who all injected amphetamines. The study was part of a PhD dissertation and was conducted over three months. It attempted to assess the relationship between the culture of the estate where the friendship group lived and their HIV risk behaviour (AMF).
- An exploration of young women's sexuality was conducted as part of a doctoral thesis. From 1991–1994 individual interviews with three groups of women (hetero-sexual women, lesbian women and single mothers) took place in Northern Ireland (MM).

FEATURES OF QUALITATIVE RESEARCH APPROACHES

Qualitative research approaches share common features. They:

Evidence-based Health Promotion. Edited by Elizabeth R. Perkins, Ina Simnett and Linda Wright.
© 1999 John Wiley & Sons Ltd.

- reject traditional scientific research models
- favour 'naturally occurring' data
- grounds emerging data in theory
- focus on meaning and function of social action
- reject traditional research models.

Traditional scientific research models, regardless of the area or issue under consideration, begin with a number of assumptions. Firstly, they assume that there is one true reality that can be known, that there is an objective social world 'out there' and if you conduct research in a scientific way then you can reflect that single social reality. This means that there is no recognition or acceptance that there may be different social realities arising from the way in which people and groups actively construct the world and their identities. Different individuals or groups may experience the world in a particular way that may be influenced by many different kinds of social experience. Secondly, within traditional scientific research aspects of people's social experience, e.g. age, gender, race, class are treated as variables and as such are often presented as unproblematic. In identifying class as one variable that might, for example, correlate with HIV risk behaviour the approach fails to give recognition to the very different experiences individuals may have of class and the complex ways in which this might relate to aspects of their behaviour. Finally, it is assumed that the way in which research presents the social world is through a relationship between two or more variables. The expected relationship between these variables is expressed in the hypothesis. The relationship between variables is seen as being the same across a variety of contexts and across time. Only research conducted in this particular way is considered as having the status of fact. Any other kind of evidence is perceived as inferior and at worst anecdotal.

One of the main models, incorporating the above features, and used extensively to gain insights into the practice of safer sex is the Health Belief Model (Rosenstock, 1974). This approach assumes that attitudes and behaviour are directly linked and that changing attitudes will change behaviour. In the model the relationship between attitudes and behaviour is presented as a little more complicated, as it includes what are termed 'modifying variables'. These are factors that may affect whether a change in attitude brings about a change in behaviour and include: perceived vulnerability, cost–benefit ratio, external prompt (e.g. seeing a poster, a television programme). In short, the model still maintains that changing attitudes is likely to change behaviour, e.g. changing attitudes towards HIV will result in more people engaging in safer sex. In order for the person to change their behaviour the model proposes that some additional things must happen, one of which is termed 'perceived vulnerability' (i.e. that a person must perceive themselves to be at risk of contracting HIV). This model has not provided a good blueprint for instilling the practice of safer sex among individuals, especially young people (Holland et al., 1990; Ingham, 1991). In particular it has been criticised by qualitative researchers for failing to recognise several important aspects of sexual behaviour. The criticisms relate back to features of a traditional scientific approach to research which were discussed earlier. The criteria are as follows.

External Reality

Qualitative perspectives reject notions of a single, objective reality and suggest that concepts of reality are multiple and socially negotiated. In terms of HIV and safer sex, concepts such as AIDS, risk and safer sex are defined and mean different things to different individuals and groups, i.e. they are relative and open to interpretation. For example, Ingham et al. (1991) noted how in their sample, personal risk assessment was on a diverse number of sources, including geographical area and familiarity.

Typical Respondent

The idea that differences among participants (e.g. class, race, sexual orientation) can be ignored is rejected within qualitative approaches. Indeed, such differences are perceived as fundamentally influencing participants' experiences of their world. For example, in the studies with young women carried out by McFadden (1994) sexual orientation coloured understandings of sexual pleasure. Among many of the young heterosexual women pleasurable sex was equated solely with their male partner's orgasm, in contrast to the lesbian women for whom sexual pleasure not only incorporated the pleasure of their partner but more significantly their own sexual enjoyment and gratification.

Scope of Findings

Qualitative approaches do not profess to uncover 'facts' which can be applied to any context but rather provide an account of issues in particular historical contexts. A qualitative approach would recognise that researching sex and sexuality needs to start with some kind of recognition of the cultural context of sexual behaviour. The society we live in means that sexual behaviour is not something people are open and willing to talk about. It can be described as a 'sensitive' research topic. A qualitative approach would also recognise and explore the different social rules that govern the way in which heterosexual men and women can and may choose to behave, e.g. men do not get called 'slags'. In addition the way in which different sexualities are marginalised, stigmatised or invisible, e.g. lesbians and gay men, would inform the research practice and findings.

Favour 'Naturally Occurring' Data

Qualitative researchers favour naturally occurring data rather than that produced from manipulating a set number of variables. As a result qualitative texts present the complexity of the naturally occurring data – the data are interesting as they provide insight into possible obstacles (social regulations, cultural norms, etc.) that individuals face in the processes of decision making and practice. In their investigation of the concept of 'rationality', Ingham et al. (1991) illustrated the many definitions and diverse obstacles that individuals face with regard to executing the so-called *rational* practices of safer sex. For one young man safer sex was perceived as the sensible thing to do but as unrealistic in intimate situations:

> Well, in cold blood and sitting here with my clothes on, it's very sensible and it's perfect and it's the thing you should do and obtain a full sexual history of your prospective partner, but you get into a dimly lighted room, wearing no quite so many clothes, with somebody you find attractive, you sort of feel a bit awkward (Ingham, 1991, p 11).

While for one young woman, safer sex was again perceived as sensible but as something that she could personally not attain:

> He came over and kissed me and I thought, 'Oh, I can't do this', you know, and he was going 'Why not, why not. . . . You can't get pregnant first time' . . . I didn't believe him but I still went ahead and did it without any sort of . . . I remember thinking 'I'm stupid', but still being that stupid, if you know what I mean (Ingham, 1991, p 9).

This presentation of complexity, multiple interpretations and contradictions gives insight into the very diverse reasons why people may not be engaging in safer sex. Qualitative methods can reveal both the limitations of concepts such as choice and how engaging in apparently irrational behaviour makes sense, from the perspective of the person involved.

Theory Emerging from Data

A qualitative approach aims to examine research data (texts, observations, interviews, field notes) with a view to theory and concepts emerging from the data (Henwood & Pidgeon, 1993). This is in contrast to quantitative approaches which have already given a predicted relationship between variables in the form of hypotheses. Consequently, the investigation centres around the pre-defined relationship between variables. In qualitative research the process of analysis involves examining the data for themes, categories, contradictions and omissions. The researcher is not aiming to impose their own categories or definitions on the data but to try and explore and examine ways in which the people researched experience, explain and talk about their lives or aspects of their lives. An example of this is provided in the later section 'Analysing Interview Data'. As a qualitative researcher is not confined by a pre-determined set of variables in the analysis, the uncovering of aspects of people's lives, experiences or perspectives can be a very exciting and interesting process. For example, in the young people and drugs study, one of the interesting themes that emerged from the interview data was the way in which young people spoke about their futures. It was clear that there were important differences in the way they spoke about their futures, that could be related to their expectations with regard to future drug use. Some groups of young people spoke about their futures with great pessimism. They seemed to feel that there was nothing for them, no future, no chance of a job or even an opportunity to move off the particular estate where they lived.

Other young people spoke about futures in terms of 'A' levels or careers. Formal education was not the only way in which the young people expressed optimistic views of their futures. Other expressions of optimism included one group who were in a band and soon to be going on tour; for others it was the expectation of getting a place of their own. There seemed to be a relationship between their sense of the possible and their views on drug use. Those who had a sense of a future, a future with potential for change, spoke about drug use as a phase. For them, drug use was perceived as something they did not expect to continue with into adulthood. This was in contrast to those who spoke about having no hope for change; they talked about the likelihood of carrying on using drugs, of doing the same things as they were now.

Focus on Meaning and Function of Social Action

Given the emphasis on the written and spoken word in qualitative approaches to research, language becomes the central focus through which the meaning and function of social action can be derived. What people say and how they say it is seen as a key way of accessing and understanding participants' experiences. For example, Sue Lees (1993) illustrated the centrality of language in shaping young women's sexual understandings and practices. Through her consideration of the vocabulary of 'slag' and 'drag' she describes the tightrope that many young women walk in trying to simultaneously be sexually attractive to males and socially respectable.

WHAT ARE QUALITATIVE RESEARCH METHODS AND WHEN CAN THEY BE USED?

One of the most striking features of qualitative research is the variety of methods that come under this umbrella term. Qualitative research can involve observational studies, interviews, texts and transcripts, focus groups and group interviews. Before going into the detail of each method it might be useful to reflect on what this section actually offers. Any one text is unable to offer a comprehensive and exhaustive understanding of qualitative methodology. That said, this section provides a useful guide whether you are a novice or a practitioner more experienced in using qualitative methods. Subsequently, we would like to point you in the direction of other texts that you may find useful at different times.

DIPPING YOUR TOES IN

Glense C & Peshkin A (1992) Becoming qualitative researchers. London: Longman.

TAKING THE PLUNGE

Morse J M & Field P A (1985) Nursing research: the application of qualitative approaches.
    London: Croom Helm.
Silverman D (1993) Interpreting qualitative data. London: Sage.

CHOOSING YOUR STROKE

Harvey L (1990) Critical social research. London: Unwin Hyman.
Reinharz S (1992) Feminist methods in social research. Oxford: Oxford University Press.
Silverman D (1997) Qualitative research: theory, method and practice. London: Sage.

Observational Studies

Observational studies can take many forms. Methods can range from using coding sheets and tape recorders to making observations in settings such as outpatient clinics (Silverman, 1987), to participant observation, whereby the researcher immerses themselves within a particular culture or sub-culture to such an extent that they are part of the group they are studying (Becker, 1964). Observation studies can provide valuable insights into cultures, sub-cultures and social events. The method allows the researcher to gain first-hand experience of the social world or situation being studied and can provide detailed descriptions that illuminate social processes. In the observation study of a group of friends who injected amphetamines, I (AMF) was able to observe the way that aspects of the wider social world were reflected in drug use. For example, there were many occasions when the members of the friendship group, through their behaviour and what they said, revealed the very insular nature of the town they lived in, a town with a ethos of 'we look after our own'. A range of examples of this include: a pregnant young woman's non-attendance at any form of ante-natal provision, instead preferring the advice of other people from the estate where she lived; a man with a severe knee injury using syringes to draw off fluid from the injured knee himself, rather than attend outpatient clinic; women not attending an open meeting with a housing officer because they thought their neighbours would think they were 'snitching' on them. The range of observations reveal a clear distinction between 'them' and 'us' on the estate where the friendship group lived, with all professionals being deeply distrusted and seen as lacking in credibility, even those providing health care.

This is reflected amongst the friendship group in terms of attitudes to drug services and drug workers. A drug problem was seen as something to be dealt with either by the individual, or with help from friends – not to be taken to some outsider. Only one of the group utilised the needle exchange and others were more happy to come to him and get clean injecting equipment via him. During one day at his house, 30 people knocked on the door looking for clean injecting equipment. The insular nature of the town was also reflected in the drug supply chain. On the estate where the friendship group lived, only one person was involved in supplying amphetamine. People would go to him, rather than go to someone else they did not know and pay less.

The central tool of data collection in the observation study was field notes. This involved writing up observations and conversations as soon as possible after having left the group. Field notes would include descriptions of people, behaviour and places and notes on events and conversations.

EXTRACT OF A FILED DIARY NOTE

Brian sat in a chair at Carl's house. He did not lounge in the seat even though it was a comfy seat, but sat quite still and upright. He was about five foot 10 inches and broad shouldered. He had until recently been involved in body building (I knew this from previous conversations). I sat down near him and began talking. I asked about his face. He had bad bruising down the left side of his face, the bruising looked severe, although there was little swelling. In our conversation he sat still, his body seemed tense and he spoke in a quiet controlled voice. I asked him what he was doing at Carl's. He said he was just picking up some speed and then he was going to see if he could find the people who had beaten him up. He said 'I'm looking for the people who did this', moving his head to indicate his face. As he said this he also stood up and from the right sleeve of his big overcoat, which he was still wearing, he slipped a metallic baseball bat. He held the bat in his hand and indicated that he intended to use it to attack the people he was looking for. Having done this (it only took a few seconds) he slipped the bat up his sleeve again and slowly sat back down again.

Interviews

Interviews provide the researcher with a means of accessing a fuller picture of participants' experiences than variable-based quantitative approaches. The question and answer sequence provides a flexible forum for discussion, allowing both the researcher and the participant to input into the data collected. Again this contrasts with pre-coded, questionnaire-based approaches, which limit respondent participation in the research process. According to Silverman (1993), when compared with quantitative approaches (e.g. survey, questionnaire), interviews offer three distinct advantages:

- they produce naturally occurring data
- they facilitate inclusion of material not anticipated by the researcher

- the data collected addresses the 'why' (e.g. why do people fail to practise safer sex) as opposed to simply the 'how many' question.

Group Interviews and Focus Groups

A group interview involves one or more interviewers talking with a number of people. It does not usually involve having an interview schedule and as such is usually relatively unstructured. In the group interviews with the young people we had four or five topics that we were interested in covering but there were no set questions for each topic and no urgency to cover every topic; it very much depended on what the young people themselves brought to the interview and what they wanted to say. Mullings (1985) outlines the advantages of this method as being the ability to present a range of perspectives and provide an insight into the dynamics of the group. In the young people and drugs study, a group interview offered several positive features in addition to the advantages identified by Mullings. Being in a group, rather than a one-to-one interview meant that there was some shift in the power dynamic. Not only were we visiting them as a group 'on their turf', but within the group individuals could see how far others were willing to go in terms of disclosure of drug use and as such negotiate boundaries. They could also interrogate us as to our motives and our own understanding and experience with drugs. Taping and transcribing the interview also meant that we could return the transcript to them, they could examine it and have some control over what we actually analysed. They could delete things they had said if they wished. They had an element of control and inclusion. The other important element, for this study, relates to one of the advantages highlighted in Mullings. Interviewing in groups might provide insight into the way in which the group's ideas and experiences might be 'dynamic', and how issues of agreement and individual differences might be negotiated.

A focus group is not the same as a group interview. It is as the title suggests 'focused'. It involves as Vaughan et al. (1996) describe, focusing on a single theme usually a 'concrete experience' (p 3) or a 'recurrent experience' (p 4). The group, usually seven to ten people (Krueger, 1994), is normally relatively homogeneous and the 'moderator' is prepared with questions and probes so as to conduct a planned interview. The starting point is the presentation of the focus by the moderator who then uses the probes to elicit the complexity of feelings, attitudes and ways of thinking about any one focus.

Texts and Transcripts

Heritage (1984) placed language as the central medium through which our social world is organised. It is through our 'talk' with others that meaning is attached to our thoughts, feelings and practices. The analysis of newspaper articles, interview dialogues and other written documents is commonplace within qualitative research and produces rich sources of data. A variety of analytic techniques, including content analysis and the more in-depth discourse analysis, can be used to extract information from the written data. Texts provide valuable sources for uncovering the multiple strategies and processes underlying social action as well as the constraints which limit self-expression and practice. For example, Gough (1998), through the analysis of texts, charted diverse constructions of 'new' sexism in the 1990s, where feminist women are criticised as 'taking things too far'. This is from one of the male participants justifying his biologically-based definition of women as 'birds':

B. What do you not like about feminist women?
K. Ahh, they're just, I don't know, it's hard to put into words but I used to, like inflame things, so many things I disagree with, like about 'em, quite a lot of it fair enough but at the same time they take it too far, I mean women should obviously be allowed to have jobs and stuff but they gotta accept there's some jobs they can't do, like you get bloody women pilots and stuff, and they can't make the fitness don't you think?
L. You can't [pause]
K. One or two campaigns like a few years ago in America the em, corps or whatever and she lasted two weeks when she got in [laughs] so she had to go through all the court battles and like every [lesbian] in the country is up in arms about it and she lets down the whole female race because she couldn't take it and there are situations where women shouldn't be in, I mean they're good in business and stuff like that, there's no problem there, but it's just sometimes they take it just too far, this equal rights stuff [pause] eh, same as vegetarians [laugh] [I don't know why they can't eat steak] like they come round to your house and it's like, can't eat that [pause] throw a few carrots in or something em, but when you go round theirs like they don't go out and buy some steak, it's just a bit of hypocrisy [pause] a lot of it [it's the greatest load of shit] some of it fair enough, I mean you know [pause] that sort of thing but when it comes to sexism and there's, like, chauvinism, quite a difference, do you know what I mean/ I disagree with a lot but you can see the good points as well – it's just the extreme versions [pause] callin' women birds, uhh, [exasperation] God the stress I get for that, sometimes say it in the wrong place . . .
L. It's degradin' though . . .
K. It's not, it's . . .
L. I, wouldn't call, well you know that don't you?
K. Yeah but callin' them birds, it's not like that, I mean a bird is a nice little, cheapy little you know, bird like you know it's sweet has a nice voice . . .
L. Sits beside you when you want it to [K. laughs] but when you want it to fly away just . . .
K. Back in the cage
L. That's not sexist at all [ironic]
(Gough, 1998)

In addition, texts and transcripts:

• are accessible by other researchers, thus allowing the possibility of additional interpretations
• enable others to scrutinise the end research product for instances of researcher bias.

See Table 15.1.1.

Table 15.1.1   The range of qualitative methods and when they might be used

Observation	Interviews	Group interviews	Focus groups	Texts and transcripts
Insights into social processes framing behaviour, particularly if they might not be accessible through words/ language	Explores participants' view of the world as experienced by them Illuminates contradictions and conflicts Flexible and adaptive	Insights into multiple perspectives Explores impact of group dynamics	Single topic Illuminates complexity of attitudes/ behaviours	Highlights social processes through language Multiple definitions framing research focus

WHY ADOPT A QUALITATIVE APPROACH?

In addition to the earlier discussion about the strengths of particular qualitative methods, these are two further important contributions that a qualitative approval can provide. First, it allows you to situate your work in its social and cultural contexts. Second, it allows the researcher to reflect on a range of research politics and philosophy.

The social, cultural and political contexts which facilitate and limit behaviours are made visible to the researcher using qualitative methodologies. The boundaries within which participants' experience their world become accessible for the researcher to share. For example, in a similar way to the issue of sexual behaviour discussed earlier, drug use is not a neutral topic; it is an activity that tends to raise emotional and moral issues for people within our society. A qualitative approach recognises the importance of wider social contexts, both in terms of the need to be aware of how these may affect the way we think about young people's drug use and in order to question 'how official definitions of problems arise' (Silverman, 1993, p 8). In undertaking the young people's drug use study the focus was not on existing 'deficit' models of young people, i.e. only young people who: have certain personality traits; come from certain types of families; do not attend school and use drugs, etc. We wanted to start from how the young people themselves perceived drugs and drug use, without any of the pre-defined conceptions.

Secondly, qualitative methodologies enable the researcher to make visible her or his research boundaries and philosophy and to explore how these may have influenced the research process. In the case of my research (MM), I came from a traditional scientific psychology background (my beliefs in facts, objectivity and my ability to change behaviour all intact!), one which had a legacy of undervaluing the experience of women (Rose, 1982). Thus I wanted a research methodology which would allow me to give recognition to women's experiences as a legitimate topic of research and also allow those experiences to be voiced by the women who owned them. Feminist methodologies which veer towards qualitative techniques and generate understanding through the, '. . . practice of integrating feeling, thinking and writing' (Rose, 1982) became appealing. In the 1990s, I was also living in a society which after giving visibility to minorities (gay men) was again trying to deny their existence (Clause 28, politicisation of single mothering, etc.). Both of these influences undoubtedly shaped my research through which I wanted to give voice to women including those women who were currently on the fringes of society.

GETTING STARTED

As with quantitative research, the researcher using qualitative approaches needs initially to reflect on the nature, purpose and outcomes of the research process. Ask yourself:

1. What information do you want from the research?
2. Why are you using qualitative rather than quantitative methods?
3. Why do you want to give a voice to this sample of participants?
4. What perspectives are you the researcher adopting (e.g. personal, political, cultural, etc.)?

Methods

As stated above, there are a variety of ways in which qualitative data can be collected. Aim to achieve 'best fit' between the type of information required and the method employed. Ask yourself whether one method (e.g. open ended interviewing) or a combination of methods (e.g. observation and interviewing) would be the best information.

The study exploring drug use in the world of young people used both group interviews and follow-up individual interviews. As we were asking about drug use, we felt that a group situation would allow the young people to hear the kind of things others would say and explore the limits of what they wished to disclose as a group. The group interviews were relatively unstructured; we had three broad areas we wished to ask about (young people and drug use, drug education, services/help they might want), but generally we wanted the group interviews to develop in any direction the young people themselves took it. We were wanting to give a voice to young people with regard to drugs and we aimed to have as few preconceived categories as possible. Individual follow-up interviews with any of the group who were willing to do so, enabled us to talk to people one-to-one, to draw and expand on data collected in the group interview, as well as to explore the degree of consensus in the group.

Ethics

The close, often prolonged contact that the qualitative researcher has with her or his participants places a special emphasis on ethical considerations. The well-being of the participants and their comfort throughout the research process are of primary importance. Briefing the participant about what will happen during the research process as well as what will happen to the data they have provided is essential. Other issues include:

- informed voluntary participation
- confidentiality.

In addition, Walker (1985, p 19) points out at the analysing stage, 'unlike the quantitative researcher he [*sic*] cannot distance himself from his data by retreating into the elegant world of mathematics' but must remember that she or he is committed to working *with* participants. So this sets in play a whole new set of questions which the researcher may consider (Reason & Rowan, 1981):

- authenticity (i.e. awareness of personal feelings)
- alienation (e.g. extent to which rules characterise the research process)
- patriarchy (i.e. consideration of sexist, racist, classist assumptions)
- dialectical (e.g. looking for contradictions, adopting a reflexive approach)
- legitimacy (i.e. honesty in relation to own research needs and interests).

ANALYSING INTERVIEW DATA

An Example of Grounded Theory Analysis

Grounded theory was introduced by Glaser and Strauss (1967) as a means of liberating researchers of sociology from the theoretical straitjacket imposed by a few grand theories. Implicit within such an approach is the rationale that the establishing of prior hypotheses when researching social phenomenon seriously reduces the complexity and diversity likely to be encountered. A researcher using grounded theory does not have to have a hypothesis to investigate so they only look at one or two features of the data collected. Grounded theory aims to explore all of the participant's dialogue, and like all qualitative approaches values the authenticity of the participant's experience and seeks to present the findings so that they reflect the language of the participant (and not the researcher). This is achieved by coding the data into categories which utilise and preserve the participant's own vocabulary. Grounded theory also encourages reflexivity, whereby the researcher writes her or himself into the inquiry process. The researcher is encouraged to keep memos throughout the analysis on her or his feelings, thoughts and ideas. Finally, grounded theory, by enabling some type of construction of reality, offers the first important step to social change.

The Process

Firstly the audio-taped conversations are transcribed and written copies produced. The transcript is then segmented into units for analysis. The size of the unit is arbitrary, some practitioners analyse line by line, others use paragraphs. These are then numbered (e.g. paragraph one, two, etc.). Having completed this, the next task is to read one paragraph and condense the content into 'meaning units' – the smallest piece of information that can make sense by itself – and then to categorise this. As the following example shows, this initial stage primarily involves restating the unit in the third person and so often results in categorisation that is long-winded and ungainly:

R.   Can you tell me about the sex education you received at school?
P.   Well, school gave some information but it was sort of a Roman Catholic school that I went to and they sort of pussyfooted around it [sex] and never came right out and explained anything. I actually got most of my information from my older sister and friends.

This was then categorised as:

[1]   P. said school provided some information on sex but describes school as pussy-footing (around sex) and not explaining it right out.
[2]   P. describes school as Roman Catholic.
[3]   P. reported getting most of her information (on sex) from older sister and friends.

As can be seen, even at this initial stage it is essential that the participant's vocabulary is preserved. It is common practice to record categorisation on numbered index cards (e.g. pg. par., etc.).

Analysis continues by working through the transcript and generating new meaning units as described. As each new card is completed, it is placed on a large surface. At this stage, those units which the researcher believes reflect similar themes or look as if they go together are placed in the same pile or cluster. Each cluster is then given a name based on the meaning, tying the units together and thus generating a higher category which subsumes all the cards in the pile. The name given to the category at this stage should remain closely related to the participant's language. Again, an example will help to illuminate this process.

[1]   P. said school sex education was sort of R.E. class and sex was presented as something respectable that happens between a man and woman.
[2]   P. said school talked about periods, puberty and growing up.
[3]   P. said school used to talk around sex without telling you anything and because everyone was young they were too embarrassed to ask any questions.

These categories can be subsumed under, 'The nature of sex education', thus preserving the essence of the above categories. At this stage it is helpful to define the new category as it facilitates the identification of further instances as the analysis continues. In doing this, the researcher is making explicit what qualifies for inclusion in the category, a decision that was previously made by the researcher on the basis of appearance and intuition.

As the analysis proceeds and the categories continue to emerge, units of meaning are compared to each category that exists, and in doing so may, if appropriate, be assigned to more than one category. In cases where no category fits the unit, a new one is created to represent it. This process of assigning units of meaning to more than one category, if applicable, is referred to as open categorising and according to Rennie et al. (1988, p 143) 'permits the researcher to preserve subtle nuances of the data'.

At this stage, a series of 'higher' descriptive categories have been generated. The researcher continues to code the transcript, always clustering (placing cards in piles) and periodically stopping to categorise and define emerging clusters, as well as considering new categories. Those conducting grounded theory are advised to review existing categories regularly, using the following guidelines:

- if a category seems too expansive, sub-divide
- if a category seems too specific, collapse and redefine
- consider previously isolated instances for inclusion in clusters.

In this example, as analysis continued, the category 'The nature of school sex education' expanded rapidly and subsequently sub-divided into 'Criticisms of school sex education', 'Sex education as a social event' and 'Informal learning at school'. Obviously this process is repeated for all transcripts.

The process of assigning units to categories is an exhaustive one and categories are said to 'saturate' when it is clear what future instances will be located in the category. This will occur at different rates for different categories. When this has been completed and all the transcripts have been categorised, the next stage is to review all of the descriptive categories generated, with a view to producing further higher categories. At this stage the aim is for the researcher to move from descriptive to conceptual language – to go beyond the categories generated and participants' terms and to develop links between categories, make inferences, to theorise. It is at this point in the analysis that the researcher participates actively, drawing on her or his knowledge, experience and imagination to create categories.

These constructed categories lean more towards explaining the links between categories than simply describing them. Perhaps another example will illustrate this; throughout the categorising of the sexuality transcripts, the young women made frequent remarks about differences in the way women and men perceive sex. These constituted two higher order categories, 'Women and sex', the properties of which included:

[1] P. said she could never sleep with someone she didn't love.
[2] P. said that for women sex is much more emotional than for men.

[3] P. said it is definitely harder for women to say they are interested in sex than it is for men.

[4] P. said that although women should be able to say they enjoy sex, they find it difficult to.

and 'Men's sexual pleasure', the properties of which included:

[1] P. said that for men sex is just physical pleasure.

[2] P. said she thought men just want to get the leg over when they can.

[3] P. said that for men sex is often just a physical thing.

[4] P. said that while for men in relationships sex is both a physical and emotional thing, for men not in relationships sex can still be a physical pleasure.

The above categories represent the contrasting pictures of what sex means to women and men that were drawn by these young women during their interviews. For women, sex was couched in terms of love, emotional commitment and caring, whilst for men it was described as primarily a physical pleasure. In light of the entire findings of the study, this is obviously a simplistic glimpse of sex in the 1990s. However, it did highlight an important omission from these young women's dialogue – sex as something that women think of in terms of pleasure and desire. Consequently at this stage such findings allowed a more abstract category, 'The elusive discourse of desire' to be inferred and which aligns closely with Fine's (1988) 'Missing discourse of desire'.

Following this process what usually results is a hierarchy of concepts in which central categories subsume lower order ones – these latter categories function as defining properties of the categories at the next highest level. As with any theorising, parsimony is a concern and the focus is to move towards a central defining category, one which is the most abstract and most densely related to the other categories and their properties.

Finally, the core categories are compared with literature on similar and different social aspects and where possible connections drawn with existing literature. In addition, at this stage it is suggested that the theory generated may be further enriched by consulting relevant others (e.g. other professionals working in the field). For example, following the analysis of the data from the interviews with young heterosexual women four main themes were evident:

- gender identity
- school sub-culture
- price of heterosexuality
- love and relationships in the 1990s.

It is important to remember that while qualitative analysis provides a number of themes around which the discussion of the data can be structured, this separation of the content is somewhat artificial as it is usually absent from participants' talk. To illustrate, when discussing their sexuality, the young heterosexual women in the study rarely made singular allusions, but rather their thoughts and experiences were part of a complex collection of personal ideas, social processes and regulations. Thus understandings of themselves as 'women' included not only their relations with the opposite sex but also women's position in society, career aspirations, their mothers' experiences, peer beliefs and practices, etc.

WHAT IS 'GOOD QUALITATIVE RESEARCH'?

As with quantitative approaches it is important that qualitative research is conducted rigorously and critically. Various methods exist which allow the researcher to ensure that her or his approach has produced relevant and informative data. The terms used for evaluating qualitative research vary and are often very different from those used for evaluating quantitative methods. Do not be put off if different authors use different terms or a different number of evaluative criteria or even if they use the same terms as quantitative researchers, i.e. reliability and validity. Many of the terms used relate to issues already discussed in the 'getting started' section as they relate to the process of analysis, for example the extent to which there is evidence of saturation or recurrent patterning. The following is presented as a series of questions you might ask yourself when reading a piece of qualitative research or reflecting on a project you may have carried out. The questions address key issues in the evaluative criteria for qualitative methodology.

Is There Evidence that the Researcher is Engaging in Reflexivity?

Reflexivity is a concept that relates to the extent to which a researcher is continually examining the ways in which their own presumptions may have impacted on the research process and findings. The researcher may attempt to demonstrate this by providing a section that is a personal reflection on the research process, a 'my story' section. Such a section might examine why they chose the research topic, how the research question came to be framed in the way that it was and what they thought and felt about doing the research. If there is not a separate section issues of reflexivity may be addressed in the discussion sections of a report. What you are asking here is to what extent there is evidence that the researcher's presumptions, categories and explanations have been open to challenges arising from the data and how honest the researcher is about what they bring to the research.

Are There any Attempts to Allow for Alternative Interpretations of the Data?

Given that qualitative research recognises that it provides one interpretation of the data, it is important that the analysis contributing to a particular interpretation of the findings is demonstrated to be systematic, with the data interrogated for exceptions/contradictions to the particular emergent categories and patterns. In any research texts there are examples of exceptions when not all of the research participants agree or think about something in the same way. Some writers may include two possible explanations and explain why they have chosen one as the most appropriate. Other writers may include relatively large extracts of text or field notes to allow the reader the opportunity to make sense of the data in a different way to that presented in the research.

If the Reader is Starting off from a Particular Explicit Perspective (e.g. Feminist, Participative, Marxist), to what Extent have they Demonstrated or Reflected these Principles in the Research Design, Process and Analysis?

Depending on the philosophical and/or political position of the researcher and the claims of the research then questions can be asked of the entire process that reflect the extent to which a piece of research can be said to: give voice to marginalised groups, reflect the epistemology of feminism and/or utilise a participatory approach. For example, the research on women's sexuality was undoubtedly influenced not only by my feminist principles, but also by my interactions with and admiration for my participants, in particular the lesbian women and single mothers.

Has there been Any Attempt at Triangulation in the Collection of Data?

Triangulation involves collecting data from different perspectives or vantage points. This may mean using different sources, different researchers, or adopting different roles; or using a variety of methods to collect data. For example, in the young people and drugs study, the use of group interviews followed at a later date by individual interviews allowed for some elements of triangulation. It was possible using these two data collection methods to examine the consistency between the kind of disclosures an individual might make in a group and what they may say in an individual interview; changes to events or stories could be monitored and noted. In addition two researchers in interviews could provide different data about the group and the interpretation of the interview. In the observational study of a group of friends who injected amphetamines, there were elements of triangulation. In addition to examining consistency in the stories and events related by differing individuals, other sources of data collection could also be utilised. Interviews were conducted with two drug workers and a health promotion officer who worked in the area; this allowed for the potential for alternative perceptions of the estate, and in particular drug use on the estate, to be presented and discussed. From a different angle, because members of the friendship group had been involved in criminal activities and ended up appearing in court, it was possible to check court reports in the local paper to verify appearances. The local paper also provided verification of some of the aspects of drug use on the estate and particularly the way in which the estate was perceived within the town.

WHAT USE IS EVIDENCE FROM QUALITATIVE STUDIES?

There are many different contributions qualitative evidence can make. It is the intention here to address some of those.

Communicating

One of the useful contributions qualitative data can make, by its emphasis on naturally occurring data and language and texts, is to give a 'voice' to participants. Practitioners are able to see, read and hear the kind of things participants might say in their own language from their own perspective. This is also useful if the research is focusing on professionals' interactions with clients/patients. An analysis can reveal the ways in which professionals speak about health and illness and contrast the ways of talking about the same issues from the perspective of client/patient. One example is how other young people can recognise and respond to the way young people talk about drugs within the young people's study. The use of quotes and text allow the young people's language and perspective to be reflected in the research report. This means that the evidence has a credibility for young people. It also means that it can reveal to practitioners ways of talking about topics/events, etc. An understanding of the way in which young people talk about something like drugs means that an attempt to communicate with people through official literature, workshops or training can begin from a position of understanding and reflecting of aspects of young people's social worlds.

Accessing Different Social Worlds

Conducting and reading qualitative research has the potential to allow you to gain an insight into and empathy for the social world of many diverse groups, whether they be young people and drug use, injecting drug use or young women and sexuality. An understanding of another's social world allows you to have an increased understanding of why someone might behave in a certain way, what that behaviour might mean to them and what thoughts and feelings might underpin different experiences. This is graphically illustrated in my own work on women's sexuality (MM). Prior to interviewing the young heterosexual women about their sexual practices I understood the greatest barriers to the practice of safer sex to be embarrassment and fear that carrying condoms could lead to them becoming known as 'slags'. Following the analysis of the data, however, I became aware of another factor, the fear of being perceived as frigid. For many of the young women interviewed, unsafe sex had taken place in situations where they had not intended to have sex, but were worried that they would lose face and be ridiculed if they did not.

Conceptualising

As the analysis of qualitative research involves working from the data and not starting with a pre-established hypothesis, it can offer evidence which challenges and changes the way we might think about or conceptualise a topic, a behaviour, etc. One example might be the way in which qualitative methods can reveal how what may first appear as an irrational behaviour can be understood as having meaning from the participants' frame of reference. For example in the observational study of a group of friends injecting amphetamines, their lifestyle and drug using behaviour on the surface appears somewhat chaotic and random. By spending time with the group and recording and analysing their drug using behaviour it is clear that their drug use is governed by certain social rules that relate to gender, place of injecting, who is present when injecting occurs, who you might consider lending your injecting equipment to, etc. This kind of understanding might allow a practitioner to work within existing social rules in order to address, for example, issues relating to HIV and safer injecting. In the young people's drug study one of the issues that emerged was young people's boundaries around drug use. Initially the young people would say they would use 'anything', but it became quite clear that they all had boundaries around drug use. Boundaries might take the form of certain drugs (e.g. heroin, solvents) or routes of administration (e.g. injecting, etc.) that they wouldn't use. Understanding young people's boundaries is useful in working within a harm reduction framework to reinforce boundaries or potentially to shift them.

Enhancing Services and Provisions

Qualitative data provides powerful insights into processes which shape individuals' behaviour, including locating the participants' frame of reference and cultural and/or political barriers to uptake of services or adopting certain preventative health behaviours. All of these have important contributions to make in enhancing service delivery and provision. For example, in our work on young people and drug use; when asked about what they wanted young people continually made reference not to aspects of provision, e.g. opening hours, location, etc., but almost always talked about a relationship, a person. They wanted someone they could trust, someone who had a credible understanding of drug issues. The study reveals that although health professionals themselves may see material aspects of a service as the key issue for service utilisation, the young people themselves prioritised the nature of the relationship between themselves and the person they were seeking help from. The young people did not identify current provision as targeted at them. Existing drug services were for 'junkies', people with dependent heroin problems. The implication being that the best kind of provision would be something specifically targeted at young people and independent from mainstream drug provision.

Supporting Training and Education

As previously stated on p 371, under 'communication', the capacity for qualitative methods to give 'voice' to differing groups means that the evidence is accessible and credible to the participant group as well as to other non-researchers. The use of quotes and extracts of texts provides an accessible input into training issues. For example, in our work on young people and drugs, following the publication of the report, both researchers engaged in a series of seminars, a part of a programme aimed at headteachers, teachers, school nurses, community police and youth workers. The local qualitative data was a useful way of communicating to these groups about the experiences of young people with regard to drug use in a more powerful way than a series of tables would have done. We were able to offer quotes and examples of text to illustrate the general findings and to provide stimulus for group discussion.

Promoting Policy and Structural Change

Due to central features of qualitative research, which reflect participants' frame of reference and give 'voice' to participants, qualitative methods can contribute to the development of policy which reflects experiences, priorities and perspectives of individuals and groups who are the target of such policies rather than those of policy makers. In addressing issues of conceptualisation and the wider social and political contexts of behaviours, qualitative research can also contribute to the development of policies that recognise the real contradictions and tensions that exist in many people's experiences. For example, the findings relating to sex education from the sexuality research contributed to changes in the policy and provision of school-based sex education in Southern Ireland in the mid-1990s.

CONCLUDING REMARKS

Qualitative data:

- accesses participants' frame of reference
- locates multiple contexts
- highlights ideologies and power issues
- provides rich descriptions of real world experience
- integrates the personal into the research process
- answers the 'why' as well as the 'how' questions.

REFERENCES

Becker H (1964) reprinted in Heller T, Gott M & Jeffrey C (Eds) (1987) Drug use and misuse: a reader. Milton Keynes: Open University Press.

Fine M (1988) Sexuality, schooling and adolescent females: the missing discourse of desire. *Harvard Educational Review*, 58, 29–93.

Glaser B G & Strauss A (1967) The discovery of grounded theory: strategies for qualitative research. New York: Aldine.

Gough B (1998) Men and the discursive reproduction of sexism: repertoires of difference and equality. *Feminism and Psychology*, 8(1), 25–49.

Henwood K L & Pidgeon N F (1993) Qualitative research and psychological theorising. In: M Hammersley (Ed), Social research: philosophy, politics and practice. London: Sage.

Heritage J (1984) Garfinkel and ethnomethodology. Cambridge: Polity Press.

Holland J, Romanzanoglu C & Scott S (1990) Managing risk and experiencing danger: tensions between government AIDS education policy and young women's sexuality. *Gender and Education*, 2(2), 125–146.

Ingham R (1991) Beliefs and behaviour: filling the void. Paper presented at ERSC sponsored seminar. 'Young People and Aids', March.

Ingham R, Woodcock A & Stenner K (1991) Getting to know you: young people's knowledge of partners at first intercourse. *Journal of Community and Applied Social Research*, 1(2), 117–132.

Krueger R A (1994) Focus groups: a practical guide for applied research. London: Sage.

Lees S (1993) Sugar and spice: sexuality and adolescent girls. London: Penguin.

McFadden M (1994) Female sexuality in the second decade of AIDS. Unpublished PhD thesis. Belfast: School of Psychology, Queen's University.

Mullings C (1985) Group interviewing. University of Sheffield: CRUS.

Reason P & Rowan J (1981) Human inquiry: a sourcebook of new paradigm research. Chichester: John Wiley.

Rennie D L, Phillips J R & Quartaro G K (1988) Grounded theory: a promising approach to conceptualisation in psychology? *Canadian Psychology*, 29(2), 139–150.

Rose H (1982) Making science feminist. Milton Keynes: Open University Press.

Rosenstock I M (1974) The health belief model and preventative health behaviour. *Health Education Monographs*, 2(4), 354–386.

Silverman D (1987) Communication and medical practice. London: Sage.

Silverman D (1993) Interpreting qualitative data. London: Sage.

Vaughan S, Schumm J S & Sinagub J (1996) Focus group interviews in education and psychology. London: Sage.

Walker R (1985) Applied qualitative research. Aldershot: Gower.

Chapter 16

Monitoring and Evaluating Progress

Linda Wright

INTRODUCTION

This chapter focuses on some of the most difficult aspects of evidence-based health promotion practice. Designing and conducting evaluation studies is full of problems for health promotion practitioners, because the traditional textbook approaches to evaluation, involving scientific measurement of outcomes, are virtually impossible to apply with any degree of rigour. Unlike needs assessment, which most practitioners will attempt without undue anxiety, evaluation raises real concern and anxiety at practitioner level, because of the potential power that evaluation evidence has to affect their work and even their livelihoods. Those who purchase and manage health promotion services need to know whether projects are achieving their intended goals, and the process by which goals are achieved. Such evidence is essential for rational and equitable use of limited resources. The problems start when those who have a stake in the evaluation have differing views on the criteria for success or when the design and methodology do not produce adequate, reliable or useful evidence to inform decision making.

Fortunately, encouraging progress has been made in the last decade to develop a rationale for health promotion evaluation and methodologies that are sensitive and appropriate to health promotion needs. This chapter offers both an overview of this progress (Section 16.3) and two case studies which describe practitioners' efforts to gather evaluation evidence.

Section 16.1, *Monitoring and Evaluation in Cardiac Rehabilitation*, describes the system adopted by a multi-disciplinary team to monitor and evaluate patient improvement and the services provided. A substantial component of cardiac rehabilitation involves health promotion activities rather than clinical interventions. Jane Powell describes the reasons for evaluating cardiac rehabilitation and how the chosen design takes account of both clinical standards for evidence and the health education requirements for evidence to inform decisions about how and when lifestyle advice is best provided.

Evidence-based Health Promotion. Edited by Elizabeth R. Perkins, Ina Simnett and Linda Wright.
© 1999 John Wiley & Sons Ltd.

Section 16.2, *The 'Get Moving!' Study*, is an account by a health promotion specialist of a local evaluation study that combined attempts to measure the processes and outcomes of a project to promote physical activity in general practice settings. The first stage evaluated the effectiveness of different approaches to changing physical activity behaviour within the general practice setting. This is an example of how an evaluation study can also contribute to needs assessment, by providing information about how to tailor the intervention. The second stage of the study focused on implementation, a neglected element of academic evaluation studies, and one of the reasons why practitioners find outcome focused evaluations so limited.

Section 16.3, *Evaluation in Health Promotion: The proof of the pudding?*, examines new developments in health promotion evaluation and discusses their relevance for practice. The message of this section is an important theme of the book – that the ultimate test for new evidence is the extent to which it can be used by health promotion practitioners, managers and planners, to promote individual and community health.

Section 16.1

Monitoring and Evaluation in Cardiac Rehabilitation

Jane Powell

INTRODUCTION

Cardiac rehabilitation is defined by the World Health Organisation (WHO, 1993) as 'the sum of activities required to influence favourably the underlying cause of the disease, as well as to ensure the patients the best possible physical, mental, and social conditions so that they may, by their own efforts, preserve or resume when lost, as normal a place as possible in the life of the community'.

Coronary heart disease (CHD) is the biggest single cause of death in the UK today. It accounts for 140 000 deaths per year. Overall, 88% of men and 90% of women have at least one of the four major risk factors: smoking, inadequate physical activity, raised blood cholesterol and raised blood pressure (Central Health Monitoring Unit, 1994). Smoking is associated with 18% of CHD deaths. To reduce ill-health and death caused by CHD, the Department of Health (1992) *Health of the Nation* document sets national targets which address the four main risk factors and aim to reduce premature death, under the age of 65, from CHD by at least 40% by the year 2000, and to reduce the death rate in people aged 65–74 by at least 30% by the year 2000.

BENEFITS OF CARDIAC REHABILITATION

There is a wide diversity in the provision of cardiac rehabilitation programmes within the UK. There are extreme discrepancies in the funding, the scope of rehabilitation programmes and auditing of programmes (Horgan et al., 1992). Programmes have been under resourced, and this appears to originate from a perception that cardiac rehabilitation is ineffective. However, recent studies have reported benefits in several areas, including the physical, psychological and social well being of the patient (Bethel & Mullee, 1990; Horgan et al., 1992; Naismith et

Evidence-based Health Promotion. Edited by Elizabeth R. Perkins, Ina Simnett and Linda Wright.
© 1999 John Wiley & Sons Ltd.

al., 1979). Antman et al. (1992) demonstrated improvements in terms of mortality. A meta-analysis of trials identified a reduction of up to 25% in all-cause mortality in post-infarction patients who attended cardiac rehabilitation, including exercise (O'Connor et al., 1989). Patients who exercise achieve their optimal functional rate more rapidly than those who do not, have fewer visits to their doctor or hospital, and are more likely to return to work (Hung et al., 1994). However, despite the evidence, Davidson et al. (1995) states that many patients who would benefit from a cardiac rehabilitation service will never participate in an adequate one. Constant evaluation of existing programmes is necessary to encourage purchasers to demand that a satisfactory service is provided.

Cardiac rehabilitation programmes have been estimated to be cost-effective: Gray et al. (1997) estimates that the mean cost per patient per programme is £370. In comparison with other medical and surgical interventions it may be considered cost-effective. The benefits gained from cardiac rehabilitation include reduction of cardiovascular risk factors, a reduction in hospital readmissions, early return to work, and improved psychological, physical and social functioning (Oldridge et al., 1988).

WHY THE NEED TO MONITOR AND EVALUATE?

Although there is now substantial evidence to demonstrate the benefits of cardiac rehabilitation, it is still difficult to show which aspect of rehabilitation is effective. The desired outcomes are long term, such as smoking cessation, regular exercise and a healthy low-fat diet. Evaluation and monitoring needs to be short- and long-term to ensure the intervention immediately post-infarction is effective.

Cardiac rehabilitation has been shown to benefit other groups of patients not just clients who have experienced a myocardial infarction (MI). These include angina sufferers, cardiac surgery and heart failure patients. However, owing to a lack of resources this wide population cannot always be targeted, and patients who are at a relatively low risk, and therefore require less monitoring and supervision, are selected for participation. This group of patients might benefit the least, in comparison to people with heart failure, who are in a higher risk group but may benefit more from involvement in rehabilitation programmes.

Secondary prevention is targeted at people who already have heart disease, such as myocardial infarction, angina, coronary artery bypass grafts, or percutaneous transluminal coronary angioplasty. Evidence shows that risk factor modification reduces the risk of recurrent cardiac events, and slows down the progression of coronary atherosclerosis, thereby, reducing hospitalisation from recurrent cardiac events (Pyorala et al., 1994).

Cardiac rehabilitation is a multi-disciplinary approach, which can incorporate a wide range of disciplines including medical and nursing personnel, physiotherapists, occupational therapists, health psychologists, pharmacists, dieticians and exercise physiologists. Due to its multi-disciplinary nature, and the resources it entails, effective audit tools need to be utilised to highlight the efficacy of such programmes, and any weaknesses. Intervention needs to be evaluated to ensure that it is having the desired effect. Evaluation is needed to assess the results of the intervention, and to determine if the objectives of the cardiac rehabilitation programme have been met. Assessing how the effects were achieved is also valuable in determining effective interventions. Effective evaluation can aid development of the programme, and provide the health care professional with job satisfaction when objectives are met.

A working party under the joint auspices of the National Institute for Nursing, the Joint Medical Practice and Audit Committee of the British Cardiac Society and the Royal College of Physicians of London, developed guidelines and audit standards for cardiac rehabilitation in the UK (Horgan et al., 1992). The working party stated that all centres treating cardiac patients should offer a cardiac rehabilitation programme, and published clinical guidelines and audit standards. Three main elements of the cardiac rehabilitation process were identified:

1. Explanation and understanding of the diagnosis and management.
2. Specific rehabilitation intervention, such as exercise and secondary prevention.
3. Long-term lifestyle changes.

THE CARDIAC REHABILITATION PROGRAMME

The programme highlighted here is set in a general hospital which treats approximately 300 heart attacks (myocardial infarctions) per year. The hospital is situated in a developing industrial community, which has a high incidence of coronary heart disease and smoking (Director of Public Health, 1996). The programme offers an educational and exercise package for clients who have had heart attacks, cardiac surgery, coronary angioplasty, and for a limited number of newly diagnosed angina sufferers. It is a multi-disciplinary approach, involving medical, nursing, physiotherapy, dieticians, occupational therapy and pharmacy personnel. The cardiac rehabilitation sister co-ordinates the programme, and is responsible for its monitoring and evaluation. The programme co-ordinator constantly assesses the programme, looking at interventions used, comparing it with other programmes and monitoring results – this is all part of the evaluation process.

The main aims of cardiac rehabilitation are to prevent reoccurrence of a cardiac event and to restore the individual to optimum physical, psychological and social well-being. The main components of the programme are:

1. *Education*: improving the patient's knowledge of the disease and disease process, management of the condition;
2. *Cardiovascular risk factor* modification: smoking, raised cholesterol, hypertension, lack of exercise.
3. *Exercise*: returning the individual to their optimum physical capabilities.

The whole programme lasts approximately 12 weeks.

The first step in rehabilitating the cardiac patient is education. This begins when they are in hospital, improving the patients' knowledge about their condition and treatment. Also important at this stage is reassurance, encouraging the development of a positive approach to recovery. Following this it is necessary to assess their coronary risk factors, and to implement appropriate action. It is important to treat the patients as individuals, and accept that not everyone requires all the intervention at hand. A patient with high cholesterol is initially referred to the dietician, as the first line approach to management. High cholesterol is determined by a blood test. The timing of the blood test is very important, as the cholesterol level falls following a myocardial infarction. The test is therefore done within the first 24 hours of onset of chest pain within the coronary care unit. The cholesterol level rises to its pre-infarct level at approximately three months, hence the indication for a three-month secondary prevention clinic. At present high cholesterol in CHD is determined as anyone with a cholesterol level greater than 5.2 (Betteridge et al., 1993). Recent studies have shown that dietary intervention led to a significant reduction in total mortality during a two-year follow-up post-MI only if accompanied by a reduction in plasma cholesterol levels (Burr et al., 1989; DeLorgeril et al., 1994). A diet which is high in fruit and vegetables, oily fish and olive oil is recommended, although the effect of diet on atherosclerosis is quite complex, and full lipid profiles are necessary to assess risk and determine appropriate lipid-lowering therapy. Full profiles include Triglyceride level, High Density (HDL) and Low Density Lipoprotein (LDL) levels, and the ratio between total cholesterol and HDL level. Although the evidence has been unclear in earlier trials, now trials such as the Scandinavian Simvastatin Survival Study have verified that lowering cholesterol can cause a reduction in fatal and non-fatal coronary events (Sivers, 1996).

Smoking is considered the main risk factor for CHD. Studies have shown that stopping smoking will reduce the risk of a further non-fatal MI and cardiovascular mortality rate by up to 50% (Wilhelmsson et al., 1975). Giving smoking cessation advice and support is cost-effective, and has been shown to produce a 5% smoking cessation sustained up to one year (British Heart Foundation, 1994). During the programme smoking cessation advice is given by the cardiac rehabilitation nurses. Individuals who are experiencing difficulties stopping are seen by the smoking cessation nurse, which is a more intense consultation.

Following discharge, the individual and partner commence an education programme; topics include diet, stress management and relaxation, medication, exercise and basic life support skills. The sessions are given by the appropriate health professional. Each session is evaluated by the group members, to determine the appropriateness of the session, what they have gained and any weaknesses of the programme. A three-week stress management course is also run by the occupational therapist. Following this, another evaluation form is completed.

On discharge follow-up is arranged at one month post-MI. Present at the clinic is the cardiologist, cardiac rehabilitation sister and the dietician. The individual undergoes an exercise stress test to determine evidence of on-going ischaemia, and the need for coronary angiography, and possible angioplasty or coronary artery bypass grafts. Their medication is reviewed to ensure they are taking the appropriate drugs. If evidence of on-going ischaemia is confirmed by the exercise test, then other drugs can be added. The cardiologist will also assess if the patient is able to attend the exercise programme. The exercise programme offers three levels; low level, intermediate and advanced. Patients are assessed to determine which level is suitable.

Modifiable risk factors are monitored including smoking, exercise, blood pressure, diet and weight. Diet is addressed more closely again. The patient is sent a diet diary to complete the week prior to the appointment. As most people have a regular diet routine, the dietician is able to ascertain if desired changes have been achieved.

Following completion of the exercise stress test, the individual is then started on a graduated exercise programme lasting approximately ten weeks. Upon completion of the programme, approximately three months post-cardiac event, the individual attends a nurse-led secondary prevention clinic, as mentioned earlier. At the clinic the patient has a repeat check of their coronary risk factors, and assessment of lifestyle changes achieved. Cholesterol level is checked again at this point. If this remains abnormal, i.e. greater than 5.2, then lipid-lowering treatment is commenced. Their smoking status is obtained, exercise level, blood pressure, diet and whether they have returned to work. All the information is entered on a database.

Liaison with the primary health care team is also vital to ensure continuity of care and a uniform approach to the patient's recovery – in effect, to provide a seamless service. The GP receives correspondance from the hospital on discharge, at one month, and again at three months post-MI. Developing alliances with the primary health care team is important to facilitate long-term monitoring and compliance with lifestyle modifications. Within the district of the hospital, a scheme called Exercise on Prescription is rapidly developing. This involves local leisure centres, who are training fitness consultants to exercise high-risk groups of patients. The scheme is overseen by the local health authority. The cardiac rehabilitation team refer clients on to the scheme upon completion of the cardiac rehabilitation programme.

MONITORING AND EVALUATION

Monitoring of these interventions takes several forms:

1. *Patient/partner evaluation form*: the form is completed following the educational part of the programme. It obtains feedback on what the patient and partner have gained from the sessions and whether they have found them useful and applicable.

2. *Monitoring return to work*: the majority of clients return to work after 6–8 weeks; any delay is noted and also the cause for the delay.
3. *Lifestyle changes made*: the main changes monitored are: cessation of smoking, dietary changes and the uptake of regular exercise.
4. *The Hospital Anxiety and Depression (HAD) scale*: this is used to assess psychosocial functioning (Zigmond & Snaith, 1983). The scale is used pre- and post-cardiac rehabilitation intervention. The scale consists of 14 items divided into two sub-scales for anxiety and depression; the patient rates each item on a four-point scale. Individuals who have scores of seven or less are non-cases, scores of 8–10 doubtful, scores of 11+ implies definite cases. This scale was found to be a reliable tool in detecting emotional disorder. It was recommended for use in patients undergoing medical treatment, to facilitate detection and management of emotional disorders.
5. Keeping a database is an integral part of auditing. The database helps to monitor the demand for the service, and to keep a record of attendance rates. All patient information is easily stored on the database and, therefore, makes it easily accessible. The database also allows easy monitoring of the individuals' risk factor modifications, thereby aiding the auditing process.
6. Nurse-led follow-up clinics have been implemented, to monitor risk factor modification. These secondary prevention clinics are an effective means of tracking coronary risk factors.

Monitoring attendance of the programme is also important, and reasons why people do not attend. Some of the reasons that have been noted are lack of transport, lack of interest and a lack of support from family. From looking at attendance rates and comparing them with lifestyle changes, one is able to get an indication of whether attendance correlates with improved lifestyle changes and early return to work. At the three-month stage of rehabilitation, the HAD scale is repeated, and compared to the earlier score.

Is cardiac rehabilitation improving psycho-social outcome? This at present is in the early stages, and it is too soon to comment. However, if levels are high on initial assessment and, for some, remain high even after rehabilitation, then this may be an indication to utilise the skills of a clinical psychologist. The HAD scale may also highlight the need to improve the level of stress management intervention. This is an example of how on-going assessment and evaluation using various tools can highlight areas ripe for development. If a higher score can be correlated with a higher incidence of readmission, then a better case is available for lobbying health service managers to improve resources.

A common model used in promoting lifestyle changes in the cardiac patient is the stages of change model (Prochaska & DiClemente, 1994). (See Chapter 4.) This model enables the health promoter to view the client who has not been able to adopt a lifestyle change not as a failure, but as someone who is going through a process of change. The cardiac rehabilitation programme applies the model to the main risk factors as a means of assessing the client and determining what stage they are at, thereby enabling appropriate intervention to be instigated. Evaluating the client in this way enables the health promoter to monitor change and the maintenance of that change. Use of the model can facilitate effective use of resources. Some individuals have multiple risk factors to change, and find it difficult to change them simultaneously. In these instances, it is necessary to change what the individual sees as their priority and this may vary from the health professionals' priority.

As well as having effective outcomes it is essential that cardiac rehabilitation interventions are also cost-effective, especially within today's climate of limited health care resources. The British Heart Foundation (1994) estimates that each year in Britain there are 330 000 people who have a myocardial infarction, and 1.9 million people have angina. Three per cent of all hospital admissions are due to CHD, and for men aged between 45 and 64, this figure rises to 10%. The high incidence of CHD has a profound effect on the health service resources, government and industry. CHD costs the health service an estimated £917 million pounds per year. In 1990/91, 53 million working days were lost due to CHD, representing over 10% of all days lost due to sickness. The majority of these days were covered by invalidity benefit, which cost the government over £463 million. It is estimated that the working days lost cost industry over £3 billion in lost production (British Heart Foundation, 1994).

The high incidence of CHD and the subsequent financial costs demand attention. Wang (1994) states that both can be reduced through comprehensive educational planning. Fulfilling a patient's educational and psychological needs will enable them to return to optimum health, and may facilitate a reduction in the number of hospital readmissions and the duration of hospital stays (Rosenberg, 1971).

Although gaining feedback from clients and partners is important, it is also worth noting that they are often reluctant to criticise the care they receive. Therefore, one cannot rely on this form of evaluation alone. Clients during the early stages are more amenable to lifestyle changes and this may lull health professionals into a false sense of achievement, as long-term monitoring of the programme suggests that the more remote the event, the more likely clients are to relapse into unhealthy behaviour patterns.

Through evaluation, barriers to cardiac rehabilitation have been highlighted, these include transport, availability, accessibility and financial barriers. Ways to overcome these barriers need to be explored in order to encourage greater attendance. At present hospital transport is utilised for those who have no means of transport and the community exercise on prescription scheme at local leisure centres is offered at reduced rates in order to overcome clients' financial restraints. Some groups equate healthy eating with increased cost and professionals need to break down such barriers and myths in order to achieve desired outcomes.

Due to the number of disciplines involved, one of the problems is developing audit systems that span the professions. This can be achieved in consultation with all those involved. If cardiac rehabilitation is to have a significant impact, then effective monitoring and evaluation of intervention is imperative.

REFERENCES

Antman E M et al. (1992) A comparison of results of meta-analyses of randomised trials and recommendations of clinical experts. Treatments of myocardial infarction. *Journal of the American Medical Association*, 268, 240–248.

Bethel H J N & Mullee M (1990) A controlled trial of community based coronary rehabilitation. *British Heart Journal*, 64, 370–375.

Betteridge D J et al. (1993) Management of hyperlipidaemia: a practice guide. *Postgraduate Medical Journal*, 69, 359.

British Heart Foundation/Coronary Prevention Group Statistics Database (1994) Coronary heart disease statistics. London: British Heart Foundation.

Burr M L et al. (1989) Effects of changes in fat, fish and fibre intakes on death and myocardial infarction: Diet and Reinfarction Trial (DART). *The Lancet*, ii, 757.

Central Health Monitoring Unit (1994) Health survey of England. London: Department of Health.

Davidson C et al. (1995) A report of a working group of the British Cardiac Society: cardiac rehabilitation services in the United Kingdom. *British Heart Journal*, 73, 201–202.

DeLorgeril M et al. (1994) Mediterranean alpha-linolenic acid-rich diet in the secondary prevention of coronary heart disease. *The Lancet*, 343, 1454.

Department of Health (1992) The Health of the Nation: a strategy for health in England. London: HMSO.

Director of Public Health (1996) A profile of Shropshire. Shropshire: Shropshire Health.

Gray A M, Bowman G S & Thompson D R (1997) The cost of cardiac rehabilitation services in England and Wales. *Journal of the Royal College of Physicians of London*, 31, 57–61.

Horgan J et al. (1992) Working party report on cardiac rehabilitation. *British Heart Journal*, 67, 412–418.

Hung J et al. (1994) Changes in rest and exercise myocardial perfusion and left ventricular function 3 to 26 weeks after clinically uncomplicated acute myocardial infarction. *American Journal of Cardiology*, 54, 943–950.

Naismith L D et al. (1979) Psychological rehabilitation after myocardial infarction. *British Medical Journal*, 1, 439–446.

O'Connor G T et al. (1989) An overview of randomised trials of rehabilitation with exercise after myocardial infarction. *Circulation*, 80, 234.

Oldridge N B et al. (1988) Cardiac rehabilitation after myocardial infarction. Combined experience of randomised clinical trials. *Journal of the American Medical Association*, 260, 945–950.

OPCS (1993) Health survey for England. In: The Health of the Nation: Briefing pack. London: HMSO.

Prochaska J O & DiClemente C (1994) The transtheoretical approach: crossing traditional foundations of change. In: J Naidoo & J Wells (Eds), Health promotion: foundations for practice. London: Baillière Tindall.

Pyorala G et al. (1994) Prevention of coronary heart disease in clinical practice. *European Heart Journal*, 15, 1300.

Rosenberg S G (1971) Patient education leads to better care for heart patients. *HSMHA Health Reports*, 86(9), 793–802.

Sivers F (1996) Evidence-based strategies for secondary prevention of coronary heart disease. In: F Sivers (Ed), *Cardiology 2000* (p 18). London: Merck Sharpe & Dohme.

Wang W T (1994) The educational needs of myocardial infarction patients. *Rehabilitation*, 9(4), 28–36.

Wilhelmsson C et al. (1975) Smoking and myocardial infarction. *The Lancet*, i, 415.

World Health Organisation (1993) Needs and action priorities in cardiac rehabilitation and secondary prevention in patients with coronary heart disease. In: D R Thompson et al. (Eds), Cardiac rehabilitation guidelines in the United Kingdom: guidelines and audit standards. *Heart*, 75, 89–93.

Zigmond A S & Snaith R P (1983) The Hospital Anxiety and Depression Scale. *Acta Psychiatrica Scandinavica*, 67, 361–370.

The 'Get Moving!' Study

Graham Simmonds

Evaluation is generally considered by health professionals to be an essential part of any project. Within the competitive, cash limited environment of today's health care few would refute the importance of knowing the extent to which a project's aims and objectives have been achieved and the process by which these outcomes were arrived at. However, health promotion practitioners who seek to apply these expectations by commissioning an evaluation, or conducting an evaluation study themselves, find that the practice of evaluation is considerably more complex than the rhetoric. The evaluation models and techniques chosen by the non-specialist practitioner evaluator will inevitably be a compromise between the ideal textbook design and the limits imposed by time, finance and expertise available. This section uses the experience of evaluating the 'Get Moving!' project to illustrate some of the issues involved in evaluating a health promotion project.

A CASE IN POINT – THE 'GET MOVING!' STUDY

An increasing number of projects nationally have focused on promoting physical activity in general practice and most have omitted rigorous evaluation (Health Education Authority, 1994). The approach adopted has usually centred on an 'exercise prescription' model where GPs are encouraged to send patients who are deemed to be inactive to leisure centres to receive motivational advice. In 1993, the Bristol Area Specialist Health Promotion Service (BASHPS, now called Health Promotion Service Avon) and Avon Health Authority were considering using this approach. However, without strong evidence available, it was decided a research project was needed to help direct future planning.

Initial funding for 'Get Moving!' was given by Avon Health Authority to BASHPS to assess the effectiveness of this method of promoting physical activity. However, when a steering group was set up, it was soon agreed that the leisure centre was not necessarily the most appropriate place for all patients. There was also an acknowledgement of the lack of research available on how best to motivate people

---

Evidence-based Health Promotion. Edited by Elizabeth R. Perkins, Ina Simnett and Linda Wright.

to change their physical activity behaviour. Therefore a more general project was developed to evaluate the effectiveness of different approaches to change physical activity behaviour within the general practice setting (phase 1). A project officer was employed to carry out this research. A description of the research design is covered later.

Upon completion of phase 1, funding became available for a second and third year. Having discovered the more effective methods to motivate patients, it became necessary to investigate how to motivate primary care staff to promote activity to patients. This was the aim of phase 2.

As with any piece of research, clarifying the main questions that needed to be answered was an essential first step. For 'Get Moving!' there were two separate questions:

- What is the most effective method of giving advice in primary health care?
- How can primary health care teams be encouraged to promote physical activity?

Having clear aims helped keep the project focused and made decisions on evaluation techniques much easier.

The people who need to be persuaded by the findings may also dictate the evaluation methods used. For example, some funding organisations are quite strict about the types of research they allow. However, you need to decide what kind of research will provide the information *you* require. In the case of this project, the health authority commissioners and the medical community were the main audience. BASHPS decided to contract the Exercise and Health Research Unit at the University of Bristol for their expertise in this area, which also added credibility to the project.

The following account outlines how decisions were made about the research design and evaluation methods of each of the two phases of the project.

Choosing what to Measure

For the 'Get Moving!' project, the question of what changes should be measured was not simple. In phase 1, some groups might have argued for measurement of fitness levels, others for reduction in morbidity and others for improvements in self-esteem. Understanding what outcome was realistic and necessary was crucial. Figure 16.2.1 outlines a sequence of health promotion outcomes that might be achieved within the short, medium and long term. Reduced morbidity and mortality are long-term goals that may take as long as ten or 20 years to achieve. In contrast, project funding may be for as little as six months or a few years at most. The results of large morbidity and mortality studies often provide a rationale for funding a short-term programme. What then has to be argued is the link between the changes a piece of work produces and the benefits shown by large studies. For

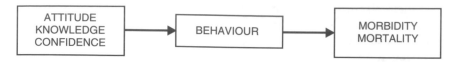

Figure 16.2.1   Sequence of research outcomes (adapted from Patton, 1997)

short- or medium-term programmes, usually the most that can be achieved is behaviour change, with the assumption that a positive change should lead in the longer term to a reduction in morbidity.

If behaviour does not change, the intervention may still have been effective. As discussed in Chapter 4, the stages of change model proposes that people move through various changes in attitude before adopting a behavioural change and many people may rotate through the cycle many times before achieving a maintained state of change (Prochaska & DiClimente, 1982). A short-term study may not lead to a behaviour change. It is therefore essential that the outcome measures used are sensitive enough to measure realistic short-term changes. Examples might be changes in awareness, attitudes, knowledge, self-esteem or self-efficacy. Basic changes on these levels will be the most likely outcome of a short-term project (Kemm & Close, 1995). During 'Get Moving!', actual activity levels did not change during phase 1; although for some intervention groups their stage of change did increase.

Phase 2 was concerned with how to encourage a team to change. This meant that a whole range of variables had to be considered, including the knowledge, skills and behaviour of the practice team as well as their internal communication networks and teamwork. A general practice is a complex social environment involving many personalities. To enter this project with a set of preconceived ideas of the issues may have missed fundamental problems. For example, use of a standard pre-/post-test questionnaire might reveal that lack of time and funding were important. However, it might not reveal the importance of a key member of staff who is in a controlling position and who needs to be convinced, or that resources produced were not used by many GPs because they were located in an adjacent room rather than handed to them directly. Consequently, having a broad approach to evaluation was necessary to understand the practice, so that these underlying issues could be explored and the phase 2 intervention tailored to the practice context.

Choosing how to Measure

Evaluation methods can take different forms, such as written, observational or verbal. In phase 1 it was necessary to assess which type of advice would be most effective when working with large numbers of people. Three alternative interventions were developed each to be given by the practice nurse. Two used the stage of change model (Prochaska & DiClemente, 1982). The interventions were

1   stage-based with verbal counselling
2   stage-based with no verbal counselling (just a leaflet)
3   general advice.

Patients were not randomised into each group, but the intervention was randomly assigned to each practice. Each patient was also given a reduced rate ticket for the local leisure centre. This dictated a larger population base, so that the results could be generalised to the entire practice and other practice populations. In order to determine whether changes seen were as a result of the intervention or caused by external factors, a control group was needed.

We were immediately confronted with an ethical dilemma. In a standard randomised control trial, one group receives either a placebo or no intervention. However, is it ethical to deny advice to one group when this could have implications for their health? One solution would have been to delay advice until after the study. However, this could have led to a situation where a practitioner might be asked for advice about physical activity. They would then have to either refuse to give advice or remove the person from the study. It was agreed that the practice nurse in the control group would use the normal intervention currently given to patients locally. This would then indicate whether the new techniques were better than the present methods

It was necessary to ensure the people delivering the advice were not affected by the information given by the other groups. Therefore they were kept unaware of the other interventions. The logical and adopted strategy was to train four separate practices. However using this option, differences between the treatment groups could be due to the differences in the staff. Alternatively, each intervention could have been carried out in one practice. However, preventing staff talking about their type of advice to other staff within the same team would have been difficult. Another option could have been to train each staff member in all of the techniques. They would then have randomly applied each intervention. Training a practitioner to give different advice to different patients would have been difficult to monitor. The practitioner might have merged various parts of each intervention, thus creating an opportunity for error in the research.

In phase 1, due to the large number of people involved (over 200), the assessment techniques had to be quick, non-invasive, and not unduly disturb the current staff. The researcher would not have time to interview each patient individually, and it would be unlikely that the practice staff could spend time recording information from the patient. The chosen solution was a closed self-completed questionnaire, which took respondents approximately ten minutes to complete. Stage of change, physical activity and self-efficacy were measured (Desharnais et al., 1986). This would provide a necessary significance (p) value to convince the medical community.

Each practice was involved in negotiations about how to administer the questionnaire. All finally decided to give it to patients in the waiting room. The validity and reliability of the questionnaire were of course important and so pre-validated questions were used. The readability and accessibility of the questions also needed careful consideration. Some people may only have ten minutes to fill out the form, and may have refused to take part in the study if they saw a weighty questionnaire. This would reduce the response rate, and also introduce a sample bias which is created when a group of the population is excluded from the project. If the people don't even register on the project, they cannot be evaluated. This group may be more or less likely to change than those who drop out, thus making the results seem better or worse than they are.

Initially, the whole practice was invited to a presentation in their workplace, with lunch provided. This was intended to get everyone on board and sell the importance of a project. If the staff involved in the research were not convinced, then the work was less likely to succeed. Working with the reception staff and developing a system that was easy for them to use was vital. Practices were regularly visited to discuss and solve any problems.

Patients were followed up at two and six months, using the initial questions as well as further questions about activity patterns and use of the local leisure centre. At this point it was tempting to add many more questions to the questionnaire. Every question had to reflect the research question. The longer the questionnaire was, the less likely a person was to fill in and return it. A pre-paid, addressed envelope was supplied and people who did not return the questionnaires were followed up twice. Again, losing people from the initial sample could create another sample bias.

Phase 2 was more concerned with the process of promoting activity in general practice. Factors included barriers, level of communication and level of promotion of activity. It would have been simple to design a questionnaire to measure these variables, give it to the practice, provide some training, and re-administer the questionnaire. However, this phase was not only interested with what training might enable primary health care workers to change, but also how to work effectively with the practice. It was important to get to know the practice and understand their situation. Personal contact was important. It was also vital to draw out underlying reasons that a questionnaire might miss. In short, the gathering of data was part of the process of change. Clearly it is difficult to generalise findings to other practices, although combined with other research, an overall picture can be created.

Although six practices were initially contacted, only one eventually signed up. The researcher visited each practice, sometimes more than once, presenting the research proposal, and then allowing the practice to decide. Negotiation was the key factor. An ideal amount of contact time was suggested, though the practice eventually agreed to less. As the process developed could be used in the future, the work had to be flexible to accommodate all possibilities. The preparation with the practice was as important as any subsequent work.

The project took a team-building and educational approach. All staff were interviewed. Encouraging the groups to be as truthful as possible was essential. Each group within the practice (practice and community nurses, GPs and receptionists) was interviewed. Again, the receptionists were an important group to involve. The groups were interviewed separately, as the hierarchy within the practice could prevent honest responses. Areas such as communication, barriers and knowledge were covered, and the same questions were asked of all groups. Avoiding asking leading questions is difficult, but researchers new to this area will find they learn this extremely quickly. The staff were also given a questionnaire to evaluate their attitude to and level of promotion of physical activity. This would provide some quantitative data to support the information gathered. General findings from the interviews were presented at a training session and time was allowed to discuss how to take this further. Any resource materials requested such as leaflets, posters and further information were supplied or produced. Follow-up interviews were then held after a few months.

Any resources developed for the practice were always done in conjunction with the practice. For example, a practice protocol was produced outlining how the practice would promote physical activity in the future. This was returned twice to the practice for amendments before it was agreed. The process of agreement was as important as the agreement itself.

This method of evaluation is time-consuming. All the interviews were taped and transcribed. Drawing out and grouping similar comments can be laborious. However, the richness of the data provides a more realistic feel of the practice. It also allowed time to go deeper into specific areas that could have been overlooked by a closed or self-completed questionnaire. The reports produced were shown to the practice before publication to ensure no confidential information was included. Care must be taken to keep individuals in the study anonymous.

In this section, I have attempted to describe how within one project, two different types of evaluation were used for different situations. It should be clear from the health promotion approach used which type of evaluation is best. Using an inappropriate method just to produce complicated statistics will create results that will be questioned. If the results are not positive, do not be afraid to publish them. Be honest in your work. It is tempting to gloss over parts that have not gone to plan, but the whole concept of the research community is to share and develop ideas. A negative result is just as useful as a positive one. Qualitative research may provide the reasons why the work did or did not go according to plan.

A FINAL RUMINATION

I have discussed the importance of funders and purchasers who need to be persuaded by evaluation evidence. Existing financial pressures on the NHS mean that health promotion may be seen as a soft target. The types of evaluation that are expected of health promotion projects should be put into perspective with the rest of the NHS. Only 53% of clinical techniques are evaluated by randomised controlled trial (Ellis et al., 1995). In this study a further 29% were accepted as having convincing non-experimental evidence. The types of work done in health promotion do not lend themselves neatly to a randomised controlled trial. Rather than forcing a project to provide quantitative results that will never be positive, other more sensitive and appropriate types of research need to be accepted. A well-done piece of qualitative research may go a long way to persuade key people of the benefits of this approach. Keep rooted in your philosophical beliefs and use them to guide you towards the best evaluation method.

KEY LEARNING POINTS

- Set clear aims and objectives.
- Be realistic – do not try to understand the world in six months.
- Understand your audience. What type of research do they need to be convinced by?
- Choose the most appropriate research method to answer your initial question. Do the questions asked really get to the crux of the issue?
- Do not be afraid of your limitations. Ask for help from colleagues or local institutions.
- Publish both positive and negative findings.

REFERENCES

Desharnais R, Bouillon J & Godin G (1986) Self-efficacy and outcome expectations as determinants of exercise adherence. *Psychological Reports*, 59, 1155–1159.

Ellis J, Mulligan I, Rowe J & Sackett D L (1995) Inpatient general medicine is evidence based. *The Lancet*, 346, 407–412.

Health Education Authority (1994) Physical activity promotion in primary health care in England. London: HEA.

Kemm J & Close A (1995) Health promotion theory and practice (p 162). London: Macmillan.

Patton M Q (1997) Utilisation-focused evaluation (p 220). London: Sage.

Prochaska J O & DiClemente C C (1982) Transtheoretical therapy: toward a more integrative model of change. *Psychotherapy: Theory, Research & Practice*, 19(3), 276–287.

Section 16.3

Evaluation in Health Promotion: The Proof of the Pudding?

Linda Wright

'The proof of the pudding is in the eating' Proverb

For health promotion practitioners and managers alike, evaluation is often used as a stick to beat up their efforts, rather than a positive encouragement to evidence-based practice. Academics castigate their attempts to do it, purchasers clamour for evidence of effectiveness, funders will not part with a penny before they have 'proof that it works' and clinicians will not accept an evaluation as valid unless it meets their standards for clinical evidence. Couple these expectations with funding and time limitations and the very word 'evaluate' is enough to send many health promoters galloping off into the distance before you have time to say randomised control trial.

Fortunately, help is at hand. There are now a few knights in shining armour: influential bodies such as the World Health Organisation (Ziglio, 1997) and the Health Education Board for Scotland (Perkins & Wright, 1998; Wimbush, 1998) and academics (e.g. Macdonald et al., 1996; Nutbeam, 1998; Nutbeam et al., 1990) who appreciate the realities of practitioner research. They advocate new approaches and tools that will both facilitate evaluation at practitioner level, and define some of its limits. Health promotion has finally begun to develop its own methodologies for evaluation, which take account of the aims, values and processes which distinguish health promotion from other health care disciplines. For example, see Beattie (1995) on evaluation of community development for health initiatives; Springett and Dugdill's (1995) framework for evaluating workplace health promotion; Shiroyama et al.'s (1995) account of evaluating health promotion projects in primary care; Hawe and colleagues' (1991) health workers' guide to evaluating health promotion and Wright and Perkins' (in press) toolbox for health promotion research and evaluation. There is a growing literature that acknowledges that standard scientific approaches to evaluation have limited value for

Evidence-based Health Promotion. Edited by Elizabeth R. Perkins, Ina Simnett and Linda Wright.
© 1999 John Wiley & Sons Ltd.

health promotion practice; they either don't work, won't work or fail to provide useful information (Nutbeam, 1996; Secker et al., 1995).

However, most of this encouraging development is being led by academics, researchers and international bodies such as WHO. In order to get these ideas into practice, health promotion practitioners need to engage in this debate actively and apply these new initiatives and theories to their own work. The 'proof of the pudding' does not rest with academic research, but with testing, through the day to day health promotion activities of health promoters from different disciplines, working in different settings. So what encouragement (see below) can health promotion practitioners gain from these recent developments?

NEW DEVELOPMENTS IN HEALTH PROMOTION EVALUATION: IMPLICATIONS FOR PRACTITIONERS

- A clearer rationale for evaluation in health promotion
- Some boundaries to practitioner level evaluation studies
- Useful criteria
- Refocus on implementation
- Acknowledgement of the importance of context and setting
- A broader repertoire of evaluation methodologies
- Utilisation focused evaluation

A CLEARER RATIONALE FOR EVALUATION IN HEALTH PROMOTION

Doing evaluation means making judgements about the value or worth of a health promotion project or activity. The purpose of evaluation is therefore bound up in the broad values and goals of health promotion and at the level of practice, with the personal beliefs, values and perceptions of the stakeholders. As Dale Webb points out (Chapter 3, Section 3.1), health promotion is a different kind of endeavour to clinical practice. It is centrally concerned with enabling and empowering individuals and communities to increase control over, and improve, their health. This means that a narrow focus on health outcomes borrowed from evidence-based medicine does not adequately encompass all, or even most, of the questions that evaluation in health promotion should legitimately address. As many have argued, health promotion is equally concerned with evaluations focused on issues such as equity, empowerment, access to health services, community involvement and healthy public policy (Macdonald et al., 1996; Whitehead, 1991; Ziglio, 1997). Indeed, at practitioner level, evaluation of the long-term health outcomes of a health promotion initiative is rarely feasible or even appropriate.

Practitioners faced with the difficulties of reconciling their stakeholders' diverse expectations of the purpose of an evaluation, particularly challenges to measure long-term health outcomes, can therefore emphasise these core health promotion values in their negotiations. Building again on core values, adopting a partici-patory approach to evaluation, involving both stakeholders and the client group has also been found to be crucial to the success of evaluation studies, in a wide variety of settings and disciplines (Patton, 1997; Springett et al., 1995).

Those concerned with delivering and planning health promotion services have a very broad range of questions for evaluation studies to answer, of which 'does it work?' is only one. In health promotion practice, evaluation is expected to be useful in informing decisions about whether to stop, continue or extend a project and how it should be changed or improved. At local level evaluations usually have several purposes, according to the values and priorities of the people involved. When planning an evaluation, checking out what your manager or funders count as success, or what they think is important for good health promotion performance, will save a lot of misunderstanding later. An open, negotiated approach to evaluation, which explicitly takes account of the stakeholders' values and expec-tations, will provide a practical framework for gathering evidence that will actually be used, rather than dumped on a shelf to gather dust.

REASONS FOR EVALUATION IN HEALTH PROMOTION PRACTICE

1. To improve the design or performance of a health promotion project, policy, activity or service.
2. To make choices between health promotion activities.
3. To aid decisions about which activities should be funded and which initiatives have greatest impact.
4. To learn how a particular health promotion project or activity might be repeated and sustained elsewhere.
5. For accountability, to find out whether an activity is conducted according to an agreed plan, objectives and time frame.
6. To find out whether a project provides value for money (cost-effectiveness).
7. To test whether new or innovative ideas will work in practice.

SOME BOUNDARIES TO PRACTITIONER LEVEL EVALUATION STUDIES

Establishing a clearer rationale for health promotion evaluations and adoption of a broader range of methodologies (see below) have helped to define the health promotion 'territory' and so set some boundaries to practitioner level evaluations. Cost, time and resource constraints also usually impose major limitations on the type of work that can be attempted. These realities are yet another reason why a participative approach to evaluation is appropriate at practitioner level. Negoti-ating what questions can be answered, within the resources available, will be central to achieving a useful evaluation and to ensuring that the evaluation and the people who conduct it are not set up to fail. There will be circumstances when it is better not to attempt to do an evaluation at all, rather than produce poor quality evidence that becomes a political liability (see below).

WHEN NOT TO DO AN EVALUATION

Do not attempt an evaluation when:

- you do not have enough time, skills or funding
- the work you are doing has been researched and documented elsewhere
- the successes and failures are well documented and the reasons are clearly understood
- the results are likely to be ignored
- you do not have the support of your manager/organisation.

If any of these apply, stick to simple monitoring for accountability. Build good record keeping and review systems into your work, and ensure that you can provide a clear explanation of your approach (including the results of previous research, if appropriate).

As noted in Chapter 12, the research literature is distinctly lacking in practical guidance on how much different kinds of evaluation studies cost and how long they take. This problem can be compounded if those involved in planning an evaluation lack practical research experience. There are obvious pitfalls that can be thought through and avoided, such as selecting measures that are unlikely to change over the term of the evaluation (see indicators below), trying to complete 50 semi-structured interviews in a week, or allowing half a day to write up a report. Unless your department or organisation has a research specialist, this is where the advice of an experienced researcher is really useful, even if you have to pay for it. This option should be considered as an alternative to commissioning an outside researcher or agency to do the whole of the evaluation. Within a participative framework, external researchers should be involved as partners to local health promotion practitioners, rather than their agents. Your responsibility will be to ensure that the researcher understands the resource constraints, the requirements of the stakeholders and the health promotion principles and values that underpin the work.

Illuminative, process evaluations are likely to be more feasible for health promotion practitioners than formal outcome studies. Apart from the cost and the methodological difficulties of outcome studies, recognition of the process of change (see Chapter 1) means that it is not even appropriate to attempt to measure a project's outcomes until it has been successfully adopted, implemented and has been running smoothly for some time. Time-limited health promotion projects of three years or less should not be evaluated using a summative outcomes model. Recognising the phases of change of a project will help you to decide what type of evaluation is appropriate and the sorts of questions it is appropriate to ask. For example, at the adoption phase of change, when you are trying to get a new project up and running, your evaluation might involve gathering evidence about who or what helped or hindered its adoption. You might also be interested in whether its consumers were ready to take it on and perceived it as relevant to their needs (see Graham Simmonds' account of evaluating the 'Get Moving!' project in Section 16.2 of this chapter). Alternatively, at the implementation phase, when the same project is running, but not yet part of established services, you might wish to gather evidence about how related services perceive it, its accessibility to the client group, or evidence of practicality – whether concrete 'how to' help is offered to its consumers.

USEFUL CRITERIA

Evaluation involves making judgements about the value of a health promotion activity or project, by comparing it with some criteria that are considered to be an indication of good performance. These criteria are usually derived from the aims and objectives of the project. If the activity or programme does not have a clear rationale with both long- and short-term objectives it becomes extremely difficult to evaluate it. If you don't know where you want to go, how will you know whether you have got there or how much further you have to go (outcome evaluation)? You will also be unable to judge whether you have set off on the right road (impact evaluation) or whether your vehicle is suitable for the journey (input and process evaluation).

Evaluation is also difficult when project managers, funders and staff disagree about the project's aims and objectives or about the relative importance of different objectives. Outcome evaluations imposed on health promotion projects by external decision makers and funders have been known to select outcome criteria that were not the stated goals of the project. For example, the Health Education Authority's Drinkwise campaign was considered by some policy makers to have failed, because it did not succeed in reducing the proportions of the adult population who drank more than the recommended sensible drinking levels. This was not a goal of the campaign, which, when evaluated according to its stated aims (raising public awareness of units and sensible drinking levels), was found to have been highly successful (Wright, 1996). This is why it is worth investing time and effort in establishing why the evaluation is wanted and negotiating this with everyone who will have an interest in its results. This process will usually reveal any differences between the various stakeholders' expectations about what the project and the evaluation should achieve. If major differences do emerge, then you will need to go back to the stakeholders and renegotiate either the focus of the evaluation, or the goals of the project, or both.

Reliance solely on the rigorous standards of evidence and inclusion criteria adopted by effectiveness reviews has excluded a lot of evidence that is useful to health promotion practice. Moreover, health status criteria for success are often only measurable in the long term and even then cannot usually be confidently attributed to the health promotion intervention.

The development of useful evaluation criteria involves building up chains of indicators for measuring change at different stages in a project's development and over different periods of time. These will link up immediate objectives (focused on implementation) with intermediate goals (focusing on impact) and long-term objectives (focused on outcomes). There are a wide range of 'off the shelf' indicators available. In particular, the national health promotion agencies have put considerable efforts into developing health promotion indicators. For example, the WHO European Office co-ordinates a collaborative cross-national study of the health behaviour of secondary school-aged children. All of the UK countries participate, via biannual national surveys of secondary school children. The data offer national frameworks of indicators for health education with 11–15-year-olds, involving measures of knowledge, motivations, skills, behaviours and health status. Currie and Todd (1990) report how this data can be used to evaluate health promotion projects. Indicators have also been developed for evaluating health promotion in different settings, e.g. the 'Health at work in the NHS' programme (Wessex Institute of Public Health Medicine, 1994); and primary health care nursing (Health Education Authority, 1997). General population surveys have also been used to establish national baseline indicators for health promotion topic areas (Health Education Board for Scotland, 1997).

These indicators *may* be transferable to evaluation of local level health promotion projects, if they are replicating work done at national level. However, generally, indicators are only valid in the contexts for which they were designed. Despite the increased acceptance of health promotion's broad goals, nationally defined indicators continue to be mainly set within a clinical health gain framework. Hayes and Willms (1990) note the paucity of indicators of healthy communities, while indicators of community participation and equity are very hard to find (Dean, 1998; Hunt, 1998). Health promotion practitioners who wish to evaluate their own efforts will continue to have to develop their own indicators that relate to the goals and processes of the project or activity being evaluated. The current British Government strategy paper, *Our Healthier Nation* (Department of Health, 1998) places less emphasis on nationally defined criteria for success than the health gain targets in the *Health of the Nation*, which have driven health promotion activities for the last decade. This means that local planners and health promotion managers currently have more freedom (and more responsibility) to define their own useful criteria for evaluating the process and outcomes of their services.

REFOCUS ON IMPLEMENTATION

Part of the revolution in health promotion evaluation has been that researchers are finally listening to what practitioners say they want from evaluation studies. In order to act on evidence that says an intervention is effective, practitioners need to know how it works in order to implement it. As noted in Chapter 12, the number of evaluation studies on dissemination, adoption and implementation are still small in comparison to the mass of outcome-focused data. However, there is a growing recognition by policy makers and funders that these types of study are important. At practitioner level, where many evaluations do ask about process, the results are rarely disseminated beyond the local area and so much valuable experience is lost. If evidence-based health promotion is to progress, then there needs to be a forum whereby practitioners' accounts of how they implemented health promotion projects are afforded equal, if not higher, priority and status than outcome reports.

ACKNOWLEDGEMENT OF THE IMPORTANCE OF CONTEXT AND SETTING

Alongside an acknowledgement of the importance of implementation evaluations has come an understanding that the multiple contexts and settings for health promotion represent an important dynamic in gathering and using evaluation evidence. These two issues are related – outcome evaluations are usually specific to a particular context and setting and provide little guidance about transferability. For example, we may have no evidence about how a peer-led sexual health project in a school might transfer to the informal setting of a youth club, or how a cardiac rehabilitation leaflet evaluated positively with hospital patients might work if used in a community setting by practice nurses.

Where local evaluation studies have explicitly aimed to identify features of settings that might affect the process or outcomes of a health promotion programme, they have produced evidence that has had important implications for practice. For example, Wilkinson et al.'s (1997) account of an action research evaluation of a workplace initiative identified local vehicles for health promotion (work canteens and vending machines, provision of bicycle sheds) and features of the workplace setting that were important for success. These included staff participation in health decisions and the need to involve general managers in small companies with no occupational health or human resources departments.

A BROADER REPERTOIRE OF EVALUATION METHODOLOGIES

The key issue for health promotion practice is the usefulness of the data, not the method by which it is obtained. This means that evaluation methodologies should be chosen to support the intended use of the evaluation, by its intended users (Patton, 1997). If practitioners adopt a participative approach to planning evaluation, then the very process of negotiation will define the questions that the evaluation should answer and these, together with the time and resources you have available, will guide your choice of methodology.

Denzin and Lincoln (1994) report that in the last 25 years a quiet 'methodological revolution' has been taking place in evaluation studies. There is now a considerable body of evaluation practice from fields largely outside health care, that has moved beyond scientific, quantitative methods to embrace more interactive qualitative approaches. Despite the widespread acceptance in academic circles that both types of methodologies are useful and can be combined (Brannen, 1992; Milburn et al., 1995), this revolution is still going on at the level of health promotion practice and the 'warring camps' (Beattie, 1995) continue to thrive at all levels. Some of the arguments practitioners might use to emphasise the limitations of the more traditional methods are given below. Because of the difficulties of meeting the stringent requirements of the randomised control trial, health promotion researchers who soldier on under the scientific outcomes banner have tended to end up with weaker evaluation designs such as quasi-experimental designs. As a result they get the worst of both worlds – design and validity criticisms from those committed to the RCT gold standard and complaints from practitioners that their results are not useful, because they do not contain sufficient information (Macdonald et al., 1996).

LIMITATIONS OF SCIENTIFIC OUTCOME METHODS FOR EVALUATING HEALTH PROMOTION PROGRAMMES

The naturalistic and multifaceted nature of health promotion programmes means that it is difficult for scientific outcomes designs:

- to meet the rigorous standards expected of a randomised control trial or even a quasi-experimental design, e.g. establish control groups, control confounding variables, achieve randomisation;
- to be certain about the relationship between cause and effect;
- to provide unequivocal evidence of effectiveness;
- to formulate indicators that are sensitive enough to measure change within the study period.

Outcome evaluation provides no information about *how* the results were achieved, thus limiting implementation, repetition of success or rejection of programmes that have not been effective.

In response to disputes about what counts as success and the frustrations of trying to apply quantitative, scientific outcome designs to health promotion evaluations, a growing number of evaluation studies are being reported which have adopted a range of alternative methodologies. These tend to be qualitative strategies, focusing on:

- involving the programme deliverers and the target groups as active participants, rather than subjects to be studied,

- the researcher as a partner rather than a detached observer,
- illumination of the process by which outcomes are achieved rather than focusing on the outcomes themselves.

Adoption of these approaches does not necessarily imply that interest in outcomes is abandoned altogether, or that quantitative data is not collected. The best evaluation designs (in terms of providing useful evidence for practice) may be those which combine several methods and collect both qualitative and quantitative data; e.g. Beattie (1995) describes the use of mixed methodologies, or pluralistic approaches in relation to evaluating community development for health programmes. However, such combined methods should not be used uncritically; see Milburn et al. (1995) for some considerations for appropriate use.

The pluralistic methodologies use frameworks based on dialogue, consultation and participation – processes that are much closer to the everyday practice of health promotion practitioners than the skills required of an evaluator working within a traditional scientific framework. Some methods can be deliberately combined with a service delivery role, such as action research (Sanford, 1981). Here the evaluator has a hands-on role and results are continually fed back into the project as a series of loops. For example, Wilkinson et al. (1997) used an action research approach to both evaluate and stimulate a workplace health promotion project in Bedfordshire. The practitioner-as-researcher approach involves project workers conducting the evaluation themselves and reflecting in and on action in a systematic way. Several methods involve collecting stories around the focus of the evaluation, which can be a natural extension of health promotion practitioners' interviewing and case reporting skills. For examples, see Margaret MacVicar's account of her students' experiences of learning about research (Chapter 13, Section 13.2); Blackburn et al.'s (1997) evaluation of disseminating research on women's smoking to health practitioners and Hesketh et al.'s (1995) evaluation of health promotion delivered by community pharmacists. For more detailed advice on qualitative evaluation methodologies see Patton (1987; 1997) and Mays and Pope (1996).

While this expanded range of methods for evaluation offers practical solutions to many of the problems facing health promotion evaluation, they are not a rapid, complete or easy answer. To use them, practitioners need help and support, of the kinds I discussed in Chapter 12. Health promotion practitioners and managers whose initial training took place over ten years ago may not have been introduced to the newer approaches and will need to be updated or offered opportunities to try them out. As I argue in Chapter 12, a strategic approach is required by service managers, planners and commissioners, to establish a framework of support and supervision for practitioners to enable them to develop their skills in evidence-based health promotion practice. In turn, to increase their acceptability to stakeholders, more published accounts are needed of pluralistic evaluations. Quality standards for this type of work have been developed by researchers and academics (Rogers et al., 1997; Secker et al., 1995) and these need to be understood and applied at practice level.

UTILISATION FOCUSED EVALUATION

One of the central themes of this book is that health promotion practitioners will only use evaluation evidence, whoever gathers it and however it is obtained, if they think it is useful. Throughout this book we have suggested ways that the much discussed evidence–practice gap can be reduced. We have aimed our book at practitioners and have deliberately set out to include evidence gathered by them. It is clear that even if health promotion practitioners gain inspiration and encouragement from our contributors, they will need the support of their managers and organisations in order to work in an evidence-based way. They will also need academics and researchers who are prepared to be flexible and creative in acknowledging the realities of health promotion practice and a forum that enables the many issues raised in this book to be critically examined and developed.

REFERENCES

Beattie A (1995) Evaluation in community development for health: an opportunity for dialogue. *Health Education Journal*, 54(4), 465–472.

Blackburn C, Graham H & Scullion P (1997) Disseminating research findings on women's smoking to health practitioners: findings from an evaluation study. *Health Education Journal*, 56, 113–124.

Brannen J (Ed) (1992) Mixing methods: quantitative and qualitative research. Aldershot: Avebury.

Currie C & Todd J (1990) Health behaviours and health indicators in schoolchildren in central region: a profile of the region and evaluation of two health promotion projects: a survey conducted as part of the Scottish WHO health behaviour in school age children. Edinburgh: The University of Edinburgh.

Dean K (1998) Measuring health behaviour and health: towards new health promotion indicators. *Health Promotion*, 3(1), 13–21.

Department of Health (1998) Our Healthier Nation. London: HMSO.

Denzin N & Lincoln Y (1994) Handbook of qualitative research. London: Sage.

Hawe P, Degeling D & Hall J (1991) Evaluating health promotion: a health worker's guide. Sydney: McLennan and Petty.

Hayes M & Willms S (1990) Healthy community indicators: the perils of the search and the paucity of the find. *Health Promotion International*, 5(2), 161–166.

Health Education Authority (1997) Promoting health through primary health care nursing: guide to quality indicators. London: HEA.

Health Education Board for Scotland (1997) Indicators for health education in Scotland. Edinburgh: Health Education Board for Scotland.

Hesketh A, Lindsay G & Harden R (1995) Interactive health promotion in the community pharmacy. *Health Education Journal*, 54(3), 294–303.

Hunt S (1998) Measuring health behaviour and health: towards new health promotion indicators. *Health Promotion*, 3(1), 23–34.

Macdonald G, Veen C & Tones K (1996) Evidence for success in health promotion: suggestions for improvement. *Health Education: Research, Theory and Practice*, 11, 367–376.

Mays N & Pope C (Eds) (1996) Qualitative research in health care. London: BMJ Publishing Group.

Milburn K, Fraser E, Secker J & Pavis S (1995) Combining methods in health promotion research: some considerations about appropriate use. *Health Education Journal*, 54(3), 347–356.

Nutbeam D (1996) Achieving 'best practice' in health promotion: improving the fit between research and practice. *Health Education: Research, Theory and Practice*, 11(3), 317–326.

Nutbeam D (1998) Evaluating health promotion: progress, problems and solutions. *Health Promotion International*, 13(1), 27–44.

Nutbeam D, Smith C & Catford J (1990) Evaluation in health education: a review of progress, possibilities and problems. *Journal of Epidemiology and Community Health*, 44, 83–89.

Patton M Q (1987) How to use qualitative methods in evaluation. London: Sage.

Patton M Q (1997) Utilization-focused evaluation. London: Sage.

Perkins E R & Wright L (1998) Developing research awareness, knowledge and skills amongst health education/promotion specialists and health promoters in Scotland. Final report of Phase 1: Training needs analysis. Edinburgh: Health Promotion Board for Scotland.

Rogers A, Popay J, Williams G & Latham M (1997) Inequalities in health and health promotion: insights from the qualitative research literature. London: Health Education Authority.

Sanford N (1981) A model for action research. In: P Reason & J Rowan (Eds), Human inquiry: a sourcebook of new paradigm research. Chichester: John Wiley.

Secker J, Wimbush E, Watson J & Milburn K (1995) Qualitative methods in health promotion research: some criteria for quality. *Health Education Journal*, 54(1), 74–87.

Shiroyama C, McKee L & McKie L (1995) Evaluating health promotion projects in primary care: recent experiences in Scotland. *Health Education Journal*, 54(2), 226–240.

Springett J & Dugdill L (1995) Workplace health promotion programmes: towards a framework for evaluation. *Health Education Journal*, 54(1), 88–98.

Springett J, Costongs L & Dugdill L (1995) Towards a framework for evaluation in health promotion: methodology, principles and practice. *The Journal*, Summer, 61–65.

Wessex Institute of Public Health Medicine (1994) Indicators and outcome measures for 'Health at work in the NHS' in Wessex. Winchester: Wessex Institute of Public Health Medicine.

Whitehead M (1991) The concepts and principles of equity and health. *Health Promotion International*, 6, 217–228.

Wilkinson E, Elander E & Woolaway M (1997) Exploring the use of action research to stimulate and evaluate workplace health promotion. *Health Education Journal*, 56(2), 188–198.

Wimbush E (1998) The research training needs of health promotion practitioners (conference paper). Second Nordic Health Promotion Research Conference, Stockholm, 9–11 September 1998.

Wright L (1996) A review of the Drinkwise campaign, 1989–94. London: Health Education Authority.

Wright L & Perkins E (in press) Toolbox for health promotion research and evaluation. Edinburgh: Health Education Board for Scotland.

Ziglio E (1997) How to move towards evidence-based health promotion interventions. *Promotion and Education*, 4, 29–32.

Bibliography

Aaron J I, Evans R E & Mela D J (1995) Paradoxical effect of a nutrition labelling scheme in a student cafeteria. *Nutrition Research*, 15, 1251–1261.

Abrams D B, Follick M J & Biener L (1988) Individual versus group self-help smoking cessation at the workplace: initial impact and 12 month outcomes. In: T Glynn (chair), Four National Cancer Institute funded self-help smoking cessation trials: interim results and emerging patterns. Symposium conducted at the annual meeting of the Association for the Advancement of Behaviour Therapy, New York.

Advisory Council on the Misuse of Drugs (1993) Drug education in schools: the need for new impetus. London: HMSO.

AIDS Advisory Committee (1995) Review of HIV and AIDS in prisons. London: HM Prison Service.

Ajzen I (1985) From intention to actions: a theory of planned behaviour. In: J Kuhl & J Beckman (Eds), Action control: from cognition to behavior. Englewood Cliffs, NJ: Prentice Hall.

Albright C L, Flora J A & Fortmann S P (1990) Restaurant menu labelling: impact of nutrition information on entree sales and patron attitudes. *Health Education Quarterly*, 17, 157–167.

Alkin M C et al. (1979) Using evaluations: does evaluation make a difference? Beverly Hills, CA: Sage.

Allen I (1987) Sex education and personal relationships. London: Policy Studies Institute.

Anderson J (1988) Coming to terms with mastectomy. *Nursing Times*, 84(4), 41–44.

Antman E M et al. (1992) A comparison of results of meta-analyses of randomised trials and recommendations of clinical experts. Treatments of myocardial infarction. *Journal of the American Medical Association*, 268, 240–248.

Antonovsky A (1996) The salutogenic model as a theory to guide health promotion. *Health Promotion International*, 11(1), 11–18.

Appleby J (1997) Health promotion: feelgood factors. *Health Service Journal*, 107(5560), 24–27.

Ashworth P (1995) The meaning of participation in 'participant observation'. *Qualitative Health Research*, 5(3), 366–387.

Atkins K, Hirst N, Lunt N & Parker G (1994) The role and self-perceived training needs of nurses employed in general practice: observation from a national census of practice nurses in England and Wales. *Journal of Advanced Nursing*, 20(1), 46–52.

Avery J & Jackson R (1993) Children and their accidents. London: Edward Arnold.

Bagnall G & Lockerbie L (1995) HIV/AIDS education: are senior pupils losing out? *Education and Health*, 13(3), 37–42.

Balding J W (1992) After the survey: nine workshops using the Health-Related Behaviour Questionnaire. Exeter: Schools Health Education Unit.

Balding J W (1994) Young people in 1993: the Health-Related Behaviour Questionnaire results for 29,074 pupils between the ages of 11 and 16. Exeter: Schools Health Education Unit.

Balding J W (1995) Young people in 1994. Exeter: Schools Health Education Unit.

Balding J W (1996) Young people in 1995. Exeter: Schools Health Education Unit.

Balding J W (1997) Young people in 1996: the Health-Related Behaviour Questionnaire results for 22,067 pupils between the ages of 12 and 15. Exeter: Schools Health Education Unit.

Balding J W, Regis D, Wise A, Bish D & Muirden J (1996) Bully off: young people that fear going to school. Exeter: Schools Health Education Unit.

Baldwin S (1990) Alcohol education and offenders. London: Batsford.

Baldwin S, Wilson M, Lancaster A & Allsop D (1988) Ending offending. Glasgow: Scottish Council on alcohol.

Bandura A (1977) Social learning theory. Englewood Cliffs, NJ: Prentice Hall.

Bandura A (1977) Self-efficacy: toward a unifying theory of behaviour change. *Psychological Review*, 84, 191–215.

Bandura A (1982) Self-efficacy mechanism in human agency. *American Psychologist*, 37, 122–147.

Barber M, Stoll I & Mortimore P (1995) Governing bodies and effective schools. OFSTED. London: HMSO.

Basch C E (1984) Research on disseminating and implementing health education programs in schools. *School Health Research*, 54, 57–66.

Batsleer J (1996) It's all right for you to talk: lesbian identification in feminist theory and youth work practice. *Youth and Policy*, 52, 12–21.

Batten E & Taylor D H (1982) Operation Smokestop: smoking cessation self-help groups in Wessex. Lifeline Report no. 5, Wessex Regional Health Authority.

Batten E, High S, Graham H, Rossi J & Ruggiero L (in preparation) Applying the transtheoretical model to a West Midlands pregnant population: 1. Reliability and validity of the model.

Batten E, High S, Graham H, Rossi J & Ruggiero L (in preparation) Applying the transtheoretical model to a West Midlands pregnant population: 2. Stage of change, parity and social circumstances.

Batten L (1985) Smokestop National Conference Proceedings. Health Education Council/ University of Southampton.

Baum F (1993) Healthy cities and change: social movement or bureaucratic tool? *Health Promotion International*, 8, 31–40.

Baum F (1995) Researching public health: behind the qualitative–quantitative methodological debate. *Social Science and Medicine*, 40(4), 459–468.

Beattie A (1991) Knowledge and control in health promotion: a test case for social policy and social theory. In: J Gabe et al. (Eds), The Sociology of the Health Service (pp 162–202). London: Routledge.

Beattie A (1995) Evaluation in community development for health: an opportunity for dialogue. *Health Education Journal*, 54(4), 465–472.

Becker M H (Ed) (1974) The belief model and personal health behaviour. Thorofare, NJ: Slack.

Becker H (1964) reprinted in T Heller, M Gott & C Jeffrey (Eds) (1987) Drug use and misuse: a reader. Milton Keynes: Open University Press.

Bee F & Bee R (1994) Training needs analysis and evaluation. London: Institute of Personnel and Development.

Benner P (1984) From novice to expert: excellence and power in clinical nursing practice. Menlo Park, CA: Addison-Wesley.

Bethel H J N & Mullee M (1990) A controlled trial of community based coronary rehabilitation. *British Heart Journal*, 64, 370–375.

Betteridge D J et al. (1993) Management of hyperlipidaemia: a practice guide. *Postgraduate Medical Journal*, 69, 359.

Bibbins L (1995) Gender, sexuality and sex education. In N Harris (Ed), Children, sex education and the law: examining the issues. London: National Children's Bureau.

Billings J & Cowley S (1995) Approaches to community needs assessment: a literature review. *Journal of Advanced Nursing*, 22, 721–730.

Blackburn C, Graham H & Scullion P (1997) Disseminating research findings on women's smoking to health practitioners: findings from an evaluation study. *Health Education Journal*, 56, 113–124.

Blakeslee T R (1980) The right brain: a new understanding of the unconscious mind and its creative powers. London: MacMillan Education.

Blakey V (1991) You don't have to say you love me. An evaluation of a drama-based sex education project for schools. *Health Education Journal*, 50(4), 161–165.

Blane D, Brunner E & Wilkinson R (1996) Health and social organization: towards a health policy for the 21st century. London: Routledge.

Blaxter M (1990) Health and lifestyles. London: Tavistock/Routledge.

Blum R (1987) Contemporary threats to adolescent health in the United States. *Journal of the American Medical Association*, 257, 3390–3395.

BMA Foundation for AIDS (1989) HIV and AIDS in Prison. London: BMA Foundation for AIDS.

BMRB (1995) Qualitative research conducted on behalf of the HEA. London: Health Education Authority.

Bonell C (1996) Outcomes in HIV prevention: report of a research project. London: The HIV Project.

Boud D, Cohen R & Walker D (Eds) (1993) Using experience for learning. Buckingham: Open University Press.

Bowen C (1997) The Bridgwater Detached (Street) Youth Work team. Somerset: Somerset County Youth Service.

Boyd M et al. (1993) The public health post at Strelley: an interim report. Nottingham: Nottingham Community Health NHS Trust.

Boydell T & Leary M (1996) Identifying training needs. London: Institute of Personnel and Development.

Bracht N, Finnegan J R, Rissel C, Weisbrod R, Gleason J, Corbett J & Veblen-Mortenson S (1994) Community ownership and program continuation following a health demonstration project. *Health Education Research*, 9, 243–255.

Bradshaw J (1992) The concept of social need. In: L Ewles & I Simnett (Eds), Promoting health: a practical guide. London: Scutari Press.

Brambleby P (1995) Tracking the financial shifts. In: C Riley, M Warner, A Pullen & C Semple Piggott (Eds), Releasing resources to achieve health gain. Oxford: Radcliffe Medical Press.

Brannen J (Ed) (1992) Mixing methods: quantitative and qualitative research. Aldershot: Avebury.

Bridges J M (1990) Literature review on the images of the nurse and nursing in the media. *Journal of Advanced Nursing*, 15(7), 850–854.

British Heart Foundation/Coronary Prevention Group Statistics Database (1995) Coronary heart disease statistics. London: British Heart Foundation.

Brown A & McCaughan N (Eds) (1991) Various articles. *Groupwork*, 4(3).

Brown S, Meald M & Sallans C (1995) Nobody listens: problems and promise for youth provision. Middlesbrough: Middlesbrough City Challenge/Middlesbrough Safer Cities.

Brummell K & Perkins E R (1995) Public health at Strelley: a model in action. Nottingham: Nottingham Community Health NHS Trust.

Bruner J S (1962) On knowing: essays for the left hand. Cambridge, MA: Harvard University Press.

Brunner E J (1996) The social and biological basis of cardiovascular disease. In: D Blane, E Brunner & R Wilkinson (Eds), Health and social organization: towards a health policy for the 21st century. London: Routledge.

Brunner E J, Marmot M G, White I R, O'Brien J R, Etherington M D, Slavin B M, Kearney E M & Davey Smith G (1993) Gender and employment grade differences in blood cholesterol, apolipoproteins and haemostatic factors in the Whitehall 11 study. *Atherosclerosis*, 102, 195–207.

Brydolf M & Segesten K (1996) Living with ulcerative colitis: experiences of adolescents and young adults. *Journal of Advanced Nursing*, 23, 39–47.

Bulmer M (Ed) (1978) Social policy research. London: Macmillan.

Burgess R, Davies L & Dilley C (1993) Drugs and offending. Northampton: CAN.

Burgess R, Houlihan A & Grant L (1998) Drugs and offending: therapeutic resources for work with prisoners. Northampton: CAN.

Burnard P (1987) Towards an epistemological basis for experiential learning in nurse education. *Journal of Advanced Nursing*, 12, 189–193.

Burns H (1996) Purchasing cost effective health care. Presentation at Making a Difference: Investing in Effective Health Promotion Conference, Durham.

Burr M L et al. (1989) Effects of changes in fat, fish and fibre intakes on death and myocardial infarction: Diet and Reinfarction Trial (DART). *The Lancet*, ii, 757.

Buzan T (1989) Use your head. Third edition. London: BBC Books.

Cale L (1997) Health education in schools: in a state of good health? *International Journal of Health Education*, 35(2), 59–62.

Campion P, Owen L & McNeill A (1994) Smoking before, during and after pregnancy in England. *Health Education Journal*, 53(2), 163–173.

Cannon N (1995) Lifescreen – calling all women. A breast screening theatre in health education project. Evaluation report commissioned by Kensington and Chelsea and Westminster Health Commissioning Agency.

Capacchione L (1988) The power of your other hand: a course in channeling the inner wisdom of the right brain. North Hollywood, CA: Newcastle Publishing.

Caplan N (1977) A minimal set of conditions necessary for the utilization of social science knowledge in policy formation at the national level. In: C H Weiss (Ed), Using social research in public policy making (pp 183–197). Lexington, MA: Lexington Heath.

Caplan R & Holland R (1990) Rethinking health education theory. *Health Education Journal*, 49, 10–12.

Care Sector Consortium (1997) National occupational standards for professional activity in health promotion and care: introductory guide. London: HMSO.

Carper B (1978) Fundamental patterns of knowing in nursing. *Advances in Nursing Science*, 1(1), 13–23.

Carr-Hill R (1984) Radicalising survey methodology. *Quality and Quantity*, 18: 275–292.

Cashdan S (1973) Interactional psychotherapy: stages and strategies in behavioural change. New York: Grune & Stratton.

Centre for Reviews and Dissemination (1993) Brief interventions and alcohol use. *Effective Health Care*. York: CRD.

Chambers M & Coates V (1993) Research in nursing, Part 2. *Senior Nurse*, 13, 1.

Champion V L & Leach A (1989) Variables related to research utilization in nursing: an empirical investigation. *Journal of Advanced Nursing*, 14, 705–710.

Chapman A (1996) Current theory and practice: a study of pre-operative fasting. *Nursing Standard*, 10(18), 33–36.

Charlton B (1993) Medicine and postmodernity. *Journal of the Royal Society of Medicine*, 83, 497–499.

Cimino J A (1996) Why can't we educate doctors to practise preventive medicine? *Preventive Medicine*, 25, 63–65.

Clark E & Sleep J (1991) The what and how of teaching research. *Nurse Education Today*, 11, 172–178.

Cochrane Collaboration (1994) Report. Oxford: UK Cochrane Centre.

Coggans N et al. (1991) National evaluation of drug education in Scotland. Research Monograph No. 4. Scotland: ISDO.

Colby J J, Elder J P, Peterson G, Knisley P M & Carleton R A (1987) Promoting the selection of healthy food through menu item description in a family style restaurant. *American Journal of Preventive Medicine*, 3, 171–177.

Committee on Medical Aspects of Food Policy (1994) Nutritional aspects of cardiovascular disease. Report on health and social subjects No. 46. London: Department of Health.

Contento I (1995) The effectiveness of nutrition education and implications for nutrition education in policy, programs and research: a review of research. *Journal of Nutrition Education*, 27, 279–420.

Coombs P H & Ahmed M (1974) Attacking rural poverty. How non-formal education can help. Baltimore: Johns Hopkins University Press.

Cooper C L & Payne R (1990) Causes, coping and consequences of stress at work. Chichester: John Wiley.

Cooper H M (1989) Integrating research: a guide for literature reviews. Second Edition. London: Sage.

Coulson-Thomas C (Ed) (1996) Business process re-engineering: myth and reality. London: Kogan Page.

Council for the Education and Training of Health Visitors (1977) An investigation into the principles of health visiting. London: CETHV.

Cox B D, Blaxter M, Buckle A L J, Fenner N P, Golding J F, Gore M, Huppert F A, Nickson J, Roth Sir M, Stark J, Wadsworth M E J & Whichelow M (1987) The health and lifestyle survey. London: Health Promotion Research Trust.

Cox B D, Huppert F A & Whichelow M J (Eds) (1993) The Health and Lifestyle Survey: seven years on. Aldershot: Dartmouth Publishing Company Ltd.

Crossthwaite C & Curtice L (1994) Disseminating research results – the challenge of bridging the gap between health research and health action. *Health Promotion International*, 9, 289–296.

Currie C & Todd J (1990) Health behaviours and health indicators in schoolchildren in central region: a profile of the region and evaluation of two health promotion projects: a survey conducted as part of the Scottish WHO health behaviour in school age children. Edinburgh: The University of Edinburgh.

Dam J T (1996) Healthy research in cities: a case study on the translation of health research into action in the Netherlands. *Health Promotion International*, 11(4), 265–276.

Darbyshire P (1986) Body image – when the face doesn't fit. *Nursing Times*, 82(39), 28–30.

Davidson C et al. (1995) A report of a working group of the British Cardiac Society: cardiac rehabilitation services in the United Kingdom. *British Heart Journal*, 73, 201–202.

Davis-Chervin D, Rogers T & Clark M (1985) Influencing food selection with point of choice nutrition information. *Journal of Nutrition Education*, 17, 18–22.

Dean K (1998) Measuring health behaviour and health: towards new health promotion indicators. *Health Promotion*, 3(1), 13–21.

De Haes W & Schurman J H (1975) Results of an evaluation study of three drug education methods. *International Journal of Health Education*, 18, 1–16.

Deitchman S J (1976) Best-laid schemes: a tale of social research and bureaucracy. Cambridge, MA: MIT Press.

DeLorgeril M et al. (1994) Mediterranean alpha-linolenic acid-rich diet in the secondary prevention of coronary heart disease. *The Lancet*, 343, 1454.

Dennehy A, Smith L & Harker P (1996) Not to be ignored: young people, poverty and health. London: Child Poverty Action Group.

Denscombe M & Aubrook L (1992) 'It's just another piece of schoolwork': the ethics of questionnaire research on pupils in schools. *British Educational Research Journal*, 18, 113–131.

Denton S & Baum M (1983) Psychological aspects of breast cancer. In: R Margalese (Ed.), Contemporary issues in clinical oncology. London: Churchill Livingstone.

Department for Education (1994) Circular 5/94. Education Act 1993: Sex Education in Schools. London: DfE.

Department for Education (1996) 1996 Education Act. London: HMSO.

Department for Education and Science (1988) The Education Reform Act. London: HMSO.

Department of Health (1989) Working for patients. London: HMSO.

Department of Health (1992) The Health of the Nation: a strategy for health in England. London: HMSO.

Department of Health (1993) The Health of the Nation – targeting practice – The contribution of nurses, midwives and health visitors. London: The Stationery Office.

Department of Health (1998) Our Healthier Nation. London: HMSO.

Denzin N & Lincoln Y (1994) Handbook of qualitative research. London: Sage.

Derogatis L R (1983) SCL-90-R. Towson Clinical Psychometric Research.

Desharnais R, Bouillon J & Godin G (1986) Self-efficacy and outcome expectations as determinants of exercise adherence. *Psychological Reports*, 59, 1155–1159.

Dewey J (1916) Democracy and education. An introduction to the philosophy of education. New York: Free Press.

Dewey J (1933) How we think. A restatement of the relation of reflective thinking to the educative process. Boston: D.C. Heath.

DiClemente C C, Prochaska J O, Fairhurst K S, Velicer W F, Velasquez M M & Rossi J S (1991) The process of smoking cessation: an analysis of pre-contemplation, contemplation and preparation stages of change. *Journal of Consulting and Clinical Psychology*, 59, 295–304.

Director of Health Care (1995) Dear Doctor letter. London: HM Prison Service.

Director of Public Health (1996) A profile of Shropshire. Shropshire: Shropshire Health.

Directorate of Health Care (1991) Circular instruction 30/91. HIV and AIDS: prison service policy and practice in England and Wales. London: HM Prison Service.

Directorate of Policy and Strategy (1995) Drug misuse in prison. London: HM Prison Service.

Directorate of Prison Medical Services (1990) HIV and AIDS: a multi disciplinary approach in the prison environment. London: HM Prison Service.

Dockrell W B (1982) The contribution of national surveys of achievement to policy formation. In: D B P Kallen et al. (Eds), Social science research and policy making (pp 55–74). Windsor: NFER-Nelson.

Dolan K (1997) Health promotion in prison. In Report of the Third European Conference on Drugs and HIV Services in Prisons. London: Cranstoun Drug Services.

Dorling D (1997) Death in Britain: how local mortality rates have changed – 1950s to 1990s. York: York Publishing Services.

Dorn N & Murji K (1992) Drug prevention: a review of the English language literature. Research Monograph No. 5. London: ISDD.

Downie R S, Fyfe C & Tannahill A (1997) Health promotion, models and values. Second edition. Oxford: Oxford University Press.

Dunne N (1994) Acting for health, acting against HIV. A report on the effectiveness of theatre in health education in HIV and AIDS education. Birmingham: The Theatre in Health Education Trust.

Ealy C D (1995) The women's book of creativity. Dublin: Gill and MacMillan.

Eaton L (1994) Health and young offenders. *Nursing Times*, 90(24), 32–33.

Effective Healthcare (1993) Brief interventions and alcohol use. Bulletin No. 7.

Egan G (1975) The skilled helper: a model for systematic helping and interpersonal relating. Monterey, CA: Brooks/Cole.

Ekins P (1994) Wealth beyond measure: an atlas of new economics. London: Gaia Books Limited.

Elliot M, Lau J et al. (1992) A comparison of results of meta-analyses and randomised control trials and recommendations of clinical experts. *Journal of the American Medical Association*, 268, 240–248.

Ellis J, Mulligan I, Rowe J & Sackett D L (1995) Inpatient general medicine is evidence based. *The Lancet*, 346, 407–412.

Ellison R C, Goldberg R J, Witschi J C, Capper A L, Puleo E M & Stare F J (1990) Use of fat modified food products to change dietary fat intake of young people. *American Journal of Public Health*, 80, 1374–1376.

ECHHO (1997) European Clearing Houses on Health Outcomes Conference: Outcomes measures make sense – do they make a difference? International Meeting in Linkoping, Sweden 12–13 June.

Evans R (1994) Why are some people healthy and others not? The determinants of health of populations. New York: De Gruyter.

Ewles L, Miles U & Velleman G (1996) Lessons learnt from a community heart disease prevention project. *Journal of the Institute of Health Education*, 34(1), 15–19.

Ewles L & Simnett I (1998) Promoting health: a practical guide. Fourth edition. London: Baillière Tindall.

Fairbairns J (1991) Plugging the gap in training needs analysis. *Personnel Management*, February, 43–45.

Fairclough N (1989) Language and power. London: Longman.

Fallowfield L & Clark A (1991) Breast cancer. London: Tavistock/Routledge.

Farnon C (1981) Let's offer employees a healthier diet. *Journal of Occupational Medicine*, 23, 273–276.

Fava J L, Velicer W F & Prochaska J O (1995) Applying the transtheoretical model to a representative sample of smokers. *Addictive Behaviors*, 20(2), 189–203.

Fine M (1988) Sexuality, schooling and adolescent females: the missing discourse of desire. *Harvard Educational Review*, 58, 29–93.

Fink A (Ed) (1995) The survey kit. London: Sage.

Fischler C (1988) Cuisines and food selection. In: Food acceptability (pp 193–206). London: Elsevier.

Fishbein M & Ajzen I (1985) Belief, attitude, intention and behaviour: an introduction to theory and research. Reading, MA: Addison-Wesley.

Fisher C (1986) On demand breastfeeding. *Midwife Health Visitor and Community Nurse*, 22, 194–198.

Fletcher S (1991) Designing competence-based training. London: Kogan Page.

Ford P & Walsh M (1994) New rituals for old: nursing through the looking glass. Oxford: Butterworth-Heinemann.

Fox N (1991) Postmodernism, rationality and the evaluation of health care. *Sociological Review*, 39, 709–744.

France A & Wiles P (1996) The Youth Action Scheme. London: Department for Education and Employment.

French B (1998) Developing the skills for evidence-based practice. *Nurse Education Today*, 18, 46–51.

Friere P (1972) Pedagogy of the oppressed. Harmondsworth: Penguin.

Fullan M G (1991) The new meaning of educational change. London: Cassell.

Furrell R, Oldfield K & Speller V (1995) Towards healthier alliances. London: Health Education Authority.

Galli N (1978) Foundations and principles of health promotion. Chichester: John Wiley.

Genius S J & Genius S K (1995) Adolescent sexual involvement: time for primary prevention. *The Lancet*, 345, 240–241.

Georgensen D & Del-Gaizo E (1984) Maximise the return on your training investment through needs analysis. *Training and Development Journal*, 38(8), 42–47.

Glanz K & Seewald-Klein T (1986) Nutrition at the worksite: an overview. *Journal of Nutrition Education*, 18, S1–S16.

Glaser B G & Strauss A L (1967) The discovery of grounded theory: strategies for qualitative research. New York: Aldine Publishing.

Glense C & Peshkin A (1992) Becoming qualitative researchers. London: Longman.

Goldberg D (1978) Manual of the GHQ. Windsor: National Foundation for Educational Research.

Goodman D et al. (1997) Designing a systems thinking intervention: a strategy for leveraging change. Cambridge, MA: Pegasus Communications, Inc.

Gordon J (1995) Home alone: an evaluation of the effectiveness of support groups for mothers. Unpublished Masters thesis.

Gordon J, Robertson R & Swan M (1995a) 'Babies don't come with a set of instructions': running support groups for mothers. *Health Visitor*, 68(4), 155–156.

Gordon J, Robertson R & Swan M (1995b) Support groups for high-dependency mothers in an inner city area of high deprivation. In: D R Trent & C A Reed (Eds), Promotion of mental health. Volume 4. Aldershot: Avebury.

Gott M & O'Brien M (1990) The role of the nurse in health promotion. *Health Promotion International*, 5, 2.

Gottleib N H, Galavotti C, McCuan R S & McAlister A L (1990) Specification of a social cognitive model predicting smoking cessation in a Mexican-American population. A prospective study. *Cognitive Therapy and Research*, 14, 529–542.

Gough B (1998) Men and the discursive reproduction of sexism: repertoires of difference and equality. *Feminism and Psychology*, 8(1), 25–49.

Graham H (1996) Researching women's health work: a study of the lifestyles of mothers on income support. In: P Bywaters & E McLeod (Eds), Working for equality in health (pp 161–178). London: Routledge.

Graham J & Bennett T (1995) Crime prevention strategies in Europe and North America. European Institute of Crime Prevention and Control Publications Series (28). New York: Criminal Justice Press.

Graham J & Bowling B (1995) Young people and crime. Home Office Research Study (145). London: Home Office Research and Statistics Directorate.

Gray A M, Bowman G S & Thompson D R (1997) The cost of cardiac rehabilitation services in England and Wales. *Journal of the Royal College of Physicians of London*, 31, 57–61.

Gray J & Muir A (1997) Evidence based healthcare. How to make health policy and management decisions. London: Churchill Livingstone.

Greater Glasgow Health Board (1996) Springburn parenting groups phase two: working with health visitors 'It Made Perfect Sense'. Unpublished Report. Glasgow: Health Promotion Department, Greater Glasgow Health Board.

Grossmann R & Scala K (1994) Health promotion and organisational development. Developing settings for health. European Health promotion Series No. 2, Vienna: WHO.

Guibord A (1917) Physical states of criminal women. *Journal of the American Institute of Criminal Law and Criminology*, 8, 82–95.

Haglund B, Weisbrod R R & Bracht N (1990) Assessing the community. Its services, needs, leadership and readiness. In: N Bracht (Ed), Health promotion at the community level (pp 91–108). Newbury Park, CA: Sage.

Haines A & Jones R (1994) Implementing findings of research. *British Medical Journal*, 308, 1488–1492.

Hallet-Carr E (1989) The historian and his facts: lectures from Trinity College Cambridge, 1961. In: R Comley et al. (Eds), Fields of writing: readings across the disciplines. New York: St Martin's Press.

Hamilton A (1995) Dudley 1995 Health File. The Annual Report of the Director of Public Health. Dudley: Dudley Health Authority.

Handy C (1985) Understanding organisations. Third edition. Harmondsworth: Penguin.

Handy C (1995) The empty raincoat: making sense of the future. London: Arrow Books.

Harding, T W & Schaller G (1992) AIDS policy for prisons or for prisoners? In: J M Dann, D J M Tarantola & T W Netter (Eds), AIDS in the world. Cambridge, MA: Harvard University Press.

Harris R (1992) Crime, criminal justice and the Probation service. London: Routledge & Kegan Paul.

Hart D & Webster R (1991) The revolving door stops: the Criminal Justice Act – new opportunities for drug users. London: SCODA.

Harvey L (1990) Critical social research. London: Unwin Hyman.

Hasenfield Y (Ed) (1992) Human devices as complex organisations. London: Sage.

Hawe P, Degeling D & Hall J (1991) Evaluating health promotion: a health worker's guide. Sydney: McLennan and Petty.

Hayes M & Willms S (1990) Healthy community indicators: the perils of the search and the paucity of the find. *Health Promotion International*, 5(2), 161–166.

Health Education Authority (1989) Diet, nutrition and 'healthy eating' in low income groups. London: HEA.

Health Education Authority (1994) Physical activity promotion in primary health care in England. London: HEA.

Health Education Authority (1996) The national catering initiative. Offering the consumer a choice. London: HEA.

Health Education Authority (1997) Promoting health through primary health care nursing: guide to quality indicators. London: HEA.

Health Education Authority (1997) Eight guidelines for a healthy diet. A guide for nutrition educators. London: HEA.

Health Education Board for Scotland (1997) Indicators for health education in Scotland. Edinburgh: Health Education Board for Scotland.

Health Visitors Association (1992) Principles into practice. London: Health Visitors Association.

Health Visitors Association (1992) The principles of health visiting: a re-examination. London: Health Visitors Association.

Health at Work in the NHS (1995) Working for health: a practical guide to developing a healthy workplace in the NHS. London: Health Education Authority.

Health at Work in the NHS (1995) Organisational stress in the National Health Service: an intervention designed to enable staff to address organisational sources of work-related stress. London: Health Education Authority.

Health at Work in the NHS (1996) Organisational stress: planning and implementing a programme to address organisational stress in the NHS. London: OPUS/HEA.

Heather N (1994) Interpreting the evidence on brief interventions for excessive drinkers: the need for caution. *Alcohol and Alcoholism*, 30(3), 287–296.

Heisenburg W (1927) Quoted in: Hallet-Carr E, The historian and his facts. Lectures from Trinity College, Cambridge, 1961. In: C Comley et al. (Eds) (1989) Fields of writing: reading across the disciplines. New York: St Martin's Press.

Hendry L, Shucksmith J & Philip K (1995) Educating for health: school and community approaches with adolescents. London: Cassell.

Henwood K L & Pidgeon N F (1993) Qualitative research and psychological theorising. In: M Hammersley (Ed), Social research: philosophy, politics and practice. London: Sage.

Henze R C (1992) Informal teaching and learning. A study of everyday cognition in a Greek community. Hillsdale, NJ: Lawrence Erlbaum.

Heritage J (1984) Garfinkel and ethnomethodology. Cambridge: Polity Press.

Hertzman C (1996) What's been said and what's been hid: population health, global consumption and the role of national health data. In: D Blane, E Brunner & R Wilkinson (Eds), Health and social organization: towards a health policy for the 21st century. London: Routledge.

Hesketh A, Lindsay G & Harden R (1995) Interactive health promotion in the community pharmacy. *Health Education Journal*, 54(3), 294–303.

Heyes J & King G (1996) Care and control: implementing a prison drug strategy. *Druglink*, pp 8–10. London: ISDD.

Hicks C (1994) Bridging the gap between research and practice in assessments of the value of a study day in developing critical research reading skills in midwives. *Midwifery*, 10, 18–25.

Hicks C, Hennessy D, Cooper J & Barwell F (1996) Investigating attitudes to research in primary health care teams. *Journal of Advanced Nursing*, 24, 1033–1041.

Higginbottom G (1994) A preliminary study into the effects of using a family health assessment tool. Unpublished thesis. Sheffield: Sheffield Hallam University.

Hirst P H (1974) Knowledge and the curriculum: a collection of philosophical papers. London: Routledge and Kegan Paul.

Hodgson R & Abbasi T (1995) Effective mental health promotion: literature review. Cardiff: Health Promotion Wales.

Hofstede G (1981) Culture and organisations. *International Studies of Management and Organisation*, X(4), 15–41.

Hofstede G (1983) The cultural relativity of organisational practices and theories. *Journal of International Business Studies*, Fall, 75–89.

Holland J, Romanzanoglu C & Scott S (1990) Managing risk and experiencing danger: tensions between government AIDS education policy and young women's sexuality. *Gender and Education*, 2(2), 125–146.

Horgan J et al. (1992) Working party report on cardiac rehabilitation. *British Heart Journal*, 67, 412–418.

Horn D & Waingrow S (1966) Some dimensions of a model for smoking behaviour change. *American Journal of Public Health*, 56, 21–26.

Hovland C I, Janis I L & Kelley H H (1963) Communication and persuasion. Yale: Yale University Press.

Hudson F & Manderfield M (1996) Vinney Green PSE Programme. Unpublished report. Bristol: Vinney Green Secure Unit.

Hudson F & West J (1996) Needing to be heard: the young person's agenda. *Education and Health*, 14(3), 43–47.

Hughes J A (1976) Sociological analysis: methods of delivery. London: Nelson.

Hung J et al. (1994) Changes in rest and exercise myocardial perfusion and left ventricular function 3 to 26 weeks after clinically uncomplicated acute myocardial infarction. *American Journal of Cardiology*, 54, 943–950.

Hung P (1992) Pre-operative fasting. *Nursing Times*, 88(48), 57–60.

Hunt M (1987) The process of translating research findings into nursing practice. *Journal of Advanced Nursing*, 12, 101–110.

Hunt S M (1993) The relation between research and policy: translating knowledge into action. In: J K Davies and M P Kelly (Eds), Healthy cities; research and practice. London: Routledge.

Hunt S M (1998) Measuring health behaviour and health: towards new health promotion indicators. *Health Promotion*, 3(1), 23–34.

Hunt S M & Macleod M (1987) Health and behavioural change: some lay perspectives. *Community Medicine*, 9, 68–76.

Huskins J (1996) Quality work with young people. London: Youth Clubs UK.

Ingham R (1991) Beliefs and behaviour: filling the void. Paper presented at ERSC sponsored seminar. 'Young People and Aids', March.

Ingham R (1993) Can we have a policy on sex? Setting targets for teenage pregnancies. Occasional paper. Institute of Health Policy Studies, University of Southampton.

Ingham R (1997) When you're young and in love. Southampton: University of Southampton.

Ingham R, Woodcock A & Stenner K (1991) Getting to know you: young people's knowledge of partners at first intercourse. *Journal of Community and Applied Social Research*, 1(2), 117–132.

Inglis B, Duffield J, Low L & Morris B (1996) Devising methods to assess training needs of health promoters in Scottish Area Health Boards. Final report for the Health Education Board for Scotland. Stirling: University of Stirling, Department of Education.

Jacobson L D & Wilkinson C E (1994) Review of teenage health: time for a new direction. *British Journal of General Practice*, 44, 420–424.

Janis I L & Mann L (1977) Decision making: a psychological analysis of conflict, choice and commitment. New York: Free Press.

Jeffery R W, French S A, Raether C & Baxter J E (1994) An environmental intervention to increase fruit and salad purchases in a cafeteria. *Preventive Medicine*, 23, 788–792.

Jeffs T & Smith M K (Eds) (1996) Using informal education. An alternative to casework, teaching and control? Milton Keynes: Open University Press.

Jeffs T & Smith M K (1996) Informal education – conversation, democracy and learning. Ticknall: Education Now Books.

Jeffs T & Smith M K (1999) 'Tainted money': ethical dilemmas in the funding of youth and community work. In: S Banks (Ed), The ethics of youth work. London: Routledge.

Jelinek M (1992) The clinician and the randomised control trial. In: J Daly, I McDonald and E. Willis (Eds), Researching health care: designs, dilemmas, disciplines (pp 76–89). London: Tavistock/Routledge.

Jenkins R (1985) Minor psychiatric morbidity in employed young men and women and its contribution to sickness absence. *British Journal of Industrial Medicine*, 42, 147–154.

Jenkins R, MacDonald A, Murray J & Strathdee G (1982) Minor psychiatric morbidity and the threat of redundancy in a professional group. *Psychological Medicine*, 12, 799–807.

Johnson D W & Johnson P F (1991) Joining together: group theory and group skills. London: Prentice Hall.

Jones A et al. (1995) Probation practice. London: Pitman.

Kanter R M (1993) Men and women of the corporation. New York: Basic Books.

Kelly J, St Lawrence J et al. (1992) Community AIDS/HIV risk reduction: the efforts of endorsement by popular people in three cities. *American Journal of Public Health*, 82, 1483–1489.

Kemm J & Booth D (1992) Promotion of healthier eating (pp 11–15). London: HMSO.

Kemm J & Close A (1995) Health promotion theory and practice (p 162). London: Macmillan.

Kendall S (1997) What do we mean by evidence? Implications for primary health care nursing. *Journal of Interprofessional Care*, 11(1), 23–34.

Kickbusch I (1989) Good planets are hard to find. WHO Healthy Cities Papers No. 5. Geneva: WHO.

Kim D (1994) Systems thinking tools: a user's reference guide. Cambridge, MA: Pegasus Communications, Inc.

King J C, Achinapura S & VanHorn L (1983) Nutrition in the workplace. *Journal of Nutrition Education*, 15, 59–64.

Kirby D (1995) Editorial. *British Medical Journal*, 311, 7002.

Kirkham M (1997) Reflection in midwifery: professional narcissism or seeing with women? *British Journal of Midwifery*, 5(5), 259–262.

Kitson A, Ahmed L B, Harvey G, Seers K & Thompson D R (1996) From research to practice: one organisational model for promoting research-based practice. *Journal of Advanced Nursing*, 23, 430–440.

Knorr K D (1977) Policymaker's use of social science knowledge: symbolic or instrumental? In: C H Weiss (Ed), Using social research in policymaking (pp 165–182). Lexington, MA: Lexington Books.

Kok G, van den Borne B & Mullen P (1997) Effectiveness of health education and health promotion: meta-analyses of effect studies and determinants of effectiveness. *Patient Education and Counselling*, 30(1), 19–27.

Kroutil L A & Eng E (1989) Conceptualizing and assessing potential for community participation: a planning method. *Health Education Research*, 4, 305–319.

Krueger R A (1994) Focus groups: a practical guide for applied research. London: Sage.

Lally J R, Mangione P L, Honig A S & Wittner D S (1988) More pride, less delinquency: findings from the ten-year follow-up study of the Syracuse University Development Research Program. *Zero-to-three*, 8(4), 13–18.

Lambert M J, Shapiro D A & Bergin A E (1986) The effectiveness of psychotherapy. In: S L Garfield & A E Bergin (Eds), Handbook of psychotherapy and behaviour change. Third edition. New York: John Wiley.

Lambert T (1996) The power of influence: intensive influencing skills at work. London: Nicholas Brealey Publishing.

Lansdown G (1996) A model for action: the Children's Rights Development Unit. Promoting the Convention on the Rights of the Child in the United Kingdom. London: Unicef.

Larson-Brown L B (1978) Point of purchase information on vended foods. *Journal of Nutrition Education*, 10, 116–118.

Lave J & Wenger E (1991) Situated learning: legitimate, peripheral participation. Cambridge: Cambridge University Press.

Lawrence R, Friedman G, DeFriese G et al. (1989) Guide to clinical preventive services: an assessment of the effectiveness of 169 interventions – report of the US Preventive Services Task Force. Maryland: Williams & Wilkins.

Leathwood P (1990) Food intake and food choice. In: Why we eat what we eat (pp 50–59). London: British Nutrition Foundation.

Lee C (1983) The ostrich position: sex, schooling and mystification. London: Unwin.

Lee C (1993) Talking tough: the fight for masculinity. London: Arrow Books.

Lee R (1996) How to find information: medicine and biology: a guide to searching the sources. London: British Library Science Reference and Information Service.

Lees S (1993) Sugar and spice: sexuality and adolescent girls. London: Penguin.

Leff N (1985) The use of policy science tools in public sector decision-making: social benefit–cost analysis in the World Bank. *Kyklos*, 37, 60–76.

Leighton-Beck L (1997) Networking: putting research at the heart of professional practice. *British Journal of Nursing*, 6(2), 120–122.

Leyden R, Gobel F & Killoran A (Eds) (1990) Health and lifestyle surveys: towards a common approach. London: Health Education Authority.

Liddell J A, Lockie G M & Wise A (1992) Effects of a nutrition education programme on the dietary habits of a population of students and staff at a centre for higher education. *Journal of Human Nutrition and Dietetics*, 5, 23–33.

Liddiard P (1988) Milton Keynes Felt Needs project. Milton Keynes: Open University Press.

Limb M (1996) Health of the nation under scrutiny. *Health Service Journal*, 106(5529), 8.

Lipsey M, Crosse S et al. (1985) Evaluation: the state of the art and the sorry state of the science. *New Directions for Programme Evaluation*, 27, 7–28.

Lipsky M (1980) Street-level bureaucracy: dilemmas of the individual in public services. New York: Russell Sage.

Loggie J, Jordan C & Dicks A (1996) Signposts to health: findings from the health-related behaviour survey. Jarrow: South Tyneside Health Commission.

Long A (1995) Assessing health and social outcomes. In: J Popay & G Williams (Eds), Researching the people's health (pp 157–182). London: Routledge.

Luck M & Jesson J (1996) Evaluation of community health development. Bath: Community Health UK.

Luker K & Kenrick M (1992) An exploratory study of the sources of influence on the clinical decisions of community nurses. *Journal of Advanced Nursing*, 17, 457–466.

Macdonald G, Veen C & Tones K (1996) Evidence for success in health promotion: suggestions for improvement. *Health Education Research, Theory and Practice*, 11, 367–376.

Macfarlane A (1993) Health promotion and children and teenagers (editorial). *British Medical Journal*, 306, 81.

MacVicar M H (1998) Intellectual development and research: student nurses' and student midwives' accounts. *Journal of Advanced Nursing*, 27, 1305–1316.

Maguire G P, Lee E G, Bevington D J, Kuchemann C S, Crabtree R J & Cornell C E (1978) Psychiatric problems in the first year after mastectomy. *British Medical Journal*, 1, 963–965.

Maguire J H (1990) Putting nursing research findings into practice: research utilisation as an aspect of the management of change. *Journal of Advanced Nursing*, 16, 614–620.

Mair G (1988) Probation day centres. London: HMSO.

Management Charter Initiative (1997) Management standards. London: Management Charter Initiative.

Mann T (1986) A guide to library research methods. New York: Oxford University Press.

Manne S L, Girasek D & Ambrosino J (1994) An evaluation of the impact of a cosmetics class on breast cancer patients. *Journal of Psychiatric Oncology*, 12(1/2), 83–97.

Marlatt G A, Baer J S, Donovan D M & Divlahan D R (1988) Addictive behaviour: etiology and treatment. *Annual Review of Psychology*, 39, 223–252.

Marmot M (1996) The social pattern of health and disease. In: D Blane, E Brunner & R Wilkinson (Eds), Health and social organization: towards a health policy for the 21st century. London: Routledge.

Martindale K (1997) Using the library. In: S Maslin-Prothero (Ed), Study skills for nurses. London: Ballière Tindall.

May A (1996) Forward thinking. *Health Service Journal*, 106(5510), 12–13.

Mayer J A et al. (1986) Promoting low-fat entree choices in a public cafeteria. *Journal of Applied Behavior Analysis*, 19, 397–402.

Mays N & Pope C (Eds) (1996) Qualitative research in health care. London: BMJ Publishing Group.

McBride C M & Pirie P L (1990) Post partum relapse. *Addictive Behaviour*, 15, 165–168.

McEwan R T, Bhopal R & Patton W (1991) Drama on HIV and AIDS: an evaluation of a theatre in education programme. *Health Education Journal*, 50(4), 155–160.

McFadden M (1994) Female sexuality in the second decade of AIDS. Unpublished PhD thesis. Belfast: School of Psychology, Queen's University.

McInerney D & Cooper C (1989) Profiting from healthy staff. *Sunday Times*, 3 September.

McLeod J (1994) Doing counselling research. London: Sage.

Meakin R P & Lloyd M H (1996) Disease prevention and health promotion: a study of medical students and teachers. *Medical Education*, 30, 97–104.

Meerabeau L (1995) The nature of practitioner knowledge. In: K Reed & S Proctor (Eds), Practitioner research in health care: the inside story. London: Chapman & Hall.

Mellanby A R, Phelps F A, Crichton N J & Tripp J H (1995) School sex education: an experimental programme with educational and medical benefit. *British Medical Journal*, 311, 414–420.

Meredith P, Emberton M & Wood C (1995) New directions in information for patients. *British Medical Journal*, 311, 4–5.

Meyrick J (Ed) (1997) Reviews of effectiveness: their contribution to evidence-based practice and purchasing in health promotion. Conference Proceedings. London: Health Education Authority.

Meyrick J & Gillies P (1998) Recognising the contribution of qualitative studies to systematic reviews and the search for evidence in health promotion: not widening the goal posts but changing the field of play (unpublished consultation paper). London: Health Education Authority.

Mikkelsen B (1995) Methods for development work and research. London: Sage.

Milburn K, Fraser E, Secker J & Pavis S (1995) Combining methods in health promotion research: some considerations about appropriate use. *Health Education Journal*, 54(3), 347–356.

Milburn T, Clark J, Forde L, Fulton K, Locke A & MacQuarrie E (1995) Curriculum development in youth work. Edinburgh: Scottish Office Education Department.

Milgram S (1965) Some conditions of obedience and disobedience to authority. *Human Relations*, 18(1), 57–76.

Miller W R & Rollnick S (Eds) (1991) Motivational Interviewing. London: Guildford Press.

Mistry T (1989) Establishing a feminist model of groupwork in the Probation service. *Groupwork*, 2(2), 145–158.

Mock J (1989) Healthy eating – caterers' response. *Nutrition and Food Science*, July/August, 6–9.

Morse J M & Field P A (1985) Nursing research: the application of qualitative approaches. London: Croom Helm.

Muir Gray J A (1997) Evidence-based health care: how to make health policy and management decisions. New York: Churchill Livingstone.

Mullen P D, Quinn V P & Ershoff D H (1990) Maintenance of non-smoking post partum by women who stopped smoking during pregnancy. *American Journal of Public Health*, 80, 992–994.

Mullings C (1985) Group interviewing. University of Sheffield: CRUS.

Mulrow C (1995) Rationale for systematic reviews. In: I Chalmers & D Altman (Eds), Systematic reviews. London: BMJ Publishing Group.

Naidoo J & Wills J (1994) Health promotion: foundations for practice. London: Baillière Tindall.

Naismith L D et al. (1979) Psychological rehabilitation after myocardial infarction. *British Medical Journal*, 1, 439–446.

National Consumer Council (1992) Your food: whose choice? (pp 1–26). London: HMSO.

Nettleton S & Burrows R (1997) Knit your own without a pattern: health promotion specialists in an internal market. *Social Policy and Administration*, 31(2), 191–201.

Nettleton S & Burrows R (1997) If health promotion is everybody's business what is the fate of the health promotion specialist? *Sociology of Health and Illness*, 19(1), 23–47.

Newburn T & Stanko E (Eds) (1994) Just boys doing business. London: Routledge.

Newell D (1992) Randomised controlled trials in health care research. In: J Daly et al. (Eds), Researching health care: designs, dilemmas, disciplines (pp 47–61). London: Routledge.

Newell S (1995) The healthy organisation. London: Routledge.

NHS Centre for Research and Dissemination (1996) Undertaking systematic reviews of research on effectiveness: CDR guidelines for those carrying out or commissioning reviews. NHS Centre for Research and Dissemination, University of York.

NHS Confederation (1997) The people's health service? NHS Confederation, Birmingham.

NHS Executive (1993) The Health of the Nation: a health strategy for England. London: HMSO.

NHS Executive (1994) Health promoting hospitals. London: Department of Health.

NHS Executive (1996) Clinical guidelines. London: HMSO.

NHS Executive (1996) NHSE aims and objectives. London: Macmillan.

NHS Executive (1996) Primary care led NHS: briefing pack. London: NHSE.

NHS Executive (1997) The new NHS: modern and dependable. London: HMSO.

NHS Executive North West (1994) Strategic statement. Warrington: NHSE NW.

Norton L S, Morgan K & Thomas S (1995) The ideal-self inventory: a new measure of self-esteem. *Counselling Psychology Quarterly*, 8(4), 305–310.

Nottingham Community Health (1992) Your family's health. Nottingham: Nottingham Community Health.

Nutbeam D (1996) Achieving 'best practice' in health promotion: improving the fit between research and practice. *Health Education Research*, 11(3), 317–326.

Nutbeam D (1998) Evaluating health promotion: progress, problems and solutions. *Health Promotion International*, 13(1), 27–44.

Nutbeam D, Smith C et al. (1993) Maintaining evaluation designs in long term community based health promotion. *Journal of Epidemiology and Community Health*, 47, 127–133.

Nutbeam D, Macaskill P, Smith C, Simpson J M & Catford J (1993) Evaluation of two school smoking education programmes under normal classroom conditions. *British Medical Journal*, 306, 102–107.

Nutbeam D, Smith C & Catford J (1990) Evaluation in health education: a review of progress, possibilities and problems. *Journal of Epidemiology and Community Health*, 44, 83–89.

Oakley A (1990) Who's afraid of the randomized controlled trial? In: W Roberts (Ed), Women's health counts (pp 167–194). London: Routledge.

Oakley A, Olivers S et al. (1996) Review of effectiveness of health promotion interventions for men who have sex with men. London: EPI Centre, London University Institute of Education.

O'Connor G T et al. (1989) An overview of randomised trials of rehabilitation with exercise after myocardial infarction. *Circulation*, 80, 234.

OFSTED (1997) The contribution of youth services to drug education. London: The Stationery Office.

OFSTED (1997) Inspecting youth work: a revised inspection schedule. London: The Stationery Office.

O'Keefe D (1993) Truancy in English secondary schools. London: Department for Education.

Oldridge N B et al. (1988) Cardiac rehabilitation after myocardial infarction. Combined experience of randomised clinical trials. *Journal of the American Medical Association*, 260, 945–950.

OPCS (1993) Health survey for England. In: The Health of the Nation: Briefing pack. London: Department of Health.

Orlans V (1991) Stress and health in UK organisations: a trade union case study. *Work and Stress*, 5(4), 325–329.

Ornstein R E (1975) The psychology of consciousness. Harmondsworth: Penguin.

Orr J (1992) Assessing individual and family health needs. In: K Luker & J Orr (Eds), Health visiting: towards community health nursing. Oxford: Blackwell.

Ovretveit J (1996) Ethics: a counsel of perfection? *IHSM Network*, 3(13), 4–5.

Owens D K & Nease R F (1993) Development of outcome-based practice guidelines – a method for structuring problems and synthesising evidence. *Journal of Quality Improvement*, 19(7), 249–263.

Parahoo K & Reid N (1988) Research skills: 5. Critical reading of research. *Nursing Times*, 84(43), 69–72.

Patton M Q (1987) How to use qualitative methods in evaluation. London: Sage.

Patton M Q (1997) Utilization-focused evaluation. London: Sage.

Pawson R & Tilley N (1997) Realistic evaluation. London: Sage.

Peckham S (1992) Unplanned pregnancy and teenage pregnancy: a review. Occasional Paper, Institute of Health Policy Studies, University of Southampton.

Penal Affairs Consortium (1997) Crime, drugs and criminal justice. London: Penal Affairs Consortium.

Perkins E R (1987) Good enough evaluation? In: G Campbell (Ed), Health education: youth and community. Lewes: Falmer Press.

Perkins, E R (1992) Teaching research to nurses: issues for tutor training. *Nurse Education Today*, 12, 252–257.

Perkins E R (1998) Public health approaches to family support: how good is the evidence? *British Journal of Community Nursing*, 13(6), 297–302.

Perkins E R & Wright L (1998) Developing research awareness, knowledge and skills amongst health education/promotion specialists and health promoters in Scotland. Final report of Phase 1: Training needs analysis. Edinburgh: Health Promotion Board for Scotland.

Perkins S (1996) HIV and custody. London: The HIV Project.

Perkins S (1997) Prisons. In: K Alcorn (Ed), AIDS reference manual. London: NAM Publications.

Perkins S (1998) Access to condoms for prisoners in the EU. London. National AIDS and Prisons Forum, supported by the European Commission.

Perkins S & Robinson B (1995) AIDS inside and out. London: HM Prison Service.

Perkins S & Robinson B (1995) Talking about AIDS. London: HM Prison Service.

Peters T J & Waterman R H (1982) In search of excellence: lessons from America's best run companies. New York: Harper & Row.

Peterson M & Johnstone B M (1995) The Atwood Hall Health Promotion Program, Federal Medical Center, Lexington, KY. *Journal of Substance Misuse Treatment*, 12(1), 43–48.

Phenix P (1964) Realms of meaning. New York: McGraw-Hill.

Poulter J (1994) Healthy eating at work. London: Health Education Authority.

Poulter J & Torrance I (1993) Food and health – the costs and benefits of a policy approach. *Journal of Human Nutrition and Dietetics*, 6, 89–100.

Power R (1989) Drugs and the media: prevention campaigns and television. In: S MacGregor (Ed), Drugs and British society. London: Routledge.

Price B (1992) Living with altered body image: the cancer experience. *British Journal of Nursing*, 1(13), 641–645.

Priestly P, McGuire J, Flegg D, Hensley V, Wellham D & Barnitt R (1984) Social skills in prisons and the community. London: RKP.

Prochaska J O & DiClemente C C (1983) Transtheoretical therapy: toward a more integrative model of change. *Psychotherapy: Theory, Research and Practice*, 19(3), 276–287.

Prochaska J O & DiClemente C C (1983) Stages and processes of self-change of smoking: toward an integrative model of change. *Journal of Consulting and Clinical Psychology*, 51(3), 390–395.

Prochaska J O & DiClemente C C (1984) The transtheoretical approach: crossing traditional foundations of change. Homewood, IL: Dorsey Press.

Prochaska J O & DiClemente C C (1992) Stages of change in the modification of problem behaviors. In: M Hersen, R M Eisler & P M Miller (Eds), Progress in behavior modification (pp 184–214). Sycamore, IL: Sycamore Press.

Prochaska J O & DiClemente C C (1992) The transtheoretical approach: crossing traditional boundaries of therapy. Malabar, FL: Kreiger Publishing.

Prochaska J O & Norcross J C (1994) Systems of psychotherapy – a transtheoretical analysis. Third Edition. Monterey, CA: Brooks/Cole.

Prochaska J O, DiClemente C C & Norcross J C (1992) In search of how people change. Application to addictive behaviours. *American Psychologist*, 47, 1102–1114.

Prochaska J O, DiClemente C C, Velicer W F, Ginpil S & Norcross J C (1985) Predicting change in smoking status for self-changers. *Addictive Behaviours*, 10, 395–406.

Prochaska J O, DiClemente C C, Velicer W F & Rossi J S (1993) Standardized, individualized, interactive, and personalized self-help programs for smoking cessation. *Health Psychology*, 12, 399–405.

Prochaska J O, Norcross J C & DiClemente C C (1994) Changing for good. New York: Morrow.

Public Health Alliance (1997) Framing the debate: crime and public health. Birmingham: PHA.

Purser R et al. (1989) Drink-related offending. Coventry: Council on Alcohol.

Putnam R D (1993) The prosperous community: social capital and public life. *American Prospect*, 13, 35–42.

Putnam R D, Leonardi R & Nanetti R Y (1993) Making democracy work. Civic traditions in modern Italy. Princeton: Princeton University Press.

Pyorala G et al. (1994) Prevention of coronary heart disease in clinical practice. *European Heart Journal*, 15, 1300.

de Raeve L (1994) Ethical issues in palliative care research. *Palliative Medicine*, 8, 298–305.

Ramsbottom D (1996) Patient or prisoner? A new strategy for health care in prisons. London: Home Office.

Ranade W (1995) From government to governance: implications for health for all. *Health For All News*, 32.

Real World Coalition (1996) The politics of the real world. A major statement of public concern from over 40 of the UK's leading voluntary and campaigning organisations. London: Earthscan.

Reason P & Rowan J (1981) Human inquiry: a sourcebook of new paradigm research. Chichester: John Wiley.

Reed J & Proctor S (1995) Practitioner research in health care: the inside story. London: Chapman & Hall.

Regis D (1996) The voice of children in health education: use of the Just a Tick method to consult children over curriculum content. In: M John (Ed), Children in our charge: the child's right to resources. London: Jessica Kingsley.

Reinharz S (1992) Feminist methods in social research. Oxford: Oxford University Press.

Rennie D L, Phillips J R & Quartaro G K (1988) Grounded theory: a promising approach to conceptualisation in psychology? *Canadian Psychology*, 29(2), 139–150.

Rich R F (1977) Use of social science information by federal bureaucrats: knowledge for action versus knowledge for understanding. In: C H Weiss (Ed), Using social research in policymaking (pp 165–182). Lexington, MA: Lexington Books.

Richmond K (1986) Introducing heart-healthy foods in a company cafeteria. *Journal of Nutrition Education*, 18, S63–S65.

Rifkin S (1990) Community participation in maternal and child health/family planning programmes. Geneva: World Health Organisation.

Robbins S P (1990) Organisation theory, structure, design and applications. Englewood Cliffs, NJ: Prentice Hall.

Roberts H & Beales J G (1993) Responding to the responders: feedback from a postal survey. In: Health education and the mass media. How to communicate effectively (pp 197–201). Amsterdam: Dutch Centre for Health Promotion and Health Education.

Roberts H, Bali B & Rushton L (1996) Non-responders to a lifestyle survey: a study using telephone interviews. *Journal of the Institute of Health Education*, 34, 57–61.

Robertson D (1995) HIV and custody. London: Health Education Authority.

Robinson J & Elkan R (1996) Health needs assessment: theory and practice. London: Churchill Livingstone.

Robinson K (1983) What is health? In: J Clark & J Henderson (Eds), Community health. Edinburgh: Churchill Livingstone.

Roe A (1982) A psychologist examines sixty-four eminent scientists. In: P Vernon (Ed), Creativity. Harmondsworth: Penguin.

Roe L, Hunt P, Bradshaw H & Rayner M (in press) Review of effectiveness of health promotion interventions to promote healthy eating. London: Health Education Authority.

Rogers A, Popay J, Williams G & Latham M (1997) Inequalities in health and health promotion: insights from the qualitative research literature. London: Health Education Authority.

Rolfe G (1994) Towards a new model of nursing research. *Journal of Advanced Nursing*, 19, 969–975.

Rollnick S, Heather N & Bell A (1992) Negotiating behaviour change in medical settings: the development of brief motivational interviewing. *Journal of Mental Health*, 1, 25–37.

Rolls E (1997) Competence in professional practice: some issues and concerns. *Educational Research*, 39(2), 195–210.

Rose G (1993) The strategy of preventive medicine. London: Oxford University Press.

Rose H (1982) Making science feminist. Milton Keynes: Open University Press.

Rosenberg S G (1971) Patient education leads to better care for heart patients. *HSMHA Health Reports*, 86(9), 793–802.

Rosenstock I M (1966) Why people use health services. *Millbank Memorial Fund Quarterly*, 44, 91–121.

Rosenstock I M (1974) The health belief model and preventative health behaviour. *Health Education Monographs*, 2(4), 354–386.

Royal College of Midwives (1988) Successful breastfeeding. London: RCM.

Royal College of Obstetrics and Gynaecology (1991) Report of the RCOG Working Party on unplanned pregnancy. London: RCOG.

Rozin P & Fallon A F (1981) The acquisition of likes and dislikes for foods. In: Criteria of food acceptance (pp 35–48). Zurich: Forster Verlag.

Sackett D L, Rosenberg W M C, Gray J A M, Haynes R B & Richardson W S (1996) Evidence based medicine: what it is and isn't. *British Medical Journal*, 312, 71–72.

Sackett S, Haynes R et al. (1991) Clinical epidemiology: a basic science for clinical medicine. Oxford: Radcliffe Medical Press.

Salant P & Dillman D A (1994) How to conduct your own survey. Chichester: John Wiley.

Sanford N (1981) A model for action research. In: P Reason & J Rowan (Eds), Human inquiry: a sourcebook of new paradigm research. Chichester: John Wiley.

Sanson-Fisher R, Hancock L et al. (1996) Developing methodologies for evaluating community-wide health promotion. *Health Promotion International*, 11(3), 227–236.

Sargant N, Field J, Francis H, Schuller T & Tuckett A (1997) The learning divide. A study of participation in adult learning in the United Kingdom. Leicester: National Institute for Adult Continuing Education.

Schachter S (1982) Recidivism and self-cure of smoking and obesity. *American Psychologist*, 37, 436–444.

Schell C & Rathe R (1992) Meta-analysis: a tool for medical and scientific discoveries. *Bulletin of the Medical Library Association*, 80(3), 219–222.

Schmitz & Fielding (1986) Point of choice nutritional labelling – evaluation in a workplace cafeteria. *Journal of Nutritional Education*, 18, 565–568.

Schon D (1983) The reflective practitioner: how professionals think in action. London: Temple Smith.

Schon D (1987) Educating the reflective practitioner: towards a new design for teaching and learning. San Francisco: Jossey-Bass.

Schramm W (Ed) (1960) Mass communications. Illinois: University of Illinois Press.

Schwartz F W & Bitzer E A (1997) Systems perspective of evaluation in health care. In: A Long & E A Bitzer (Eds), Health outcomes and evaluation: context, concepts and successful applications. Leeds: ECHHO.

Schweinhart L J & Weikhart D P (1993) A summary of significant benefits: the High/Scope Perry Pre-School Study through age 27. Ypsilanti, MI: High/Scope Press.

Scott K (1994) Qualitative research conducted on behalf of the HEA. London: Health Education Authority.

Scriven A & Orme J (Eds) (1996) Health promotion: professional perspectives. Basingstoke: Macmillan/Open University Press.

Secker J, Wimbush E, Watson J & Milburn K (1995) Qualitative methods in health promotion research: some criteria for quality. *Health Education Journal*, 54(1), 74–87.

Secretary of State for Health (1997) The New NHS: modern, dependable. London: The Stationery Office.

Secretary of State for Health (1998) Our Healthier Nation: a contract for health. A Consultation Paper. London: The Stationery Office.

Seedhouse D (1986) Health – the foundations of achievement. New York: John Wiley.

Seedhouse D (1997) Health promotion: philosophy, prejudice and practice. Chichester: John Wiley.

Sex Education Forum (1997a) Factsheet 12, Education Act 1996 – briefing paper on sex education. London: Sex Education Forum.

Sex Education Forum (1997b) Factsheet 13, Sex Education Matters. London: National Children's Bureau.

Shapiro H (1994) Druglink factsheet 6: Drug testing. London: ISDD.

Shapiro S, Skinner E, Kessler L, Cottler L & Regier D (1984) Utilisation of health and mental health services. *Archives of General Psychiatry*, 41, 971–978.

Sharp D & Lowe G (1989) Adolescents and alcohol – a review of the recent British research. *Journal of Adolescence*, 12, 295–307.

Shepherd R (1990) Overview of factors influencing food choice. In: Why we eat what we eat (pp 12–30). London: British Nutrition Foundation.

Shiroyama C, McKee L & McKie L (1995) Evaluating health promotion projects in primary care: recent experiences in Scotland. *Health Education Journal*, 54(2), 226–240.

Silverman D (1987) Communication and medical practice. London: Sage.

Silverman D (1993) Interpreting qualitative data. London: Sage.

Silverman D (1997) Qualitative research: theory, method and practice. London: Sage.

Sim J (1990) Medical power in prisons. Milton Keynes: Open University Press.

Simnett I (1995) Managing health promotion. Chichester: John Wiley.

Simnett I, Jones L, Perkins E R & Wall D (1997) Helping patients change their behaviour: a resource pack for hospital doctors. Birmingham: West Midlands Board of Postgraduate Medical and Dental Education, University of Birmingham, Medical School.

Sivers F (1996) Evidence-based strategies for secondary prevention of coronary heart disease. In: F Sivers (Ed), Cardiology 2000 (p 18). London: Merck Sharpe & Dohme.

Smee C (1995) Introduction. In: Riley et al. Releasing resources to achieve health gain. London: Radcliffe Medical Press.

Smith C & Nutbeam D (1990) Assessing non-response bias: a case-study from the 1985 Welsh Heart Health Survey. *Health Education Research*, 5, 381–386.

Smith G & Cantley C (1985) Assessing health care: a study in organisational evaluation. Milton Keynes: Open University Press.

Smith M (1994) Local education. Buckingham: Open University Press.

Smith M K (1997) Introducing informal education. The informal education homepage, http//:www.infed.org/i-intro.htm

Smith M L, Glass G V & Miller T L (1980) The benefits of psychotherapy. Baltimore: Johns Hopkins University.

Smith P & Cantley R (1985) Assessing health care: a study in organisational evaluation. Milton Keynes: Open University Press.

Smith P (1992) The emotional labour of nursing. Basingstoke: Macmillan.

Smith P (1996) Measuring outcome in the public sector. London: Taylor & Francis.

Snee K (1991) Neighbourhood needs. *Community Outlook*, 1(2), 38–39.

Snyder M P, Story M & Trenkner L L (1992) Reducing fat and sodium in school lunch programs: the LUNCHPOWER! intervention study. *Journal of the American Dietetic Association*, 92, 1087–1091.

Sorenson G, Morris D M, Hunt M K, Hebert J R, Harris D R et al. (1992) Work-site nutrition intervention and employees dietary habits: the Treatwell program. *American Journal of Public Health*, 82, 877–880.

Speller V & Webb D (1997) Looking at the quality of health promotion interventions in the systematic review process: redressing the balance. In: J Meyrick (Ed), Reviews of effectiveness: their contribution to evidence based practice and purchasing in health promotion. London: Health Education Authority.

Speller V, Learnmouth A & Harrison D (1997) The search for evidence of effective health promotion. *British Medical Journal*, 315, 361–363.

Springett J & Dugdill L (1995) Workplace health promotion programmes: towards a framework for evaluation. *Health Education Journal*, 54(1), 88–98.

Springett J, Costongs L & Dugdill L (1995) Towards a framework for evaluation in health promotion: methodology, principles and practice. *The Journal*, Summer, 61–65.

Standing Committee on Postgraduate Medical and Dental Education (SCOPME) (1994) Teaching hospital doctors to teach. London: SCOPME.

Stead M & Hastings G (1995) Developing options for a programme on adolescent smoking in Wales. Technical report no. 16. Cardiff: Health Promotion Wales.

Stevens A & Raftery J (1990) Health care needs assessment. In: Moving forward – needs, services and contracts. A DHA Project Paper. Leeds: NHS Management Executive.

Stewart R (1998) More art than science? *Health Service Journal*, 108, 28–29.

Strauss A & Corbin J (1990) Basics of qualitative research: grounded theory and procedures and techniques. Newbury Park, CA: Sage.

Swanson J M, Albright J, Steirn C, Schaffner A & Costa L (1992) Strategies for teaching nursing research. Program efforts for creating a research environment in a clinical setting. *Western Journal of Nursing Research*, 14(2), 241–245.

Syme S L (1996) To prevent disease: the need for a new approach. In: D Blane, E Brunner & R Wilkinson (Eds), Health and social organization: towards a health policy for the 21st century. London: Routledge.

Tones K & Tilford S (1994) Health promotion: effectiveness, efficiency and equity. London: Chapman & Hall.

Tones B K, Tilford S & Robinson Y K (1989) Health education: effectiveness and efficiency. London: Chapman & Hall.

Toth B (1996) Public participation: an historical perspective. In: C Coast et al. (Eds), Priority setting: the health care debate. London: Routledge.

Towner E, Dowswell T & Jarvis S (1993) Reducing childhood accidents. The effectiveness of health promotion interventions: a literature review. London: Health Education Authority.

Training and Development Lead Body (1995) N/SVQ Level 4: Learning development. Rotherham: Cambertown Ltd.

Tripp J & Mellanby A (1995) Sex education – whose baby? *Current Paediatrics*, 5, 272–276.

Vang J (1997) Swedish policy on the evaluation of hospital performance. Workshop on evaluating hospital effectiveness and efficiency. Milan (Italy) 30 Sept–2 Oct. Geneva: WHO.

Vass A (1990) Alternatives to prison. London: Sage.

Vaughan S, Schumm J S & Sinagub J (1996) Focus group interviews in education and psychology. London: Sage.

de Vaus D A (1991) Surveys in social research. London: George Allen and Unwin.

Veen C, Vereijken A et al (1994) An instrument for analysing effectiveness studies on health promotion and health education. Development, use and recommendations. Utrecht: International Union for Health Promotion and Health Education.

Velicer W F, DiClemente C C, Prochaska J O & Brandenburg N (1985) A decisional balance measure for assessing and predicting smoking status. *Journal of Personality and Social Psychology*, 48, 1279–1289.

Velicer W F, Rossi J S, Ruggiero L & Prochaska J O (1994) Minimal interventions appropriate for an entire population of smokers. In: R Richmond (Ed), Interventions for smokers: an international perspective (pp 69–92). Baltimore: Williams and Wilkins

Wadsworth Y (1984) Do it yourself social research. Melbourne, Australia: Victoria Council of Social Services.

Wagner D (1997) The new temperance: the American obsession with sin and vice. Boulder, CL: Westview Press.

Wagner J L & Winett R A (1988) Promoting one low fat high fiber selection in a fast food restaurant. *Journal of Applied Behavior Analysis*, 21, 179–185.

Walker R (1985) Applied qualitative research. Aldershot: Gower.

Walsh D (1996) Evidence-based practice: whose evidence and on what basis? *British Journal of Midwifery*, 4(9), 454–457.

Walshe K & Ham C (1997) Who's acting on the evidence. *Health Service Journal*, 107(5547), 22–25.

Wang W T (1994) The educational needs of myocardial infarction patients. *Rehabilitation*, 9(4), 28–36.

Warr P B (1987) Work, unemployment and mental health. Oxford: Oxford University Press.

Weare K (1986) What do medical teachers understand by health promotion? *Health Education Journal*, 45(4), 235–238.

Weare K (1992) The contribution of education to health promotion. In: R Bunton & G Macdonald (Eds), Health promotion: disciplines and diversity, London: Routledge.

Weare K (in press) What kinds of medical education are needed to promote health? To what extent are we achieving them? In: N Temple & H Diehl (Eds), Prevention of disease in the western world. Athabasca, Canada: Humana Press.

Webb D (1997) Measuring effectiveness in health promotion. Southampton: University of Southampton.

Weiss C H & Bucuvalas M J (1980) Social science research and decision making. New York: Columbia University Press.

Weiss C H (1991) Policy research: data, ideas or arguments? In: P Wagner et al. (Eds), Social sciences and modern states. Cambridge: Cambridge University Press.

Wellings K, Field J, Johnson A M & Wadsworth J (1994) Sexual behaviour in Britain: The National Survey of Sexual Attitudes and Lifestyles. Harmondsworth: Penguin.

Wessex Institute of Public Health Medicine (1994) Indicators and outcome measures for 'Health at work in the NHS' in Wessex. Winchester: Wessex Institute of Public Health Medicine.

Whitaker R C, Wright J A, Finch A J & Psaty B M (1993) An environmental intervention to reduce dietary fat in school lunches. *Pediatrics*, 91, 1107–1111.

Whitaker R C, Wright J A, Koepsell T D, Finch A J & Psaty B M (1994) Randomised intervention to increase children's selection of low-fat foods in school lunches. *Journal of Pediatrics*, 125, 535–540.

White A, Freeth S & O'Brien M (1992) Infant feeding 1990. London: HMSO.

Whitehead M (1991) The concepts and principles of equity and health. *Health Promotion International*, 6, 217–228.

Whitehead M (1997) How useful is the 'stages of change' model? *Health Education Journal*, 56, 111–112.

Whyman R (1996) Screen For Your Life. A report of a theatre in health education project used to improve breast screening uptake (unpublished). Walsall: Walsall Community Arts Team.

Wilhelmsson C et al. (1975) Smoking and myocardial infarction. *The Lancet*, i, 415.

Wilkinson E, Elander E & Woolaway M (1997) Exploring the use of action research to stimulate and evaluate workplace health promotion. *Health Education Journal*, 56(2), 188–198.

Wilkinson R (1996) Income distribution and life expectancy. *British Medical Journal*, 304, 165–168.

Williams C & Poulter J (1991) Formative evaluation of a workplace menu labelling scheme. *Journal of Human Nutrition and Dietetics*, 4, 251–262.

Williams S & Macintosh J (1996) Problems in implementing evidence-based health promotion material in general practice. *Health Education Journal*, 55, 24–30.

Williams S & McIntosh J (1996) Problems in implementing evidence-based health promotion material in general practice. *Health Service Journal*, 55, 24–30.

Wilmott Y (1992) Career opportunities in the nursing service for prisoners. *Nursing Times*, 88(37).

Wimbush E (1998) The research training needs of health promotion practitioners (conference paper). Second Nordic Health Promotion Research Conference, Stockholm, 9–11 September 1998.

World Bank (1993) World development report. Investing in health. New York: Oxford University Press.

World Health Organisation (1946) Constitution. New York: WHO.

World Health Organisation (1978) Primary health care. A joint report by the Director-General of the World Health Organisation and the Executive Director of United Nations Children's Fund. Geneva: WHO.

World Health Organisation (1984) Health promotion. A discussion document on concepts and principles. Geneva: WHO.

World Health Organisation (1993) Needs and action priorities in cardiac rehabilitation and secondary prevention in patients with coronary heart disease. In: D R Thompson et al. (Eds), Cardiac rehabilitation guidelines in the United Kingdom: guidelines and audit standards. *Heart*, 75, 89–93.

World Health Organisation (1996) European health care reforms. Analysis of current strategies. Summary. Copenhagen: WHO.

WHO Global Programme on AIDS (1993) WHO guidelines on HIV infection and AIDS in prisons. Geneva: WHO.

Wright G & Slattery J (1986) Talking about healthy eating. Special report. Bradford: University of Bradford, Food Policy Research Unit.

Wright L (1996) A review of the Drinkwise campaign, 1989–94. London: Health Education Authority.

Wright L (in press) Young people and alcohol: a literature review (provisional title). London Health Education Authority.

Wright L & Perkins E (in press) Toolbox for health promotion research and evaluation. Edinburgh: Health Education Board for Scotland.

Wright P (1993) An illuminative appraisal of the uses of drama in health promotion. Unpublished MSc dissertation. Birmingham: University of Central England.

Wright P (1996) A qualitative study of lay and professional perceptions of breast health and the use of theatre as an effective method of health education (unpublished). Dudley: Dudley Health Authority.

Yates S (1994) Promoting mental health behind bars. *Nursing Standard*, 8(52), 18–21.
York Community Health Services (1992) Family health matters. York: York Health Authority.
Ziglio E (1997) How to move towards evidence-based health promotion interventions *Promotion and Education*, 4, 29–32.
Zigmond A S & Snaith R P (1983) The Hospital Anxiety and Depression Scale. *Acta Psychiatrica Scandinavica*, 67, 361–370.

Index

Index compiled by Caroline Sheard